Advances in Veterinary Science
and Comparative Medicine

Volume 35

Immunomodulation in Domestic Food Animals

Advances in Veterinary Science and Comparative Medicine

Edited by

C. E. Cornelius
California Primate Research Center
University of California, Davis
Davis, California

R. R. Marshak
New Bolton Center
University of Pennsylvania
Kennett Square, Pennsylvania

E. C. Melby
SmithKline Beecham
Animal Health Products Research and Development
West Chester, Pennsylvania

Advisory Board

Kalman Perk
André Rico
Irwin Arias
Bennie Osburn
W. Jean Dodds

Advances in Veterinary Science
and Comparative Medicine

Volume 35

Immunomodulation in Domestic Food Animals

Edited by

Frank Blecha

Department of Anatomy and Physiology
College of Veterinary Medicine
Kansas State University
Manhattan, Kansas

and

Bernard Charley

Station de Recherches de Virologie et d'Immunologie Moléculaires
Institut National de la Recherche Agronomique
Centre de Recherches de Jouy-en-Josas
Jouy-en-Josas, France

Academic Press, Inc.
Harcourt Brace Jovanovich, Publishers
San Diego   New York   Boston
London   Sydney   Tokyo   Toronto

This book is printed on acid-free paper. ∞

COPYRIGHT © 1990 BY ACADEMIC PRESS, INC.
All Rights Reserved.
No part of this publication may be reproduced or transmitted in any form or by any means, electronic or mechanical, including photocopy, recording, or any information storage and retrieval system, without permission in writing from the publisher.

ACADEMIC PRESS, INC.
San Diego, California 92101

United Kingdom Edition published by
ACADEMIC PRESS LIMITED
24-28 Oval Road, London NW1 7DX

LIBRARY OF CONGRESS CATALOG CARD NUMBER: 53-7098

ISBN   0-12-039235-6   (alk. paper)

PRINTED IN THE UNITED STATES OF AMERICA
90 91 92 93   9 8 7 6 5 4 3 2 1

CONTENTS

CONTRIBUTORS ix
FOREWORD xi
PREFACE xiii

Part I: Introduction

Rationale for Using Immunopotentiators in Domestic Food Animals
FRANK BLECHA AND BERNARD CHARLEY

I. Introduction 3
II. Why Are Immunomodulators Needed? 4
III. Specific versus Nonspecific Immunomodulation 5
IV. Summary 14
    References 14

Model Systems to Study Immunomodulation in Domestic Food Animals
JAMES A. ROTH AND KEVAN P. FLAMING

I. Introduction 21
II. Stress Models 23
III. Glucocorticoid Immunosuppression Models 26
IV. Infectious Disease Model Systems 32
V. Summary 36
    References 36

Mechanisms of Action of Some Immunomodulators Used in Veterinary Medicine
P. J. QUINN

I. Introduction 43
II. Structure and Function of the Immune System 44

CONTENTS

III. Immunomodulation.. 53
IV. Physiologically Important Immunomodulators............................ 58
V. Synthetic Compounds with Immunomodulatory Activity.................... 72
VI. Microbial Products as Immunomodulators................................ 80
VII. Liposomes... 85
VIII. Concluding Comments... 86
References.. 89

Part II: Chemical Immunomodulation

Chemically Induced Immunomodulation in Domestic Food Animals
Marcus E. Kehrli, Jr. and James A. Roth

I. Introduction.. 103
II. Chemical Immunomodulation in Domestic Food Animal Species............. 105
III. Chemical Immunomodulators Which Have Apparently Not Been Evaluated in Domestic Food Animals... 112
IV. Summary.. 115
References... 116

Classical and New Approaches to Adjuvant Use in Domestic Food Animals
Kristian Dalsgaard, Luuk Hilgers, and Gérard Trouve

I. Introduction.. 121
II. Aluminum Salts.. 122
III. Oil Emulsions... 124
IV. Surface Active Agents.. 128
V. ISCOMS... 138
VI. Muramyldipeptides... 141
VII. Polymeric Adjuvants... 142
VIII. General Conclusions... 145
References... 147

A Thymosin–Tuftsin Conjugate as a New Potential Immunomodulator in Cattle
David Nemat Khansari and Parviz Jafari

I. Introduction.. 161
II. Tuftsin: A Macrophage Activator...................................... 163

III. Thymosin-α: A T Cell Activator 165
IV. Thymosin–Tuftsin Conjugate (IMP-1) 168
V. Conclusion 173
References 174

Part III: Cytokine Immunomodulation

The Molecular Biology of Large Animal Cytokines
CHARLES MALISZEWSKI, BYRON GALLIS, AND PAUL E. BAKER

I. Cytokine Biology 181
II. Recombinant Bovine and Porcine Cytokines 189
III. Conclusions 205
References 207

Interferon Immunomodulation in Domestic Food Animals
H. BIELEFELDT-OHMANN AND S. R. MARTINOD

I. Introduction 215
II. Modulation of Nonspecific Antimicrobial Defense Mechanisms 216
III. Modulation of the Specific Cellular Immune Response 218
IV. Enhancement of Antimicrobial Mechanisms in the Gut 221
V. Immunoenhancement in Noninfectious Diseases 222
VI. Concluding Remarks 224
References 225

In Vivo Use of Interleukins in Domestic Food Animals
FRANK BLECHA

I. Introduction 231
II. Rationale for Using Interleukins in Domestic Food Animals 235
III. *In Vivo* Studies with Interleukins in Domestic Food Animals 237
IV. Conclusions and Prospects 245
References 246

Part IV: Physiologically Regulated Immunomodulation

Nutritional Modulation of Immunity in Domestic Food Animals
P. G. Reddy and R. A. Frey

- I. Introduction 255
- II. Protein and Energy 257
- III. Fat-Soluble Vitamins 262
- IV. Water-Soluble Vitamins 266
- V. Minerals 268
- VI. Conclusion 274
- References 275

Neuroendocrine–Immune Interactions
Keith W. Kelley and Robert Dantzer

- I. Introduction 283
- II. Characteristics of the Neuroendocrine–Immune System 284
- III. Conclusions 297
- References 299

Potential for Improving Animal Health by Modulation of Behavior and Immune Function
John J. McGlone

- I. Introduction 307
- II. Behavior of Farm Animals 308
- III. Social Behavior and Immune Function 309
- IV. Nonsocial Behaviors and Immune Function 311
- V. Brain-Immune Interactions 312
- VI. Concluding Remarks 313
- References 314

Index 317

CONTRIBUTORS

Numbers in parentheses indicate the pages on which the authors' contributions begin.

PAUL E. BAKER, Immunex Research and Development, Seattle, Washington 98101 (181)

H. BIELEFELDT-OHMANN,[1] Veterinary Infectious Disease Organization, University of Saskatchewan, Saskatoon, Saskatchewan S7N 0W0, Canada (215)

FRANK BLECHA, Department of Anatomy and Physiology, College of Veterinary Medicine, Kansas State University, Manhattan, Kansas 66506 (3, 231)

BERNARD CHARLEY, Station de Recherches de Virologie et d'Immunologie Moléculaires, Institut National de la Recherche Agronomique, Centre de Recherches de Jouy-en-Josas, 78350 Jouy-en-Josas France (3)

KRISTIAN DALSGAARD, Animal Biotechnology Research Center, State Veterinary Institute for Virus Research, Lindholm, DK-4771, Kalvehave, Denmark (121)

ROBERT DANTZER, Psychobiologie des Comportements Adaptatifs, Institut National de la Recherche Agronomique and, Institut National de la Santé et de la Recherche Medicale, 33077 Bordeaux, France (283)

KEVAN P. FLAMING, Department of Veterinary Microbiology and Preventive Medicine, Iowa State University, Ames, Iowa 50011 (21)

R. A. FREY, Department of Anatomy and Physiology, College of Veterinary Medicine, Kansas State University, Manhattan, Kansas 66506 (255)

---

[1] *Present address:* Menzies School of Health Research, Casuarina, Darwin, Australia.

CONTRIBUTORS

BYRON GALLIS, Immunex Research and Development, Seattle, Washington 98101 (181)

LUUK HILGERS, Duphar B. V., Animal Division, Veterinary Vaccines, Weesp, Holland (121)

PARVIZ JAFARI, Immunobiological Laboratories, Inc., New York, New York 10018 (161)

MARCUS E. KEHRLI, JR., Metabolic Diseases and Immunology Research Unit, National Animal Disease Center, USDA-Agricultural Research Service, Ames, Iowa 50010 (103)

KEITH W. KELLEY, Laboratory of Immunophysiology, Department of Animal Sciences, University of Illinois, Urbana, Illinois 61801 (283)

DAVID NEMAT KHANSARI, Immunobiological Laboratories, Inc., New York, New York 10018 (161)

CHARLES MALISZEWSKI, Immunex Research and Development, Seattle, Washington 98101 (181)

S. R. MARTINOD, Biovet Unit, Ciba-Geigy Ltd., Centre de Recherches Agricoles, St. Aubin, Switzerland (215)

JOHN J. MCGLONE, Department of Animal Science, Texas Tech University, Lubbock, Texas 79409 (307)

P. J. QUINN, Department of Veterinary Microbiology and Parasitology, University College Dublin, Ballsbridge, Dublin 4, Ireland (43)

P. G. REDDY, Department of Anatomy and Physiology, College of Veterinary Medicine, Kansas State University, Manhattan, Kansas 66506 (255)

JAMES A. ROTH, Department of Veterinary Microbiology and Preventive Medicine, Iowa State University, Ames, Iowa 50011 (21, 103)

GÉRARD TROUVE, SEPPIC, Lacaze Basse, F-81105 Castres Cedex, France (121)

FOREWORD

Immunology is one of the newest and most important basic and applied biological sciences. The impact immunology has had on agriculture, biological sciences, human and veterinary medicine, and elsewhere is remarkable considering its very short history. Although observations on disease resistance and host defense were recorded as early as the 13th century, it has only been during the present century and specifically the last 50 years, that information has been generated to provide the basis for the present day specialty of immunology. Increased awareness of mechanisms involved in immunity have come from studies on cellular and molecular aspects of immunity. These studies have also provided information required to develop methods and products for controlling or regulating the immune response. Immunomodulation, which involves increasing and/or decreasing immune responses, is essential to improve protective immunity and reduce immune mediated disease (e.g., allergy, autoimmunity).

The ability to modulate the immune response for the purpose of enhanced resistance to a wide range of pathogens is an important goal of the immunologist and microbiologist. The ability to modulate immunity for the benefit of the host would provide cost effective products for use in food animals. Vaccine technology has improved significantly since it was first introduced, however, constantly changing requirements in food animal production require additional changes, and further improvement in the development and delivery of vaccines are necessary to reduce disease losses not controlled by current vaccines. Protection from complex diseases, especially those affecting young animals where the immune system has not reached maturity, will require methods and products that currently do not exist. Improvement of vaccines will require new adjuvants. Adjuvant technology has improved with the discovery of new chemicals, synthetics, and natural products, but much work remains to be done to find optimal cost effective and acceptable products. The discovery of the role that cytokines play in immunomodulation provides an opportunity, through genetic engineering technology, to use certain cytokines as adjuvants in food animals. An increased understanding of their role in the immune system will lead to the most appropriate use of cytokines for enhancing disease resistance.

Understanding the interaction of the immune system with various organ systems is important for the development of an effective immune response. One system receiving attention because of its influence on immunity is the neuroendocrine system. Stress from a variety of factors, especially from management practices of food producing animals, profoundly affects the immune system. It has been known for years that temperature changes, shipping, and crowding have profound effects on increased susceptibility to disease. Some of the effects are undoubtedly related to exposure to new or high concentrations of pathogens, but also of importance are the modulating effects of stress on immunity. An understanding of the interaction between neuroendocrine function and immunity will lead to management practices that have the effect of enhancing immunity to various infectious diseases and providing information on proper timing of vaccination for optimal protective immunity.

The role nutrition plays in modulation of the immune system is also of great interest, especially as it relates to food animal production. Nutrients can significantly effect the development and/or maintenance of the immune system, therefore, optimal nutrition is a requirement for optimal immunity to be realized. Under certain circumstances immunomodulation can be achieved through nutritional therapy. It is critical to understand that immunity can be enhanced or suppressed with the use of certain nutrients in the diet or given by injection. The specific nutrients and the range of levels must be known to ensure that nutrition is not having a negative impact on disease resistance, but instead ensuring optimal or enhanced immunity.

This book for the first time provides valuable information on mechanisms of immunologic control and on the possible methods and products that can be used to modulate the immune response of animals. It also provides a detailed description of the numerous factors that effect an immune response and how management of these factors can be used to the advantage or disadvantage of food animal production.

RONALD D. SCHULTZ
SCHOOL OF VETERINARY MEDICINE
UNIVERSITY OF WISCONSIN-MADISON

PREFACE

The purpose of this volume is to compile recent developments in the immunology and regulation of the immune response in domestic food animals. Given the rapid rate of progress in the field, this is a difficult task; we feel however, that it is a necessary one.

The subject of this book concerns the regulation of the immune response in food animals and means of enhancing that response to decrease susceptibility to disease. The book is divided into four parts. Part I provides an overview of the basic concepts of immunomodulation and the rationale for manipulating the immune response in food animals. Part II contains information on immunopotentiation using chemicals and a thorough discussion of adjuvant use. The molecular biology and *in vivo* use of cytokines in food animals is presented in Part III. Finally, Part IV discusses physiologically regulated immunomodulation, including nutritional modulation of the immune response and neuroendocrine-immune interactions.

Our task of compiling this book was made easier by the willingness of the authors to provide timely, concise reviews of their areas of expertise. We are sincerely grateful to each author for the time and energy that was required to prepare their contribution.

FRANK BLECHA
BERNARD CHARLEY

Part I
Introduction

Rationale for Using Immunopotentiators in Domestic Food Animals

FRANK BLECHA* AND BERNARD CHARLEY[†]

*Department of Anatomy and Physiology, College of Veterinary Medicine, Kansas State University, Manhattan, Kansas 66505, and
†Station de Recherches de Virologie et d'Immunologie Moléculaires Institut National de la Recherche Agronomique, Centre de Recherches de Jouy-en-Josas, 78350 Jouy-en-Josas, France

I. Introduction
II. Why Are Immunomodulators Needed?
III. Specific versus Nonspecific Immunomodulation
   A. The Neonatal Period
   B. Stress-Induced Immunosuppression
   C. Pathogen-Induced Immunosuppression
IV. Summary
   References

I. Introduction

Prevention and treatment of disease are primary concerns of everyone involved in the production of domestic food animals. Producers, veterinarians, and production animal specialists, such as nutritionists and reproductive physiologists, can all cite specific economic endpoints that are directly related to the incidence and intensity of disease in food production animals. Indeed, even the consumer of animal agricultural products is greatly affected by the cost of maintaining an abundant supply of healthy food animal products. Consequently, much effort and expense are directed toward minimizing the incidence of disease in domestic food animals. One means of decreasing the impact of disease in food animals is increasing the animal's ability to withstand infections.

Regulation of the immune response is extremely complex. Nevertheless, we are slowly beginning to understand how the immune system, indeed the whole animal, orchestrates the body's response to an invading pathogen. With the knowledge, however incomplete, of how the immune system responds to disease-causing organisms, we can devise ways of intervening in the regulation of the immune system, particularly by modulating the host's immune response.

Immunomodulation, as the term implies, can be used to designate either a suppression or an augmentation of an immune response. The necessity and capability of suppressing the function of the immune system are well recognized in such areas as organ transplantation and autoimmune disorders. However, in general, medically induced immunosuppression is not a practical concern in domestic food animals. Conversely, augmentation of immunity has received much attention in domestic food animals and provides a means of increasing the host's resistance to disease. Various chemicals and biological substances have been used and evaluated as immunomodulators in domestic food animals and will be discussed in the following chapter of this book. Other synonyms for immunomodulators that are frequently used include immunostimulators, immunopotentiators, immunotherapeutic agents, and biological response modifiers.

II. Why Are Immunomodulators Needed?

Vaccination of domestic food animals against economically important pathogens is effective and has increased the efficiency of food animal production. However, even with the successes attained in food animal production through vaccination programs, tremendous economic losses still occur in animal agriculture that are directly related to the health of the animal. Two important examples of diseases that still cause large economic losses, bovine respiratory disease and mastitis, will be used to illustrate this point.

Respiratory disease of cattle continue to present a serious economic burden to the producer. The annual economic loss to the North American cattle industry from bovine respiratory disease has been estimated to range from $250 million to $1 billion (Babiuk *et al.*, 1987). The etiology of bovine respiratory disease is very complex and multifactorial; the interactions of viruses, bacteria, and stress greatly contribute to the disease process (Loan, 1984). Vaccines against viruses and bacteria involved in bovine respiratory disease are available and used. However, bovine respiratory disease still accounts for 65% of the health problems and deaths among feedlot cattle (Edwards, 1987). In addition to losses due to death, economic losses caused by bovine respiratory disease include reduced growth performance and increased treatment costs. These losses emphasize the need for alternative or complementary therapeutic approaches, such as immunomodulators, that may be well suited for the multifactorial etiology involved in the disease.

In economical terms, mastitis is the most devastating disease affecting dairy cows. In the United States, losses attributed to mastitis approach $2 billion each year; 70% of this economic loss is due to a reduced milk yield as a result of subclinical mastitis (National Mastitis Council, 1987). Similarly, a French epidemiological survey found that mastitis was by far the most frequent pathology affecting dairy cows (Barnouin *et al.*, 1986). Vaccination against bacteria that cause intramammary infections has been attempted as a means of decreasing mastitis. However, even in studies that have shown beneficial effects of immunization against mastitis, vaccination did not prevent new intramammary infections (Pankey *et al.*, 1985). Antibiotic therapy is used in the control of mastitis. However, because *Staphylococcus aureus* mastitis responds poorly to antibiotic therapy and because of the problem of antibiotic residues in milk, the effectiveness of antibiotic therapy in mastitis prevention and treatment is limited.

These specific examples emphasize the need to continue to search for more effective ways to minimize the impact of disease on animal production. Augmentation of the animal's immune response with the intent of increasing resistance to disease-causing organisms should decrease the economic loss due to disease in food animal production. Immunomodulation may provide an effective means of enhancing the ability of domestic food animals to withstand disease.

III. Specific versus Nonspecific Immunomodulation

When one considers the possibility of enhancing an animal's immune response, a question that must be addressed is whether specific or nonspecific immunomodulation is desired or required. Specific immunomodulation involves the potentiation of the host's immune system toward a unique, specific antigen. Vaccination programs are perhaps the best example of producing specific immunity in domestic food animals. Nonspecific immunomodulation generally is an attempt to heighten immunologic capabilities at a time when an animal may be exposed to one or several pathogens and/or be immunocompromised. Both of these concepts will be discussed further.

The distinction between adjuvants and specific immunomodulators is blurred and may be only a matter of semantics. Classical and new adjuvants offer the capability of enhancing specific immunity and are discussed in great detail in Chapter 5 of this volume. However, some substances that are not generally thought of as adjuvants, such as the interleukins and interferons, also induce a state of specific immunomodulation. For example, peripheral blood mononuclear cells from cattle injected with recombinant bovine interleukin-2 display enhanced cytolytic capabilities against bovine herpesvirus-infected target cells (Reddy et al., 1989a). However, protection against a bovine herpesvirus challenge was observed only in animals that received a vaccination against the virus in conjunction with injections of interleukin-2. Thus, in this case both nonspecific and specific immunomodulation was produced in cattle that were administered interleukin-2, but only specific immunomodulation resulted in protection against a viral challenge.

Theoretically, the capability of potentiating the host's immune response at a time when it might be immature, compromised, or overcome with pathogens should enhance the animal's ability to resist disease. This is the rationale for nonspecifically augmenting an animal's immune response. Nonspecific immunomodulation has potential in at least 3 different conditions: (1) during the neonatal period when the immune system may not be fully developed; (2) during periods of stress-induced immunosuppression; and (3) during virus- or bacteria-induced immunosuppression.

A. The Neonatal Period

Because of a very efficient placental barrier, pig, horse, and ruminant fetuses are generally very well protected from *in utero* antigenic stimuli. Therefore, although fully immunocompetent at birth, domestic food animal newborns differ from other mammalian neonates in being immunologically "virgin" (Kim, 1975; Salmon, 1984) and the development of totally effective immune defenses requires 2 to 3 weeks. During this critical neonatal period the young animal is highly susceptible to microbial infections.

Postnatal development of immune functions has been most extensively studied in the pig (Sterzl and Silverstein, 1967; Kim, 1975). Most immune parameters that have been studied appeared to be very low at birth and reached adult values at about 1 month of age. Thus, the percentage of T and B lymphocytes in peripheral blood, as estimated by E-rosettes and anti-Ig immunofluorescence techniques, was shown to increase from 3 to 4% at birth to adult values by 35 days of age (Reyero et al., 1978). A similar age-related increase has been described for serum concentrations of the third component of complement (C3) in pigs (Tyler et al., 1988).

Because of the high incidence and economic impact of respiratory and intestinal infections in young domestic animals, it is important to review studies related to the postnatal development of the mucosa-associated immune system in the pig. At birth, the intestinal, nasal, and tracheobronchial mucosa are devoid of plasma cells. Plasma cells first appear in the respiratory tract at 6–7 days of age and reach adult values at 3–4 weeks of age. This postnatal development was described for cells containing IgA as well as IgM and IgG (Bradley et al., 1976). In the intestinal lamina propria, cells with cytoplasmic IgM appeared at 4–5 days after birth, earlier than the plasma cells containing IgG and IgA. In immunologically mature pigs, IgA plasma cells predominate, however in young animals the predominant isotype secreted by lamina propria plasma cells is IgM, and adult values are not attained until 4–9 weeks of age (Allen and Porter, 1977). Similarly, porcine gut-associated lymphoid tissue is poorly developed at birth and matures during the first month of life, showing an increase in number of small intestinal intraepithelial lymphocytes and the development in size and structure of the Peyer's patches (Chu et al., 1979; Pabst et al., 1988).

Inside the lung, residing at the air–tissue interface and directly exposed to inhaled microorganisms or air pollutants, the alveolar macrophage functions as the primary defense against respiratory infections (Hocking and Golde, 1979). Functional properties of alveolar macrophages, including their immunological and antiinfectious features, have been studied in domestic food animals (Khadom et al., 1985; Charley, 1985). Rothlein et al. (1981) have studied the postnatal development of alveolar macrophages in Minnesota miniature swine. These researchers showed that lavage fluids from the lungs of newborn piglets were devoid of macrophages. However, within 2 to 3 days after birth, macrophages gradually appear inside the lung airspaces and adult values are reached at 2 weeks of age. Furthermore, macrophages collected from piglets less than 1 week old showed immature function, i.e., lower phagocytic capacity and enzyme content than adult cells. The postnatal development of lung macrophages appears to depend upon nonspecific antigenic stimulation since germ-free piglets have a much lower number of alveolar macrophages than specific-pathogen-free piglets (Rothlein et al., 1981). Additionally, alveolar macrophages from young piglets have been shown to be more permissive to pseudorabies virus, yielding higher virus progeny titers, than cells from older animals (Iglesias et al., 1989).

A last example of an immune defect occurring during the neonatal period is given by studies on porcine natural killer (NK) cells. Natural killer cell activity in the peripheral blood of newborn pigs is much lower (often undetectable) than the activity of adult cells. This NK cell defect has been observed regardless of the target cell system used: human tumor cells (Huh et al., 1981), virus-infected cells (Cepica and Derbyshire, 1984a; Yang and Schultz, 1986), or porcine tumor B-cells (Onizuka et al., 1987). Of particular interest are the observations that postnatal development of NK cells activity, which requires 2–3 weeks in specific-pathogen-free miniature swine (Huh et al., 1981) and in conventionally reared Large-White pigs (Charley et al., 1985), is delayed in germ-free miniature piglets (Huh et al., 1981). These data imply that microbial flora play a role in the maturation process of NK cell activity in neonates. Due to the high incidence of intestinal infections in young domestic food animals it is worth noting that porcine intestinal intraepithelial lymphocytes show high NK cell activity against transmissible gastroenteritis virus (TGEV)-infected pig kidney cells, whereas the same cells isolated in young piglets have no NK cell activity (Cepica and Derbyshire, 1984a). This observation has led to the hypothesis that a NK cell defect could in part explain the great susceptibility of piglets to coronavirus-induced transmissible gastroenteritis. Indeed, adoptive transfer of adult pig leukocytes established functional NK cell activity in recipient piglets and reduced their susceptibility to a TGEV challenge (Cepica and Derbyshire, 1984b).

The examples described above illustrate the existence of several different immune defects (see Table I) in neonatal domestic food animals. This lower functional immune status during the neonatal period could explain some of the neonates' susceptibility to infectious diseases, especially intestinal infections. Thus, the potential exists to increase the neonates' immune functions by using immunomodulators. A few studies have been conducted exploring means of enhancing the young animals' immune functions. For example, newborn piglets' NK cell activity was shown to be responsive in vitro to interferon (Charley et al., 1985), and in vivo to poly I:C (Lesnick and Derbyshire, 1988) or bacterial extracts (Kim, 1984). Additionally, isoprinosine has been shown to enhance the immunocompromised immune status of artificially reared neonatal pigs (Hennessy et al., 1987). In the following chapters several immunomodulating strategies will be reviewed and should help to define possible immunotherapeutic approaches to enhance young domestic food animals' resistance to disease.

TABLE I

IMMUNOLOGICAL IMPAIRMENT OF NEWBORN PIGLETS: A SUMMARY OF IMMATURE IMMUNE FUNCTIONS

Immunological compartment	Nature of the immune "defect"	Reference
Blood	Low percentage of T and B lymphocytes	Reyero et al. (1978)
	Low concentration of C3	Tyler et al. (1988)
	Low primary antibody response	Metzger et al. (1978)
	Low NK cell activity	Huh et al. (1981); Cepica and Derbyshire (1984a)
Intestine	Low number of plasma cells	Allen and Porter (1977)
	Low number of intraepithelial lymphocytes	Chu et al. (1979)
	Low number of Peyer's patches	Pabst et al. (1988)
	Low NK cell activity	Cepica and Derbyshire (1984b)
Lung	Low number of plasma cells	Bradley et al. (1976)
	Low number of alveolar macrophages	Rothlein et al. (1981)
	Immature alveolar macrophages	Rothlein et al. (1981)
	Macrophages highly permissive to pseudorabies virus	Iglesias et al. (1989)

B. STRESS-INDUCED IMMUNOSUPPRESSION

Many diseases of domestic food animals are known to involve an interaction of host exposure to stressful stimuli and viral and bacterial challenge. This concept seems to be especially relevant when one considers the etiology of respiratory and enteric diseases (Loan, 1984; Filion et al., 1984). The idea that stressed animals are more susceptible to disease generally relies on the assumption that alterations in immunocompetence have occurred (Table II). Indeed, some researchers have suggested that changes in immune function may be a useful indicator of stress in domestic food animals (Kelley, 1985; Siegel, 1985). Over the last decade several review articles have been written on the topic of stress and immunity in farm animals (Kelley, 1980, 1982, 1984, 1985,

TABLE II

EXAMPLES OF THE INFLUENCE OF STRESS ON SUSCEPTIBILITY TO INFECTIOUS DISEASE, HUMORAL IMMUNITY, AND CELL-MEDIATED IMMUNITY IN DOMESTIC FOOD ANIMALS

Stressor	Observation	Reference
Susceptibility to Infectious Disease		
Cold	Increased susceptibility to TGE virus	Shimizu et al. (1978)
Draft and cold	Increased susceptibility to *H. pleuropneumoniae*	Verhagen et al. (1987)
Exertion (swimming)	Increased susceptibility to *Pasteurella multocida* when also exposed to ammonia	Neumann et al. (1987)
Transport	Increased susceptibility to infections	Staples and Haugse (1974); Mormede et al. (1982); Filion et al. (1984)
Regrouping	Increased susceptibility to Newcastle disease, hemorrhagic enteritis, Marek's disease	Gross and Colmano (1969); Gross (1972); Gross et al. (1988)
Humoral Immunity		
Cold	Increased antibody production	Blecha and Kelley (1981); Kelley et al. (1981)
Transport	Decreased antibody production	Hartmann (1988)
Early weaning	Decreased antibody production	Blecha and Kelley (1981); Haye and Kornegay (1979)
Cell-Mediated Immunity		
Cold or heat	Decreased DTH response	Regnier and Kelley (1981)
Transport	Decreased lymphocyte proliferation	Blecha et al. (1984); Murata et al. (1987)
Early weaning	Decreased lymphocyte proliferation	Blecha et al. (1983); Hennessy et al. (1987)
Restraint	Decreased DTH and thymus weight	Westly and Kelley (1984)
	Decreased IL-2 production	Klemcke et al. (1987)
Exertion (treadmill)	Decreased lymphocyte proliferation	Blecha and Minocha (1983)

1988; Albani-Vangili, 1985; Siegel, 1985; Blecha, 1988a; Griffin, 1989). If stress-induced changes in host immunity predisposes animals to disease, then methods of modulating the immune response in stressed animals should increase disease resistance (Blecha, 1988b).

When one attempts to intervene in an animal's response to a stressor, several different approaches can be envisioned (Fig. 1). Perhaps the best means of reducing the impact of stress on animal health is by providing a less stressful environment. However, deciding which environment or management condition is the least stressful is not a simple or easy task (Curtis *et al.*, 1989; McGlone and Hellman, 1988). Thus, several environments and management conditions have been evaluated for their influence on immune function (Blecha *et al.*, 1983; Blecha *et al.*, 1984, 1985, 1986; McGlone and Blecha, 1987; Minton *et al.*, 1988) and for their impact on the physiology of the animal (Dantzer and Mormede, 1983).

Another approach has been investigated as a method of reducing the influence of stress on susceptibility to disease: blocking the physiologic response to the stressor. The association between stress, neuroendo-

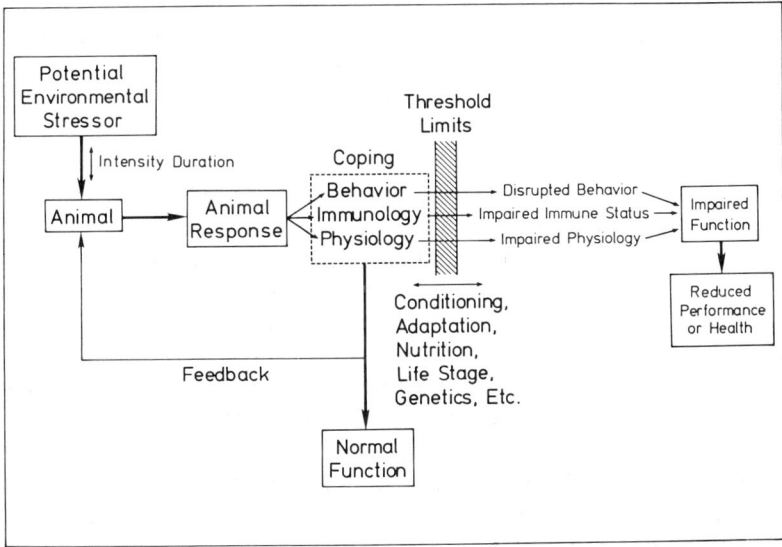

FIG. 1. Responses of animals to potential environmental stressors. Possibilities of improving performance and health in stressed animals can be envisioned by manipulating the behavior, immunology, or physiology of the animal. Taken from Hahn and Nienaber (1989), with permission.

crine responses, and alterations in immune function or disease susceptibility has been recognized for several years (Munck *et al.,* 1984; Kelley, 1988; Griffin, 1989). When increased concentrations of glucocorticoids have been associated with lower immune responses, administration of drugs that block the synthesis of corticosterone, such as metyrapone, resulted in an abrogation of the stress-induced immunosuppression (Blecha *et al.,* 1982). Recently, adrenal blocking chemicals (metyrapone and dichlorodiphenyldichlorethane) have been shown to increase the resistance of stressed chickens to viral and respiratory infections (Gross, 1989). Finally, when stress-induced immunosuppression has occurred, neurohormones, such as melatonin (Maestroni *et al.,* 1988), immunomodulating drugs (Hennessy *et al.,* 1987; Blecha, 1988b; Komori *et al.,* 1987), and cytokines (Conlon *et al.,* 1985) have been used to "up-regulate" or restore the immune response. It is likely that a combination of the approaches indicated above will provide the best means of reducing stress-induced disease problems in domestic food animals.

C. Pathogen-Induced Immunosuppression

Animals exposed to infectious disease often show depressed immune function. This is the case for several parasitic, bacterial, and viral infections. Pathogenic bacteria have been shown to affect immune responsiveness of infected animals. Thus, *Pasteurella hemolytica* or *Haemophilus pleuropneumoniae,* which both cause acute pneumonia in cattle and pigs, have been reported to exert toxic effects on lung macrophages and to alter macrophage phagocytic functions (Markham and Wilkie, 1980; Bendixen *et al.,* 1981). During bacteria-induced mastitis, suppressed responses in lymphocyte proliferation and neutrophil phagocytic functions have been reported (Nonnecke and Harp, 1988; Reddy *et al.,* 1989b). Immunosuppression of the host is also a frequent consequence of viral infections. Several examples of virus-related immunosuppression are well documented in domestic food animals (Table III), including viral diseases of great economic importance such as infectious bovine rhinotracheitis (bovine herpesvirus type-1) and pseudorabies, which cause severe pneumonia and death in cattle and pigs, respectively. As a consequence of virus-induced alteration of immune function, animals become very susceptible to secondary bacterial infections. The detrimental effects of these virus–bacteria synergistic interactions are of particular importance in the case of respiratory infections. Thus, following an initial viral multiplication in the lung, pathogenic bacteria proliferate, inducing the development of more se-

TABLE III

EXAMPLES OF VIRUS-RELATED IMMUNOSUPPRESSION IN DOMESTIC FOOD ANIMALS

Virus	Virus group	Host	Effects on the immune system	Reference
Pseudorabies	Herpesvirus	Pig	Decreased lymphocyte proliferation and IL-2 production	Flaming et al. (1989)
Bovine herpesvirus-1	Herpesvirus	Cattle	Decreased cell-mediated cytotoxicity; increased susceptibility to secondary infections; decreased IL-1 production; decreased lymphocyte proliferation	Babiuk et al. (1988)
			Decreased alveolar macrophage function	Blecha et al. (1987); Ghram et al. (1989); Carter et al. (1989); Brown and Ananaba (1988)
Parainfluenza-3 virus	Paramyxovirus	Cattle	Decreased lymphocyte proliferation	Ghram et al. (1989)
Rinderpest	Morbillivirus	Cattle	Lysis of infected lymphoid cells; decreased antibody response	Bielefeldt-Ohmann and Babiuk (1986)
Bovine leukemia virus	Retrovirus	Cattle	Decreased lymphocyte proliferation	Bielefeldt-Ohmann and Babiuk (1986)
Hog cholera virus	Pestivirus	Pig	Leukopenia; decreased lymphocyte proliferation; decreased antibody response	Charley et al. (1980); Van Oirschot (1983)
Bovine viral diarrhea	Pestivirus	Cattle	Decreased polymorphonuclear cell function	Roth and Kaberle (1983)
Transmissible gastroenteritis virus	Coronavirus	Pig	Lysis of infected alveolar macrophages	Laude et al. (1984)

vere and acute lung lesions (Jakab, 1982; Babiuk et al., 1988). If pathogen-induced immunosuppression can be moderated by immunomodulating substances, then the prospects for domestic food animals to withstand disease should be increased. Stimulation of defense mechanisms, especially lung immune defenses, will likely require activation of local lymphoid cells such as alveolar macrophages (Charley, 1986). Targeting of immunomodulators to the critical organs will require special delivery systems, such as encapsulation in liposomes (Fogler et al., 1980), which should be considered in the field of domestic food animal immunoenhancement.

IV. Summary

In the production of domestic food animals several situations exist where disease decreases production efficiency. Some of these diseases are exacerbated by a lowered or compromised immune response of the host. If immunomodulators can be used to augment immune function at critical periods during the production of food animals, such as the neonatal period, and prior to or during exposure to stressors or pathogenic organisms, then the economic loss caused by infectious disease should be reduced.

References

Albani-Vangili, R. (1985). Stress e immunita. *Obiettivi Vet.* **6,** 23–30.
Allen, W. D., and Porter, P. (1977). The relative frequencies and distribution of immunoglobulin-bearing cells in the intestinal mucosa of neonatal and weaned pigs and their significance in the development of secretory immunity. *Immunology* **32,** 819–824.
Babiuk, L. A., Lawman, M. J. P., and Gifford, G. A. (1987). Bovine respiratory disease: Pathogenesis and control by interferon. *In* "A Seminar in Bovine Immunology," pp. 12–23. Veterinary Learning Systems Co., Lawrenceville, New Jersey.
Babiuk, L. A., Lawman, M. J. P., and Bielefeldt-Ohmann, H. (1988). Viral-bacterial synergistic interaction in respiratory disease. *Adv. Virus Res.* **35,** 219–249.
Barnouin, J., Fayet, J. C., Brochart, M., Bouvier, A., and Paccard, P. (1986). Enquête éco-pathologique continue. 1. Hiérarchie de la pathologie observée en élévage bovin laitier (résumé). *Ann. Rech. Vét.* **17,** 227–230.
Bendixen, P. H., Shewen, P. E., Rosendal, S., and Wilkie, B. N. (1981). Toxicity of *Haemophilus pleuropneumoniae* for porcine lung macrophages, peripheral blood monocytes, and testicular cells. *Infect. Immun.* **33,** 673–676.
Bielefeldt-Ohmann, H., and Babiuk, L. A. (1986). Viral infections in domestic animals as models for studies of viral immunology and pathogenesis. *J. Gen. Virol.* **66,** 1–25.
Blecha, F. (1988a). Stress et immunité chez l'animal. *Recl. Med. Vet.* **164,** 767–772.
Blecha, F. (1988b). Immunomodulation: A means of disease prevention in stressed livestock. *J. Anim. Sci.* **66,** 2084–2090.

Blecha, F., and Kelley, K. W. (1981). Cold stress reduces the acquisition of colostral immunoglobulin in piglets. *J. Anim. Sci.* **52,** 594-600.

Blecha, F., and Minocha, H. C. (1983). Suppressed lymphocyte blastogenic responses and enhanced *in vitro* growth of infectious bovine rhinotracheitis virus in stressed feeder calves. *Am. J. Vet. Res.* **44,** 2145-2148.

Blecha, F., Kelley, K. W., and Satterlee, D. G. (1982). Adrenal involvement in the expression of delayed-type hypersensitivity to DNFB in stressed mice. *Proc. Soc. Exp. Biol. Med.* **169,** 247-252.

Blecha, F., Pollmann, D. S., and Nichols, D. A. (1983). Weaning pigs at an early age decreases cellular immunity. *J. Anim. Sci.* **56,** 396-400.

Blecha, F., Boyles, S. L., and Riley, J. G. (1984). Shipping suppresses lymphocyte blastogenic responses in Angus and Brahman × Angus feeder calves. *J. Anim. Sci.* **59,** 576-583.

Blecha, F., Pollmann, D. S., and Nichols, D. A. (1985). Immunologic reactions of pigs regrouped at or near weaning. *Am. J. Vet. Res.* **46,** 1934-1937.

Blecha, F., Pollmann, D. S., and Kluber, E. F. (1986). Decreased mononuclear cell response to mitogens in artificially reared neonatal pigs. *Can. J. Vet. Res.* **50,** 522-525.

Blecha, F., Anderson, G. A., Osorio, F., Chapes, S. K., and Baker, P. E. (1987). Influence of isoprinosine on bovine herpesvirus type-1 infection in cattle. *Vet. Immunol. Immunopathol.* **15,** 253-265.

Bradley, P. A., Bourne, F. J., and Brown, P. J. (1976). The respiratory tract immune system in the pig. I. Distribution of immunoglobulin-containing cells in the respiratory tract mucosa. *Vet. Pathol.* **13,** 81-89.

Brown, T. T., and Ananaba, G. (1988). Effect of respiratory infections caused by bovine herpesvirus-1 or parainfluenza-3 virus on bovine alveolar macrophage functions. *Am. J. Vet. Res.* **49,** 1147-1451.

Carter, J. J., Weinberg, A. D., Pollard, A., Reeves, R., Magnuson, J. A., and Magnuson, N. S. (1989). Inhibition of T-lymphocyte mitogenic responses and effects on cell functions by bovine herpesvirus 1. *J. Virol.* **63,** 1525-1530.

Cepica, A., and Derbyshire, J. B. (1984a). Antibody-dependent and spontaneous cell-mediated cytotoxicity against Transmissible Gastroenteritis virus infected cells by lymphocytes from sows, fetuses and neonatal piglets. *Can. J. Comp. Med.* **48,** 258-261.

Cepica, A., and Derbyshire, J. B. (1984b). The effect of adoptive transfer of mononuclear leukocytes from an adult donor on spontaneous cell-mediated cytotocity and resistance to Transmissible Gastroenteritis in neonatal piglets. *Can. J. Comp. Med.* **48,** 360-364.

Charley, B. (1985). Le macrophage alvéolaire de porc: Revue bibliographique. *Comp. Immunol. Microbiol. Infect. Dis.* **2,** 99-108.

Charley, B. (1986). Effects of immunopotentiating agents on alveolar macrophage properties. *Comp. Immunol. Microbiol. Infect. Dis.* **9,** 155-159.

Charley, B., Corthier, G., Houdayer, M., and Rouzé, P. (1980). Modifications des réactions immunitaires au cours de la peste porcine classique. *Ann. Rech. Vét.* **11,** 27-33.

Charley, B., Petit, E., and La Bonnardiére, C. (1985). Interferon-induced enhancement of newborn pig natural killing (NK) activity. *Ann. Rech. Vét.* **16,** 399-402.

Chu, R. M., Glock, R. D., Ross, R. F., and Cox, D. F. (1979). Lymphoid tissues of the small intestine of swine from birth to one month of age. *Am. J. Vet. Res.* **40,** 1713-1719.

Conlon, P. J., Washkewicz, T. L., Mochizuki, D. Y., Urdal, D. L., Gillis, S., and Henney, C. S. (1985). The treatment of induced immune deficiency with interleukin-2. *Immunol. Lett.* **10,** 307-314.

Curtis, S. E., Hurst, R. J., Widowski, T. M., Shanks, R. D., Jensen, A. H., Gonyou, H. W., Bane, D. P., Muehling, A. J., and Kesler, R. P. (1989). Effects of sow-crate design on health and performance of sows and piglets. *J. Anim. Sci.* **67,** 80-93.

Dantzer, R., and Mormede, P. (1983). Stress in farm animals: A need for reevaluation. *J. Anim. Sci.* **57,** 6–18.
Edwards, A. J. (1987). New directions in bovine veterinary practice. In "A Seminar in Bovine Immunology," pp. 25–29. Veterinary Learning Systems Co., Lawerenceville, New Jersey.
Filion, L. G., Willsom, P. J., Bielefeldt-Ohmann, H., Babiuk, L. A., and Thomson, R. G. (1984). The possible role of stress in the induction of pneumonic pasteurellosis. *Can. J. Comp. Med.* **48,** 268–274.
Flaming, K. P., Blecha, F., Fedorka-Cray, P. J., and Anderson, G. A. (1989). Influence of isoprinosine on lymphocyte function in virus-infected feeder pigs. *Am. J. Vet. Res.* **50,** 1653–1657.
Fogler, W. E., Raz, A., and Fidler, I. J. (1980). In situ activation of murine macrophages by liposomes containing lymphokines. *Cell. Immunol.* **53,** 214–219.
Ghram, A., Reddy, P. G., Morrill, J. L., Blecha, F., and Minocha, H. C. (1989). Bovine herpesvirus-1 and parainfluenza-3 virus interactions: Clinical and immunological responses in calves. *Can. J. Vet. Res.* **53,** 62–67.
Griffin, J. F. T. (1989). Stress and immunity: A unifying concept. *Vet. Immunol. Immunopathol.* **20,** 263–312.
Gross, W. B. (1972). Effect of social stress on the occurrence of Marek's disease in chickens. *Am. J. Vet. Res.* **33,** 2275–2279.
Gross, W. B. (1989). Effect of adrenal blocking chemicals on viral and respiratory infections of chickens. *Can. J. Vet. Res.* **53,** 48–51.
Gross, W. B., and Colmano, G. (1969). The effect of social isolation on resistance to some infectious diseases. *Poult. Sci.* **48,** 514–520.
Gross, W. B., Domermoth, C. H., and Siegel, P. B. (1988). Genetic and environmental effects on the response of chickens to avian adenovirus group II infection. *Avian Pathol.* **17,** 767–774.
Hahn, G. L., and Nienaber, J. A. (1989). Air temperature selection guides for growing-finishing swine based on performance and carcass composition. *U.S. Meat Anim. Res. Cent. Swine Res. Prog. Rep.* No. 3.
Hartmann, H. (1988). Critères biochmiques et hématologiques du stress et leurs relations avec les mécanismes de défense *Recl. Med. Vet.* **164,** 743–750.
Haye, S. N., and Kornegay, E. T. (1979). Immumoglobulin G, A and M antibody response in sow-reared and artificially reared pigs. *J. Anim. Sci.* **48,** 1116–1122.
Hennessy, K. J., Blecha, F., Pollmann, D. S., and Kluber, E. F. (1987). Isoprinosine and levamisole immunomodulation in artificially reared neonatal pigs. *Am. J. Vet. Res.* **48,** 477–480.
Hocking, W. G., and Golde, D. W. (1979). The pulmonary alveolar macrophage. *N. Engl. J. Med.* **301,** 580–587.
Huh, N. D., Kim, Y. B., Koren, H. S., and Amos, D. B. (1981). Natural killing and antibody-dependent cellular cytotoxicity in specific-pathogen-free miniature swine and germ-free piglets. II. Ontogenic development of NK and ADCC. *Int. J. Cancer* **28,** 175–178.
Iglesias, G., Pijoan, C., and Molitor, T. (1989). Interactions of pseudorabies virus with swine alveolar macrophages I: Virus replication. *Arch. Virol.* **104,** 107–115.
Jakab, G. J. (1982). Viral–bacterial interactions in pulmonary infection. *Adv. Vet. Sci. Comp. Med.* **26,** 155–171.
Kelley, K. W. (1980). Stress and immune function: A bibliographic review. *Ann. Rech. Vet.* **11,** 445–478.
Kelley, K. W. (1982). Immunobiology of domestic animals as affected by hot and cold weather. *Proc. Livest. Environ. Symp., 2nd,* pp. 470–482.

Kelley, K. W. (1984). Stress et immunité des animaux domestiques. *Point Vét.* **16,** 49–55.
Kelley, K. W. (1985). Immunological consequences of changing environmental stimuli. *In* "Animal Stress" (G. P. Moberg, ed.), pp. 193–223. Am. Physiol. Soc., Bethesda, Maryland.
Kelley, K. W. (1988). Cross-talk between the immune and endocrine systems. *J. Anim. Sci.* **66,** 2095.
Kelley, K. W., Osborne, C. A., Evermann, J. F., Parish, S. M., and Hinrichs, D. J. (1981). Whole blood leukocyte vs separated mononuclear cell blastogenesis in calves: Time-dependent changes after shipping. *Can. J. Comp. Med.* **45,** 249–258.
Khadom, N. J., Dedieu, J. F., and Viso, M. (1985). Bovine alveolar macrophages: A review. *Ann. Rech. Vet.* **16,** 175–183.
Kim, Y. B. (1975). Developmental immunity in the piglet. *In* "Immunodeficiency in Man and Animals" (D. Bergsma, ed.), pp. 549–557. Sinauer, Sunderland, Massachusetts.
Kim, Y. B. (1984). The effects of OK-432 on porcine NK and K cell system. *In* "Clinical and Experimental Studies in Immunotherapy" (T. Hoshino and A. Uchida, eds.), pp. 32–41. Excerpta Medica, Amsterdam.
Klemcke, H., Blecha, F., and Nienaber, J. (1987). Rapid effects of adrenocorticotropic hormone (ACTH) and restraint stressor on porcine lymphocyte function. *J. Anim. Sci.* **65,** Suppl. 1, 224.
Komori, T., Nakano, T., and Ohsugi, Y. (1987). Alleviation of depressed immunity caused by restraint-stress, by the immunomodulator, lobenzarit disodium (disodium 4-chloro-2, 2'-iminodibenzoate) *Int. J. Immunopharmacol.* **9,** 433–441.
Laude, H., Charley, B., and Gelfi, J. (1984). Replication of Transmissible Gastroenteritis coronavirus (TGEV) in swine alveolar macrophages. *J. Gen. Virol.* **65,** 327–332.
Lesnick, C. E., and Derbyshire, J. B. (1988). Activation of natural killer cells in newborn piglets by interferon induction. *Vet. Immunol. Immunopathol.* **18,** 109–117.
Loan, R. W. (1984). "Bovine Respiratory Disease: A Symposium." Texas A&M Univ. Press, College Station.
Maestroni, G. J. M., Conti, A., and Pierpaoli, W. (1988). Role of the pineal gland in immunity. III. Melatonin antagonizes the immunosuppressive effect of acute stress via an opiatergic mechanism. *Immunology* **63,** 465–469.
Markham, R. J. F., and Wilkie, B. N. (1980). Interaction between *Pasteurella hemolytica* and bovine alveolar macrophages: Cytotoxic effect on macrophages and impaired phagocytosis. *Am. J. Vet. Res.* **41,** 18–22.
McGlone, J. J., and Blecha, F. (1987). The welfare of sows and piglets: An examination of behavioral, immunological and productive traits in four management systems. *Appl. Anim. Behav. Sci.* **18,** 269–286.
McGlone, J. J., and Hellman, J. M. (1988). Local and general effects on behavior and performance of two- and seven-week-old castrated and uncastrated piglets. *J. Anim. Sci.* **66,** 3049–3058.
Metzger, J. J., Ballet-Lapierre, C., and Houdayer, M. (1978). Partial inhibition of the humoral immune response of pigs after early postnatal immunization. *Am. J. Vet. Res.* **39,** 627–631.
Minton, J. E., Nichols, D. A., Blecha, F., Westerman, R. B., and Phillips (1988). Fluctuating ambient temperatures for weaned pigs: Effects on growth performance and immunological and endocrinological functions. *J. Anim. Sci.* **66,** 1907–1914.
Mormede, P., Soissons, J., Bluthe, R. M., Raoult, J., LeGarff, G., Levieux, D., and Dantzer, R. (1982). Effect of transportation on blood serum composition, disease incidence, and production traits in young calves. Influence of the journey duration. *Ann. Rech. Vet.* **13,** 369–384.

Munck, H., Guyre, P., and Holbrook (1984). Physiological functions of glucocorticoids in stress and their relation to pharmacological actions. *Endocr. Rev.* **5,** 25–44.

Murata, H., Takahashi, H., and Matsumoto, H. (1987). The effects of road transportation on peripheral blood lymphocyte subpopulations, lymphocyte blastogenesis and neutrophil function in calves. *Br. Vet. J.* **143,** 166–174.

National Mastitis Council (1987). "Current Concepts of Bovine Mastitis," pp. 6–8. National Mastitis Council, Arlington, Virginia.

Neumann, R., Mehlhorn, G., Buchholz, I., Johannsen, U., and Schimmel, D. (1987). Experimentelle untersuchungen zur wirkung einer chronischen aerogenen schadgasbelastung des saugferkels mit ammoniak unterschiedlicher konzentrationen. II. Die reaktion zellularer und humoraler infectionsabwehrmechanismen NH_3-exponieter saugferkel unter den bedingungen einer experimentallen *Pasteurella-multocida*-infektion mit und ohne thermo-motorische belasturg. *J. Vet. Med., Reihe B* **34,** 241–253.

Nonnecke, B. J., and Harp, J. A. (1988). Effects of *Staphylococcus aureus* on bovine mononuclear leukocyte proliferation and viability: Modulation by phagocytic leukocytes. *J. Dairy Sci.* **71,** 835–842.

Onizuka, N., Maede, Y., Ohsugi T., and Namioka, S. (1987). Nonspecific cell-mediated cytotoxicity of peripheral blood lymphocytes derived from suckling piglets. *Jpn. J. Vet. Res.* **35,** 41–48.

Pabst, R., Geist, M., Rothkötter, H. J., and Fritz, F. J. (1988). Postnatal development and lymphocyte production of jejunal and ileal Peyer's patches in normal and gnotobiotic pigs. *Immunology* **64,** 539–544.

Pankey, J. W., Boddie, N. T., Watts, J. L., and Nickerson, S. C. (1985). Evaluation of protein A and commercial bacterin as vaccines against *Staphylococcus aureus* mastitis by experimental challenge. *J. Dairy Sci.* **68,** 726–731.

Reddy, P. G., Blecha, F., Minocha, H. C., Anderson, G. A., Morrill, J. L., Fedorka-Cray, P. J., and Baker, P. E. (1989a). Bovine recombinant interleukin-2 augments immunity and resistance to bovine herpesvirus infection. *Vet. Immunol. Immunopathol.* **23,** 61–74.

Reddy, P. G., Blecha, F., McVey, D. S., Shirley, J. E., Morrill, J. L., and Baker, P. E. (1989b). Bovine recombinant granulocyte-macrophage colony-stimulating factor augments functions of neutrophils from mastitic cows. *J. Dairy Sci.* **72,** Suppl. 1, 11.

Regnier, J. A., and Kelley, K. W. (1981). Heat- and cold-stress suppresses *in vivo* and *in vitro* cellular immune responses of chickens. *Am. J. Vet. Res.* **41,** 294–299.

Reyero, C., Thalhammer, J. G., Reszler, G., and Stöckl, W. (1978). Development of peripheral B and T lymphocytes in piglets. *Z. Immunitaetsforsch.* **154,** 409–415.

Roth, J. A., and Kaeberle, M. L. (1983). Suppression of neutrophil and lymphocyte function induced by a vaccinal strain of bovine viral diarrhea virus with and without the administration of ACTH. *Am. J. Vet. Res.* **12,** 2366–2372.

Rothlein, R., Gallily, R., and Kim, Y. B. (1981). Development of alveolar macrophages in specific pathogen-free and germ-free Minnesota miniature swine. *J. Reticuloendothel. Soc.* **30,** 483–495.

Salmon, H. (1984). Immunité chez le foetus et le nouveau-né: Modèle porcin. *Reprod. Nutr. Dev.* **24,** 197–206.

Shimizu, M., Shimizu, Y., and Kodama, Y. (1978). Effects of ambient temperatures on induction of transmissible gastroenteritis in feeder pigs. *Infect. Immun.* **21,** 747–752.

Siegel, H. S. (1985). Immunological responses as indicators of stress. *World's Poult. Sci. J.* **41,** 36–44.

Staples, G. E., and Haugse, G. N. (1974). Losses in young calves after transportation. *Br. Vet. J.* **130,** 374–378.

Sterzl, J., and Silverstein, A. M. (1967). Developmental aspects of immunity. *Adv. Immunol.* **6,** 337–459.

Tyler, J. W., Cullor, J. S., Osburn, B. I., and Parker, K. (1988). Age-related variations in serum concentrations of the third component of complement in swine. *Am. J. Vet. Res.* **49,** 1104–1106.

Van Oirschot, J. T. (1983). Congenital infections with nonarbotogaviruses. *Vet. Microbiol.* **8,** 321–361.

Verhagen, J. M. F., Groen, A., Jocobs, J., and Boon, J. H. (1987). The effect of different climatic environment on metabolism and its relation to time of *Haemophilus pleuropneumoniae* infection in pigs. *Livest. Prod. Sci.* **17,** 365–379.

Westly, H. J., and Kelley, K. W. (1984). Physiologic concentrations of cortisol suppress cell-mediated immune events in the domestic pig. *Proc. Soc. Exp. Biol. Med.* **177,** 156–164.

Yang, W. C., and Schultz, R. D. (1986). Ontogeny of natural killer cell activity and antibody dependent cell mediated cytotoxicity in pigs. *Dev. Comp. Immunol.* **10,** 405–418.

Model Systems to Study Immunomodulation in Domestic Food Animals

JAMES A. ROTH AND KEVAN P. FLAMING

Department of Veterinary Microbiology and Preventive Medicine, Iowa State University, Ames, Iowa 50011

I. Introduction
II. Stress Models
   A. Weaning
   B. Transport Stress
III. Glucocorticoid Immunosupression Models
IV. Infectious Disease Model Systems
   A. Bovine Respiratory Disease
   B. Mastitis
V. Summary
   References

I. Introduction

Immunosuppression is considered to be an important component in the pathogenesis of many infectious disease syndromes that affect domestic food producing animals. There are many potential causes for immunosuppression, including stress, viral infection, inadequate nutrition, hormonal fluctuations, and exposure to environmental toxins. In addition, immune function in very young and elderly animals is normally suboptimal compared to that of healthy young adult animals. A number of immunomodulators have recently been evaluated for their ability to overcome some of these immunosuppressive conditions. Results of these experiments indicate that effective immunomodulators could be used to enhance suboptimal immune function and thereby increase resistance to infectious diseases (Blecha, 1988a). This chapter will focus on the use of immunosuppressive conditions as model systems for evaluating immunomodulators.

Initially, there are a number of factors to consider when developing or using immunomodulators.

1. In order to effectively use an immunomodulator, the cellular and molecular basis for the immunosuppression and the action of the immunomodulator should be understood.
2. Immunosuppressive conditions may have differing physiologic origins, just as immunomodulators act through different pathways.
3. An immunomodulator may act by reversing a specific defect induced by the immunosuppressant or it may cause general nonspecific enhancement of immune function. Therefore, depending upon the mechanism of action, an immunomodulator may act to overcome suppression induced by some factors and have no activity against other factors.
4. The model systems used to evaluate immunomodulators should involve immunosuppression, since the purpose of an immunomodulator is to correct defective immune function.
5. Immunomodulators should also be evaluated in healthy, nonimmunosuppressed animals to detect any potential adverse effects.
6. Significant species differences in response to immunomodulators exist. Therefore, it is important to evaluate immunomodulators in a target species whenever possible.
7. Timing of administration and dosage may be critical to obtaining a beneficial effect with an immunomodulator.

The activity of an immunomodulator may be evaluated by adding the immunomodulator to cells in *in vitro* assays or by administering the immunomodulator to an animal. In some cases an immunomodulator may have very different activities *in vitro* and *in vivo*. For example, some immunomodulators may work by inducing the animal to secrete various cytokines, while others must be metabolized to become active. These immunomodulators would act indirectly to cause changes in the immune function. In this situation, the results of an *in vitro* assay for immunomodulator activity would be negative, whereas *in vivo* administration of the immunomodulator may have a positive effect. Conversely, immunomodulators may have activity *in vitro* but no demonstrable activity after administration *in vivo*. This could occur for a number of reasons, including inability to achieve sufficient immunomodulator concentration *in vivo*, inadequate distribution of the immunomodulator *in vivo*, or rapid metabolic degradation of the compound *in vivo*. These problems illustrate the need to validate *in vitro* results by administering immunomodulators to animals *in vivo*.

Dosage and timing of administration of immunomodulators are also important factors to be considered. Some immunomodulators have a narrow, therapeutic dose range (Roth and Frank, 1989). In some cases, immunomodulators have been noted to lose biologic activity at higher dosages (Kaeberle and Roth, 1984), and in other cases, they have been noted to have undesirable side effects at doses that are only marginally higher than the effective dosage (Roth and Frank, 1989; Roth and Kaeberle, 1985b). The timing of administration of an immunomodulator relative to the time of occurrence of immunosuppression also may be important. Some immunomodulators must be given before the onset of the immunosuppressive event (Babiuk *et al.*, 1987); others are capable of reversing immunosuppression once it has occurred (Chiang *et al.*, 1990). The biological kinetics of the immunomodulator should be established in order to determine optimal dosage, onset, and duration of action. Such kinetic determinations require the use of quantitative assays to determine the function of cells that play an important role in host defense mechanisms.

II. Stress Models

Both physical and psychological distress are capable of altering immune function in animals (Kelley, 1980, 1982, 1984, 1985; Siegel, 1985; Albani-Vangili, 1985; Blecha, 1988b). Some of the events associated with distress that are believed to be important in altering immune function are increased secretion of glucocorticoids, endorphins, enkephalins, and catecholamines. These molecules are capable of directly altering host defense mechanisms. The distress associated with weaning and transportation in piglets and calves has been used in various model systems to evaluate immunomodulators; researchers have also shown that young calves and piglets have suboptimal immune function compared to normal adults (Reyero *et al.*, 1979; Hauser *et al.*, 1986).

A. Weaning

Weaning is certainly a stressful event for domestic animals. Piglets, for example, are shifted from a liquid diet to solid food, handled extensively, regrouped, and separated from their sow. Blecha and associates (1985) have documented a decrease in cellular immune function associated with weaning pigs. Other investigators have used this critical time in the pig's life as a model to evaluate the effectiveness of immunomodulators. Peplowski et al. (1981) described an increase in hemagglutination titers associated with supplemental (dietary or injectable) vitamin E and/or selenium treatment in pigs that were placed on trial immediately after weaning at 4–5 weeks of age. Blodgett et al. (1986) similarly evaluated the effects of several levels of dietary selenium on the immunoglobulin response to injected antigens and the dermal response to phytohemagglutinin of recently weaned swine. No significant effects were found at the levels tested. Another experiment by Flaming et al. (1988) used weaning at 3 weeks of age as a simple model of immunosuppression to evaluate the immunomodulator imuthiol. Their results showed a decrease in *in vitro* lymphocyte blastogenic responses associated with drug treatment and both positive and negative drug-associated effects on *in vivo* phytohemagglutinin intradermal test responses.

Other investigators have added additional stressors to the weanling pig in their experimental designs. Yen and Pond (1987) subjected pigs that had just been weaned to crowding stress to evaluate the effects of dietary supplementation with vitamin C or carbadox. Kornegay et al. (1986) evaluated supplemental vitamin C and E on growth performance and immune function in pigs that were kept at either a "comfortable" or "cold" nursery temperature. Hennessy et al. (1987) used artificial rearing, beginning at 48 hours of age, as their model to evaluate the effects of isoprinosine and levamisole on immune responses in pigs. Other workers (Reyero et al., 1979) also have investigated the effect of levamisole on the immune responses of young pigs (1 week and 3–4 months old) that were raised under normal husbandry practices.

The weanling pig as a model of immunosuppression offers several advantages. The drug of interest can be evaluated in a possible target animal, with a model system that has a direct application and considerable economic importance. The methodology required is relatively simple, easily repeatable, and suitable for large numbers of animals. The subjects are small in size, making trials with expensive or scarce drugs more practical. Additionally, the large litter size of pigs allows one to often assign littermates to each treatment, thereby reducing genetic differences between treatments. However, suitable housing must be available, and should be as uniform as possible to minimize environmental differences between experimental units. A limitation of the weanling pig model is that it is difficult to obtain a sufficient volume of blood on a daily basis to adequately evaluate neutrophil function.

Weaning was also a part of the stress applied to calves in an experiment designed to evaluate the effectiveness of thiabendazole in stressed animals (Roth et al., 1984). Four- to six-month-old calves were taken off pasture, weaned, the bull calves were castrated, and all calves were inoculated with several different antigens. The cattle were then confined to a feedlot. Antibody production to the injected antigens was monitored to determine immune responsiveness.

The calf weaning model has several disadvantages when compared to the pig weaning model. Calves are more genetically heterogenous and of a wider age and size range. Weather can be a much larger and more variable stress factor for calves on pasture than for swine raised in confinement. Calves are also larger, more expensive to obtain, and require more drug per animal. An advantage of the weanling calves model is that it is easier to get large volumes of blood repeatedly.

B. Transport Stress

Another model of immunosuppression due to stress that has been used is the transport of cattle to a feedlot. Blecha et al. (1984) have documented suppression of blastogenesis in response to mitogens subsequent to transport stress. Brazle et al. (1984) reported an experiment that evaluated receiving diet and levamisole treatment in feeder calves exposed to transport stress. Subsequent to feedlot arrival the animals were exposed to 16 hours of rain followed by cold winds, certainly not an easily repeated experimental protocol. This same type of model was used by Irwin et al. (1980) in a field trial evaluating the clinical efficacy of a single arrival treatment with levamisole HCl, levamisole PO_4, or thiabendazole on the incidence of shipping fever in 1464 cattle within 30 days of feedlot arrival. However, untreated controls were not included in this study.

The transport model in cattle has the advantage of providing direct clinical application in a target species with potentially great economic benefits. Large volumes of blood may be easily obtained on a regular basis from cattle. The methodology is straight forward, but due to many uncontrolled factors (weather, pretransport status, degree of exposure to infectious agents, age, and broad genetic differences) this model may produce variable results. The costs of obtaining and maintaining cattle of this size, and the amount of drug needed often limit the number of animals that may be used. Additionally, large feedlot trials are not suitable for experimental drugs that necessitate the destruction of the animals without the possibility of salvage.

III. Glucocorticoid Immunosuppression Models

Glucocorticoids are secreted in response to stress, and are known to increase the susceptibility of animals to infectious diseases (Roth, 1985; Roth and Kaeberle, 1982). Glucocorticoids are antiinflammatory and can suppress lymphocyte, macrophage, and neutrophil function in a dose-dependent manner in some species. They have been used as a reproducible method for induction of immunosuppression and subsequent evaluation of the activity of immunomodulators.

The mechanism of immunosuppression induced by glucocorticoids has been well characterized. Glucocorticoids are known to induce the synthesis of protein inhibitors of phospholipase A_2 in many cell types (lipomodulin, macrocortin) (Blackwell *et al.*, 1983; Hirata *et al.*, 1980). The phospholipase A_2 inhibitors limit the release of arachidonic acid from membrane phospholipids and therefore inhibit the formation of prostaglandins, thromboxanes, leukotrienes, and hydroxyeicosatetraenoic acids (HETEs). This activity inhibits a step in signal transduction that is known to be important in response to external stimuli (Valone, 1984). Glucocorticoids (hydrocortisone) also induce monocytes to secrete a protein factor that inhibits the activity of neutrophils (Stevenson, 1977; Frank and Roth, 1986). The combined activities of the inhibition of arachidonic acid metabolism and the glucocorticoid-induced monocyte factor will mimic *in vitro* the *in vivo* suppression of neutrophil function, which is observed after administration of glucocorticoids in cattle (Webb and Roth, 1987).

Glucocorticoids have been shown to inhibit antibody responses to specific antigens and lymphocyte blastogenic activity in response to mitogens (Pruett *et al.*, 1987; Kaeberle and Roth, 1984; Roth *et al.*, 1984; Blecha and Minocha, 1983) in cattle. The decreased blastogenic activity is associated with a decrease in the synthesis of IL-2 by lymphocytes after glucocorticoid treatment *in vivo* (Blecha and Baker, 1986).

Important species differences in response to glucocorticoids exist in domestic food producing animals. The pig seems to be much more resistant than cattle to immunosuppression by dexamethasone. Dexamethasone administered intramuscularly to pigs at 2.0 mg/kg of body weight did not consistently alter the lymphocyte and neutrophil functions that are inhibited in cattle given 0.04 mg/kg of body weight dexamethasone intramuscularly (Roth and Kaeberle, 1982). Chickens are sensitive to glucocorticoid-induced immunosuppression. Exogenous cortisol administered to chickens was associated with a decreased antibody response to sheep red blood cells, and was used as a model system to evaluate the ability of ascorbic acid to overcome the steroid-induced immunosuppression (Pardue and Thaxton, 1984). Dietary supplementation with ascorbic acid significantly ameliorated the immunosuppressive effect of cortisol.

The glucocorticoid immunosuppression model used most extensively for evaluation of immunomodulators is dexamethasone administered to cattle. Dexamethasone is approximately 25 times as potent as cortisol as an antiinflammatory agent. Advantages of the dexamethasone immunosuppression model for use in cattle are:

1. It is easily reproducible. The degree of immunosuppression can be controlled by changing the dosage and duration of administration.
2. Dexamethasone suppresses a wide range of host defense mechanisms in cattle (Roth and Kaeberle, 1981, 1982; Kaeberle and Roth, 1984; Pruett *et al.*, 1987). Therefore, an immunomodulator can be tested to determine if it normalizes a wide range of host defense mechanisms.
3. Dexamethasone administered every 24 hours causes a continuous immunosuppression. Therefore the duration of action of an immunomodulator to reverse an immunosuppression can be determined by monitoring cell function on a daily basis.
4. The administration of dexamethasone causes very little distress to the animals and the same animals can be used for multiple experiments.

The dexamethasone immunosuppression model may mimic the suppression occurring in stressed animals with elevated plasma cortisol concentration; however, the results obtained when evaluating immunomodulators in the dexamethasone immunosuppression model may not be relevant to the use of the immunomodulator on other causes of immunosuppression. Yet, because of the many advantages of this system, one may try to determine the optimal dosage and timing of administration in this model before evaluating the immunomodulator in other more cumbersome and expensive immunosuppression models.

The following series of experiments illustrate the usefulness of the dexamethasone model for titrating an effective dose, determining the time of administration and duration of action, gaining information about the mechanism of immunomodulator action, and gaining experience with an immunomodulator in a bacterial challenge model.

Dexamethasone-induced immunosuppression has been used as a model for evaluating several potential immunomodulators in cattle in our laboratory (Roth *et al.*, 1984, 1989, 1990; Kaeberle and Roth, 1984; Roth and Kaeberle, 1984, 1985a,b; Roth and Frank, 1989; Chiang *et al.*, 1990. Our typical approach is to first test several dosages of an immunomodulator in normal nonimmunosuppressed cattle to screen for biologic activity, optimal dose, and for detrimental effects in normal cattle. A typical experiment would have 4 groups with 5 or 6 animals per group. One group would serve as the untreated controls; each of the other groups would receive a single administration of a dosage of the selected immunomodulator.

The factors normally evaluated include: body temperature, total and differential white blood cell count, lymphocyte blastogenic responsiveness to mitogens, and several aspects of neutrophil function (random migration under agarose, chemotaxis, ingestion of *Staphylococcus aureus*, activity of the myeloperoxidase-hydrogen peroxide-halide antibacterial system, superoxide anion generation, antibody-dependent and antibody-independent cell-mediated cytotoxicity). These parameters would be evaluated on two occasions prior to administration of drug and then 3 days in a row beginning 24 hours after drug administration. If biologic activity of the compound is detected, then the drug would be tested in dexamethasone-treated animals using a 2 × 2 factorial arrangement. This experiment would include a group of control animals, a group of animals immunosuppressed by administering dexamethasone (0.04 mg/kg of body weight intramuscularly daily for 3 to 4 consecutive days), a group which received the immunomodulator, and a group which received dexamethasone and the immunomodulator. The immunomodulator may be administered before, concurrently with, or after administration of the first dose of dexamethasone. This model enables one to determine:

1. The degree of suppression of immune function induced by dexamethasone by a comparison of the results of the dexamethasone and control groups.
2. The alteration of immune function in normal nonimmunosuppressed animals induced by the immunomodulator using a comparison of the responses in the control group and the group that receives immunomodulator.
3. The ability of the immunomodulator to overcome the immunosuppression induced by dexamethasone; this ability is quantitated by comparing immune function in the group that received dexamethasone plus immunomodulator to the immune function in the group that received dexamethasone alone, and to the control group (i.e., the factorial interaction).

We have used variations of this model system to test the immunomodulatory activity of levamisole (Roth and Kaeberle, 1984), thiabendazole (Roth et al., 1984; Kaeberle and Roth, 1984), ascorbic acid (Roth and Kaeberle, 1985b), decoquinate (Roth et al., 1989), avridine (Roth and Kaeberle, 1985a), recombinant bovine interferon gamma (Roth and Frank, 1989; Chiang et al., 1990), and recombinant human interleukin-2 (rhIL-2) (Roth et al., 1990). Levamisole and human IL-2 had no influence on the dexamethasone-induced immunosuppression. Some of the compounds (thiabendazole, ascorbic acid, and decoquinate) had limited abilities to overcome the influence of dexamethasone on bovine neutrophil or lymphocyte function. The avridine and recombinant bovine interferon gamma, however, significantly improved several aspects of neutrophil function in dexamethasone-treated cattle.

Avridine is a lipoidal amine compound that has been shown to be an interferon inducer and an adjuvant capable of enhancing humoral and cell-mediated immune responses (Hoffman et al., 1973; Waldman and Ganguly, 1978; Niblack et al., 1979; Anderson and Reynolds, 1979). Woodard et al. (1983) demonstrated that neutrophils from cattle treated with avridine had increased bactericidal activity. The avridine had more dramatic effects in the dexamethasone-treated animals than it had previously shown in normal nonimmunosuppressed animals (Roth and Kaeberle, 1985a). Four out of five of the neutrophil function assays were improved or returned toward normal by avridine administration in the dexamethasone-treated animals. Lymphocyte blastogenic responses to phytohemagglutinin were also significantly enhanced by avridine administration prior to the administration of dexamethasone.

Since avridine had previously been shown to act as an interferon inducer, it is likely that the avridine, when administered *in vivo*, caused the animals to secrete interferon and perhaps other cytokines. These endogenous cytokines may have been responsible for the immunomodulatory activity. To test this hypothesis, peripheral blood mononuclear leukocytes (PMNL) isolated from cattle (which had been previously infected with the Bovine herpesvirus-1 [BHV1] virus) were incubated with inactivated BHV1 virus in order to induce the lymphocytes to secrete lymphokines. The PMNL culture supernate, which had been tested and found to contain interferon, was incubated with neutrophils *in vitro* to determine its influence on neutrophil function. In general, the PMNL supernatant had approximately the same biologic activity on neutrophils as did the avridine administration *in vivo* (Lukacs et al., 1985).

In order to determine if it was the gamma interferon within the lymphocyte supernatant which had the biologic activity, recombinant bovine interferon gamma was obtained from Genentec Inc. (South San Francisco, CA) and evaluated for its activity on neutrophil function *in vitro* (Steinbeck et al., 1986). The recombinant bovine interferon gamma, when incubated with neutrophils *in vitro,* had a very similar influence on neutrophil function to that of the lymphocyte supernatant *in vitro* and avridine *in vivo* (Steinbeck et al., 1986; Lukacs et al., 1985; Roth and Kaeberle, 1985b).

These results implied that the biologic activity of avridine could have been due primarily to the induction of gamma interferon. If this was the case, then the administration of recombinant bovine interferon gamma should have similar *in vivo* biologic activity as avridine. Three dosages of recombinant bovine interferon gamma (CIBA-GEIGY Limited, Basel, Switzerland) were evaluated in normal nonimmunosuppressed animals (Roth and Frank, 1989). The optimal dosage was selected and tested in an experiment having 5 controls, 5 animals immunosuppressed with dexamethasone, 5 animals treated with 0.5 mg of recombinant bovine interferon gamma, and 5 animals given dexamethasone plus 0.5 mg of recombinant bovine interferon gamma. The dexamethasone and recombinant bovine interferon gamma were each administered 2 days in a row. Neutrophil and lymphocyte function were evaluated twice before drug administration (to ensure that there were no major differences between groups before treatment) and 2 days in a row beginning 24 hours after the first administration of drug. The experiment was replicated in an additional twenty head of cattle so that there were ten animals per treatment group. The interferon gamma was found to have nearly the same activity in dexamethasone-treated animals as did the avridine (Roth and Kaeberle, 1985a; Roth and Frank, 1989).

Since the recombinant bovine interferon gamma was successful in improving several of the dexamethasone-induced defects in neutrophil function, it was decided to test the recombinant bovine interferon gamma in a bacterial infection model that depended upon dexamethasone immunosuppression as an important component of the pathogenesis. The bacterial challenge model used involved the intrabronchial administration of 5×10^9 colony-forming units of *Haemophilus somnus* and the intramuscular injection of dexamethasone daily for 3 days starting 1 day before *H. somnus* infection (Chiang et al., 1990). This challenge regimen was selected because the bacterial challenge inoculum would not produce severe pneumonia in normal nonimmunosuppressed calves, but would produce severe pneumonia in dexamethasone-treated animals. Therefore, an immunomodulator that could overcome the influence of dexamethasone should significantly decrease the severity of pneumonia.

In addition to the immunosuppression induced by dexamethasone, this model system involves at least two other factors that contribute to the pathogenesis. Young calves (less than 5 months of age) are known to have suboptimal neutrophil function (Hauser et al., 1986; Slauson et al., 1987). Secondly, H. somnus is known to have surface components that inhibit phagosome–lysosome fusion in neutrophils (Chiang et al., 1986; Hubbard et al., 1986; Bertram et al., 1986; Canning et al., 1986) and is therefore able to resist killing by the neutrophil (Czuprynski and Hamilton, 1985). Therefore, stress-induced increases in cortisol concentration, suboptimal function of neutrophils in young calves, and H. somnus virulence factors that suppress neutrophil function may all contribute to the pathogenesis of H. somnus pneumonia. If an immunomodulator can improve neutrophil function (and/or other host defense mechanisms) in the face of any or all of these factors, it should reduce the severity of pneumonia.

Twenty-four Holstein steers (1–2 months of age) were used for this experiment, 6 served as nontreated controls, 6 received recombinant bovine interferon gamma (2 μg/kg body weight) subcutaneously daily for 2 days starting 1 day before infection with H. somnus, 6 received dexamethasone (0.04 mg/kg of body weight by intramuscular injection

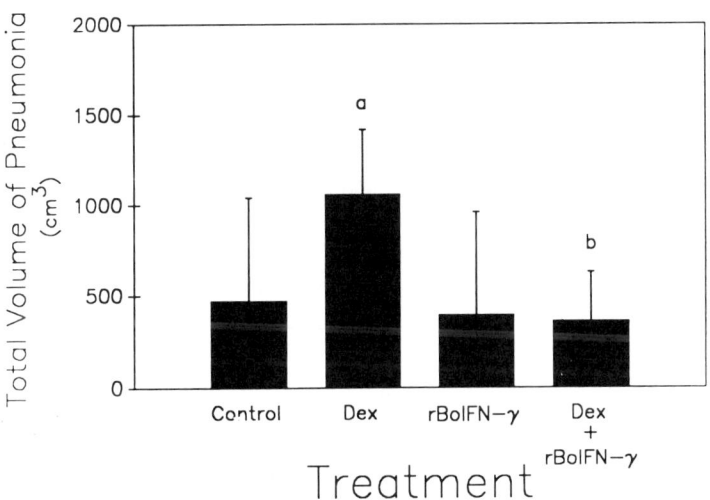

FIG. 1. Total volume of pneumonia (mean ± SEM) in 2- to 3-month-old calves 7 days after intrabronchial inoculation of 5×10^9 colony-forming units of H. somnus. Calves were given saline (controls), dexamethasone (0.04 mg/kg for 3 days intramuscularly), recombinant bovine interferon gamma (rBoIFN-γ)(2.0 μg/kg for 2 days subcutaneously), or both dexamethasone and rBoIFN-γ. There were 6 animals per group. a, The indicated value is significantly different from control, $p < 0.05$; b, the indicated value is significantly different from Dex, $p < 0.05$. Drug administration was initiated 24 hours before inoculation with H. somnus (Chiang et al., 1989).

daily for 3 days starting 1 day before experimental infection), and 6 received both the dexamethasone and recombinant bovine interferon gamma dosage regimens. The animals were monitored for one week, then necropsied to determine the extent of bacterial pneumonia. Two of the six dexamethasone-treated animals died due to bacterial pneumonia before the scheduled necropsy. The dexamethasone-treated group had a significantly increased total volume of affected lung tissue when compared to the control animals (Fig. 1). The group that received gamma interferon had a severity of pneumonia essentially only equal to that in the control animals. This was a mild pneumonia that was resolving at the time of necropsy, 7 days postchallenge. The group that received dexamethasone plus recombinant bovine interferon gamma had pneumonic lesions essentially equivalent to those of the control group; the dexamethasone plus recombinant bovine interferon gamma group did not have the severe pneumonia observed in the dexamethasone treated group. Therefore, the recombinant bovine interferon gamma overcame the increased susceptibility to bacterial pneumonia induced by the administration of dexamethasone. This clearly demonstrates that gamma interferon can have a role in the prevention of bacterial pneumonia associated with immunosuppression without the involvement of a viral component.

IV. Infectious Disease Model Systems

Prevention or therapy of infectious disease is the ultimate goal of most immunomodulation research in food producing animals. Therefore, infectious disease models are the most convincing for demonstrating the efficacy of immunomodulators. Both naturally occurring infectious disease and infectious disease challenge models may be used. Naturally occurring diseases are difficult to predict and to control, leading to variable and sometimes contradictory results. Therefore, large numbers of animals are required when naturally occurring disease is used for evaluating immunomodulators. Using healthy animals challenged with an infectious agent to evaluate the efficacy of an immunomodulator allows for a better controlled experiment so that fewer animals are used than if the researcher depended upon a natural disease outbreak. Animal to animal and experiment to experiment variability is still a problem with infectious disease challenge models. This variability is primarily due to host factors, which vary from individual to individual, and differences in the infectious challenge inoculum. The challenge inoculum must be adjusted so that infection is established and perhaps disease is produced; however, if the challenge inoculum is too high, it may overwhelm the ability of any immunomodulator to improve host resistance.

Before considering an infectious disease as a possible model system, one should understand the pathogenesis of the infectious disease to determine if prevention or therapy with an immunomodulator is a viable option, to predict the type of immunomodulator that may be effective, and to predict the optimal time of administration of the immunomodulator. Since challenge models that result in the production of clinical disease cause more distress to the animal than evaluating immunomodulators in either normal animals or in animals treated with mildly immunosuppressive drugs, it is best to do dose titration and mechanism of action studies prior to evaluating the immunomodulator in infectious disease challenge models.

Infectious disease models that have been used for evaluating immunomodulators in food producing animals include: bovine respiratory disease after stress (discussed in section II of this chapter, Stress Models), challenge with bovine herpesvirus 1 (BHV1) with or without subsequent challenge with *Pasteurella haemolytica* (Blecha et al., 1987; Babiuk et al., 1985, 1987; Roney et al., 1985; Czarniecki et al., 1985; Lawman et al., 1987; Bielefeldt-Ohmann and Babiuk, 1985a), mastitis (Kehrli et al., 1989c; Buddle et al., 1988; Flesh et al., 1982; Ishikawa et al., 1982; Onodera et al., 1980; Ovadia et al., 1978; Ziv et al., 1981; Anderson, 1984), bovine leukemia virus infection (Van Der Maaten et al., 1983), bovine viral diarrhea (BVD) virus infection (Saperstein et al., 1983), Marek's disease virus infection in chickens (Confer and Adldinger, 1981), *Haemophilus somnus* in calves (Chiang et al., 1990), and pseudorabies in pigs (Flaming et al., 1989).

A. BOVINE RESPIRATORY DISEASE

Challenge inoculation with BHV1 is the infectious disease challenge system that has been used the most extensively for evaluating immunomodulators in domestic food producing animals (Blecha et al., 1987; Babiuk et al., 1985, 1987; Roney et al., 1985; Czarniecki et al., 1985; Lawman et al., 1987; Bielefeldt-Ohmann and Babiuk, 1985a). Bovine herpesvirus 1 is an important contributor to the pathogenesis of the bovine respiratory disease complex. This virus, along with the BVD virus, bovine respiratory syncytial virus (BRSV), and parainfluenza 3 virus, has been shown to be immunosuppressive in cattle and to predispose calves to bacterial pneumonia (Jericho et al., 1982; Jericho and Langford, 1978; Potgieter et al., 1984, 1988; Roth, 1984). If a calf is infected with any one of these four viruses, then challenge exposed 3–6 days later with a relatively low dose of *P. haemolytica* (or *H. somnus* for BRSV), the calf will develop a bacterial pneumonia. The preexisting viral infection impairs host defense mechanisms sufficiently to allow an otherwise nonpathogenic challenge dose to produce severe pneumonia. Viral immunosuppression is believed to play an important role in the pathogenesis of naturally occurring outbreaks of bacterial pneumonia in cattle (Roth, 1984). Therefore, infection with any one of these viruses should serve as a useful model for evaluating immunomodulators.

Immunomodulators have been evaluated in animals challenge exposed with BHV1 only and in animals challenged with BHV1 followed by *P. haemolytica* (Blecha et al., 1987; Babiuk et al., 1985, 1987; Roney et al., 1985; Czarniecki et al., 1985; Lawman et al., 1987; Bielefeldt-Ohmann and Babiuk, 1985a). Infection with BHV1 has been shown to decrease neutrophil, lymphocyte, and macrophage function (Bielefeldt-Ohmann and Babiuk, 1985b, 1986; Blecha et al., 1987; Filion et al., 1981; Lawman et al., 1987). Treatment of cattle with human leukocyte interferon alpha (Roney et al., 1985) or recombinant bovine interferon alpha prior to infection with BHV1 has been shown to significantly reduce the severity of clinical signs due to BHV1 infection (Lawman et al., 1987; Bielefeldt-Ohmann and Babiuk, 1985a; Babiuk et al., 1985, 1987). Treatment with recombinant bovine interferon alpha prior to BHV1 challenge significantly improved certain aspects of neutrophil and lymphocyte function in BHV1 infected animals (Lawman et al., 1987; Babiuk et al., 1985; Bielefeldt-Ohmann and Babiuk, 1985a) and significantly reduced morbidity and mortality in calves challenged with *P. haemolytica* after the BHV1 challenge (Babiuk et al., 1985, 1987; Czarniecki et al., 1985). In order for the recombinant bovine interferon alpha to be effective, it had to be given prior to the BHV1 challenge. The recombinant bovine interferon alpha treatment did not significantly decrease BHV1 shedding from the nasal cavity, therefore it would appear that the recombinant bovine interferon alpha reduced the clinical signs due to its immunomodulatory activities rather than to a direct antiviral effect.

Isoprinosine was also evaluated for its influence in BHV1-infected cattle. Isoprinosine administration enhanced IL-2 production by lymphocytes from infected cattle, but it did not reverse the immunosuppressive effect of BHV1 on lymphocyte blastogenesis or the clinical course of the viral infection (Blecha et al., 1987).

The bovine viral diarrhea virus also is known to be immunosuppressive in cattle (Roth et al., 1981, 1986; Potgieter et al., 1984; Muscoplat et al., 1973). Levamisole was evaluated in calves experimentally infected with BVD virus (Saperstein et al., 1983). Levamisole was given subcutaneously daily for 3 consecutive days of each week for 7 weeks, beginning 1 week after infection. The course of the infection was mild and all calves recovered clinically between postinfection day 13 and 23. There was no difference in severity of infection or speed of recovery between the levamisole-treated calves and control calves. Cell function assays were not done in this experiment.

B. Mastitis

An increased incidence of mastitis has been associated with impaired host defense mechanisms in both cattle and swine (Lofstedt et al., 1983; Kehrli and Goff, 1989; Kehrli et al., 1989a,b; Ishikawa and Shimizu, 1983; Nagahata et al., 1988; Kashiwazaki, 1984). This leads to the hypothesis that immunosuppression may contribute to the pathogenesis of mastitis and that immunomodulators may reduce the susceptibility to mastitis. Sows that had decreased neutrophil random migration, ingestion of bacteria, and iodination were more susceptible to postpartum mastitis caused by *Escherichia coli* (Lofstedt et al., 1983). Dairy cows were found to have decreased lymphocyte blastogenic responsiveness to mitogens and decreased neutrophil random migration, chemotaxis, chemiluminescence, cytochrome c reduction, and iodination during the first week after parturition (Kehrli et al., 1989a,b; Kehrli and Goff, 1989; Nagahata et al., 1988). This periparturient period is associated with a high incidence of mastitis caused by opportunistic environmental pathogens (mostly coliform bacteria and streptococci other than *Streptococcus agalactiae*) (Hill et al., 1979; Hill, 1981).

Several studies have focused on the use of levamisole for prevention or treatment of bovine mastitis (Flesh et al., 1982; Ishikawa et al., 1982; Onodera et al., 1980; Ovadia et al., 1978; Ziv et al., 1981). The results of these studies and the characteristics of the model systems used were reviewed by Anderson (1984). He concluded that the prospect of using levamisole beneficially in mastitis was limited. However, based on the understanding of the pathogenesis of mastitis and the actions of levamisole, drying off and parturition are two times when levamisole may have rational application in mastitis prevention.

Experimentally induced *Staphylococcus aureus* mastitis has been shown to inhibit lymphocyte blastogenesis (Nonnecke and Harp, 1985) and has been used as a model of evaluating potential immunomodulators in cows (Kehrli et al., 1989c) and ewes (Buddle et al., 1988). The immunomodulator evaluated in cattle with experimentally induced

S. *aureus* mastitis was a thymosin alpha 1 containing colostral whey product, which was administered by subcutaneous injection daily for 3 consecutive days. This product produced some changes in blood leukocyte count and neutrophil random migration, and partially overcame the suppression of lymphocyte blastogenesis in response to mitogens induced by S. *aureus* infection. However, it did not reduce the number of bacteria shed into the milk. In fact, the immunomodulator treatment was associated with a moderate increase in bacterial shedding in the milk.

Glucan, a polysaccharide with immunostimulating activity isolated from the cell wall of *Saccharomyces cerevisiae*, has been evaluated for its ability to prevent or reduce S. *haemolyticus*-induced mastitis in ewes (Buddle et al., 1988). The ewes were given glucan by subcutaneous injection adjacent to the supramammary lymph node at various times prior to the intramammary infusion of S. *haemolyticus*. Glucan treatment did not prevent or cure the infection, but the milk bacterial counts from all of the glucan-treated groups were significantly reduced compared to controls.

V. Summary

Development of immunomodulators for use in food producing animals is an active area of research. This research has generally incorporated aspects of immunosuppression in model systems. This methodology is appropriate because most of the research has been aimed at developing immunomodulators for certain economically significant diseases in which immunosuppression is believed to be an important component of their pathogenesis. The primary focus has been on stress-associated diseases (especially bovine respiratory disease), infectious diseases in young animals, and mastitis. The model systems used have limitations, but they have demonstrated that immunomodulators are capable of significantly increasing resistance to these important infectious disease syndromes. As our understanding of molecular immunology increases and as more potential immunomodulators become available, the use of relevant model systems should greatly aid advancement in the field of immunomodulation.

REFERENCES

Albani-Vangili, R. (1985). Stress e immunita. *Obiettivi Vet.* **6**, 23.
Anderson, A. O., and Reynolds, J. A. (1979). Adjuvant effects of the lipid amine CP-20,961. *J. Reticuloendothel. Soc.* **26**, 667–680.

Anderson, J. C. (1984). Levamisole and bovine mastitis. *Vet. Rec.* **114**, 138–140.
Babiuk, L. A., Bielefeldt-Ohmann, H., Gifford, G., Czarniecki, C. W., Scialli, V. T., and Hamilton, E. B. (1985). Effect of bovine alpha$_1$ interferon on bovine herpesvirus type 1-induced respiratory disease. *J. Gen. Virol.* **66**, 2383–2394.
Babiuk, L. A., Lawman, M. J. P., and Gifford, G. A. (1987). Use of recombinant bovine alpha$_1$ interferon in reducing respiratory disease induced by bovine herpesvirus type 1. *Antimicrob. Agents Chemother.* **31**, 752–757.
Bertram, T. A., Canning, P. C., and Roth, J. A. (1986). Preferential inhibition of primary granule release from bovine neutrophils by an extract from *Brucella abortus*. *Infect. Immun.* **52**, 285–292.
Bielefeldt-Ohmann, H., and Babiuk, L. A. (1985a). *In vitro* and systematic effects of recombinant bovine interferons on natural cell-mediated cytotoxicity in healthy and bovine herpesvirus-1-infected cattle. *J. Interferon Res.* **5**, 551–564.
Bielefeldt-Ohmann, H., and Babiuk, L. A. (1985b). Viral-bacterial pneumonia in calves: Effect of bovine herpesvirus-1 on immunologic functions. *J. Infect. Dis.* **151**, 937–947.
Bielefeldt-Ohmann, H., and Babiuk, L. A. (1986). Alteration of alveolar macrophage functions after aerosol infection with bovine herpesvirus type 1. *Infect. Immun.* **51**, 344–347.
Blackwell, G. J., Carnuccio, R., Dirosa, M., Blackwell, G. J., Carnuccio, R., Dirosa, M., Flower, R. J., Ivanyi, J., Langham, C. S. J., Parente, L., Persico, P., and Wood, J. (1983). Suppression of arachidonate oxidation by glucocorticoid-induced antiphospholipase peptides. *Adv. Prostaglandin, Thromboxane, Leukotriene Res.* **11**, 65–71.
Blecha, F. (1988a). Immunomodulation: A means of disease prevention in stressed livestock. *J. Anim. Sci.* **66**, 2084–2090.
Blecha, F. (1988b). Stress et immunité chez l'animal. *Recl. Med. Vet.* **164**, 767–772.
Blecha, F., and Baker, P. E. (1986). Effect of cortisol *in vitro* and *in vivo* on production of bovine interleukin-2. *Am. J. Vet. Res.* **47**, 841–845.
Blecha, F., and Minocha, H. C. (1983). Suppressed lymphocyte blastogenic responses and enhanced *in vitro* growth of infectious bovine rhinotracheitis virus in stressed feeder calves. *Am. J. Vet. Res.* **44**, 2145–2148.
Blecha, F., Boyles, S. L., and Riley, J. G. (1984). Shipping suppresses lymphocyte blastogenic responses in Angus and Brahman X Angus feeder calves. *J. Anim. Sci.* **59**, 576–583.
Blecha, F., Pollmann, S., and Nichols, D. A. (1985). Immunologic reactions of pigs regrouped at or near weaning. *Am. J. Vet. Res.* **46**, 1934–1937.
Blecha, F., Anderson, G. A., Osorio, F., Chapes, S. K., and Baker, P. E. (1987). Influence of isoprinosine on bovine herpesvirus type-1 infection in cattle. *Vet. Immunol. Immunopathol.* **15**, 253–265.
Blodgett, D. J., Schurig, G. G., and Kornegay, E. T. (1986). Immunomodulation in weanling swine with dietary selenium. *Am. J. Vet. Res.* **47**, 1517–1519.
Brazle, F. K., Blecha, F., Riley, J., and Mclaren, J. B. (1984). Receiving diets and levamisole treatments for stressed feeder calves. *J. Anim. Sci.* **59, Suppl. 1**, 381(Abstr. 382).
Buddle, B. M., Pulford, H. D., and Ralston, M. (1988). Protective effect of glucan against experimentally induced staphylococcal mastitis in ewes. *Vet. Microbiol.* **16**, 67–76.
Canning, P. C., Roth, J. A., and Deyoe, B. L. (1986). Release of 5'-guanosine monophosphate and adenine by *Brucella abortus* and their role in the intracellular survival of the bacteria. *J. Infect. Dis.* **154**, 464–470.
Chiang, Y.-W., Kaeberle, M. L., and Roth, J. A. (1986). Identification of the suppressive components in *Haemophilus somnus* fractions which inhibit bovine polymorphonuclear leukocyte function. *Infect. Immun.* **52**, 792–797.

Chiang, Y.-W., Roth, J. A., and Andrews, J. J. (1990). Influence of recombinant bovine interferon gamma and dexamethasone on pneumonia attributable to *Haemophilus somnus* in calves. *Am. J. Vet. Res.* **51,** 759–762.

Confer, A. W., and Adldinger, H. K. (1981). The *in vivo* effect of levamisole on phytohaemagglutinin stimulation of lymphocytes in normal and Marek's disease virus inoculated chickens. *Res. Vet. Sci.* **30,** 243–245.

Czarniecki, C. W., Anderson, K. P., Fennie, E. B., Bielefeldt-Ohmann, H., and Babiuk, L. A. (1985). Bovine interferon-alpha$_1$1 is an effective inhibitor of bovine herpes virus-1 induced respiratory disease. *Antiviral Res., Suppl.* **1,** 209–215.

Czuprynski, C. J., and Hamilton, H. L. (1985). Bovine neutrophils ingest but do not kill *Haemophilus somnus in vitro*. *Infect. Immun.* **50** 431 436.

Filion, L. G., Mcguire, R. L., and Babiuk, L. A. (1981). Nonspecific suppressive effect of bovine herpesvirus type 1 on bovine leukocyte functions. *Infect. Immun.* **42,** 106–112.

Flaming, K. P., Thaler, R. C., Blecha, F., and Nelssen, J. L. (1988). Influence of sodium diethyldithiocarbamate (Imuthiol) on lymphocyte function and growth in weanling pigs. *Comp. Immunol. Microbiol. Infect. Dis.* **11,** 181–187.

Flaming, K. P., Blecha, F., and Anderson, G. A. (1989). Influence of isoprinosine on lymphocyte function in virus-infected feeder pigs. *Am. J. Vet. Res.* **50,** 1653–1657.

Flesh, J., Harel, W., and Nelken, D. (1982). Immunopotentiating effect of levamisole in the prevention of bovine mastitis, fetal death and endometritis. *Vet. Rec.* **111,** 56–57.

Frank, D. E., and Roth, J. A. (1986). Factors secreted by untreated and hydrocortisone-treated monocytes that modulate neutrophil function. *J. Leukocyte Biol.* **40,** 693–707.

Hauser, M. A., Koob, M. D., and Roth, J. A. (1986). Variation of neutrophil function with age in calves. *Am. J. Vet. Res.* **47,** 152–153.

Hennessy, K. J., Blecha, F., Pollmann, D. S., and Kluber, E. F. (1987). Isoprinosine and levamisole immunomodulation in artificially reared neonatal pigs. *Am. J. Vet. Res.* **48,** 477–480.

Hill, A. W. (1981). Factors influencing the outcome of *Escherichia coli* mastitis in the dairy cow. *Res. Vet. Sci.* **31,** 107–112.

Hill, A. W., Shears, A. L., and Hibbitt, K. G. (1979). The pathogenesis of experimental *Escherichia coli* mastitis in newly calved dairy cows. *Res. Vet. Sci.* **26,** 97–101.

Hirata, F., Schiffmann, E., Venkatasubramanian, K., Salomon, D., and Axelrod, J. (1980). A phospholipase A_2 inhibitory protein in rabbit neutrophils induced by glucocorticoids. *Proc. Natl. Acad. Sci. U.S.A.* **77,** 2533–2536.

Hoffman, W. W., Korst, J. J., Niblack, J. F., and Cronin, T. H. (1973). N,N-Dioctadecyl-N_1,N_1-bis(2-hydroxyethyl) propanediamine: Antiviral activity and interferon stimulation in mice. *Antimicrob. Agents Chemother.* **3,** 498–502.

Hubbard, R. D., Kaeberle, M. L., Roth, J. A., and Chiang, Y. W. (1986). *Haemophilus somnus*-induced interference with bovine neutrophil functions. *Vet. Microbiol.* **12,** 77–85.

Irwin, M. R., Melendy, D. R., and Hutcheson, D. P. (1980). Reduced morbidity associated with shipping fever pneumonia in levamisole phosphate-treated feedlot cattle. *Southwest Vet.* **33,** 45–49.

Ishikawa, H., and Shimizu, T. (1983). Depression of B-lymphocytes by mastitis and treatment with levamisole. *J. Dairy Sci.* **66,** 556–561.

Ishikawa, H., Shimizu, T., Hirano, H., Saito, N., and Nakano, T. (1982). Protein composition of whey from subclinical mastitis and effect of treatment with levamisole. *J. Dairy Sci.* **65,** 653–658.

Jericho, K. W. F., and Langford, E. V. (1978). Pneumonia in calves produced with aerosols of bovine herpesvirus 1 and *Pasteurella haemolytica*. *Can. J. Comp. Med.* **42** 269–277.

Jericho, K. W. F., Darcel, C. Q., and Langford, E. V. (1982). Respiratory disease in calves produced with aerosols of parainfluenza-3 virus and *Pasteurella haemolytica*. *Can. J. Comp. Med.* **46**, 293–301.

Kaeberle, M. L., and Roth, J. A. (1984). Effects of thiabendazole on dexamethasone-induced suppression of lymphocyte and neutrophil function in cattle. *Immunopharmacology* **8**, 129–136.

Kashiwazaki, Y. (1984). Lymphocyte activities in dairy cows with special reference to outbreaks of mastitis in pre- and postpartus. *Jpn. J. Vet. Res.* **32**, 101.

Kehrli, M. E., Jr., and Goff, J. P. (1989). Periparturient hypocalcemia in cows: Effects on peripheral blood neutrophil and lymphocyte function. *J. Dairy Sci.* **72**, 1188–1196.

Kehrli, M. E., Jr., Nonnecke, B. J., and Roth J. A. (1989a). Alterations in bovine neutrophil function during the periparturient period. *Am. J. Vet. Res.* **50**, 207–214.

Kehrli, M. E., Jr., Nonnecke, B. J., and Roth, J. A. (1989b). Alterations in bovine lymphocyte function during the periparturient period. *Am. J. Vet. Res.* **50**, 215–220.

Kehrli, M. E., Jr., Nonnecke, B. J., Wood, R. L., and Roth, J. A. (1989c). In vivo effects of a thymosin alpha$_1$-containing colostral whey product on neutrophils and lymphocytes from lactating cows without and with experimentally induced *Staphylococcus aureus* mastitis. *Vet. Immunol. Immunopathol.* **20**, 149–163.

Kelley, K. W. (1980). Stress and immune function: A bibliographic review. *Ann. Rech. Vet.* **11**, 445–478.

Kelley, K. W. (1982). Immunobiology of domestic animals as affected by hot and cold weather. *Int. Livest. Environ. Symp., 2nd*, pp. 470–482.

Kelley, K. W. (1984). Stress et immunité des animaux domestiques. *Point Vet.* **16**, 49.

Kelley, K. W. (1985). Immunological consequences of changing environmental stimuli. *In* "Animal Stress" (G. P. Moberg, ed.), pp. 193–223. Am. Physiol. Soc., Bethesda, Maryland.

Kornegay, E. T., Meldrum, J. B., Schurig, G., Lindemann, M. D., and Gwazdauskas, F. C. (1986). Lack of influence of nursery temperature on the response of weanling pigs to supplemental vitamins C and E. *J. Anim. Sci.* **63**, 484–491.

Lawman, M. J. P., Gifford, G., Gyongyossy-Issa, M., Dragan, R., Heise, J., and Babiuk, L. A. (1987). Activity of polymorphonuclear (PMN) leukocytes during bovine herpes virus-1 induced respiratory disease: Effect of recombinant bovine interferon alpha$_1$1. *Antiviral Res.* **8**, 225–238.

Lofstedt, J., Roth, J. A., Ross, R. F., and Wagner, W. C. (1983). Depression of polymorphonuclear leukocyte function associated with experimentally induced *Escherichia coli* mastitis in sows. *Am. J. Vet. Res.* **44**, 1124–1128.

Lukacs, K., Roth, J. A., and Kaeberle, M. L. (1985). Activation of neutrophils by antigen-induced lymphokine with emphasis on antibody-independent cytotoxicity. *J. Leukocyte Biol.* **38**, 557–572.

Muscoplat, C. C., Johnson, D. W., and Stevens, J. B. (1973). Abnormalities of *in vitro* lymphocyte responses during bovine viral diarrhea virus infection. *Am. J. Vet. Res.* **34**, 753–755.

Nagahata, H., Makino, S., Takeda, S., Takahashi, H., and Noda, H. (1988). Assessment of neutrophil function in the dairy cow during the perinatal period. *J. Vet. Med. (Tokyo)* **35**, 747–751.

Niblack, J. F., Otterness, I. G., Hemsworth, G. R., Wolff, J. S., III, Hoffman, W. W., and Kraska, A. R. (1979). CP-20,961: A structurally novel, synthetic adjuvant. *J. Reticuloendothel. Soc.* **26**, 665–666.

Nonnecke, B. J., and Harp, J. A. (1985). Effect of chronic staphylococcal mastitis on mitogenic responses of bovine lymphocytes. *J. Dairy Sci.* **68**, 3323–3328.

Onodera, T., Tsukamoto, T., and Kube, T. (1980). Efficacy of levamisole treatment of bovine chronic mastitis. *J. Jpn. Vet. Med. Assoc.* **33**, 375.

Ovadia, H., Flesh, J., and Nelken, D. (1978). Prevention of bovine mastitis by treatment with levamisole. *Isr. J. Med. Sci.* **14**, 394–396.

Pardue, S. L., and Thaxton, J. P. (1984). Evidence for amelioration of steroid-mediated immunosuppression by ascorbic acid. *Poult. Sci.* **63**, 1262–1268.

Peplowski, M. A., Mahan, D. C., Murray, F. A., Moxon, A. L., Cantor, A. H., and Ekström, K. E. (1981). Effect of dietary and injectable vitamin E and selenium in weanling swine antigenically challenged with sheep red blood cells. *J. Anim. Sci.* **51**, 344–351.

Potgieter, L. N. D., Mccracken, M. D., Hopkins, F. M., Walker, R. D., and Guy, J. S. (1984). Experimental production of bovine respiratory tract disease with bovine viral diarrhea virus. *Am. J. Vet. Res.* **45**, 1582–1585.

Potgieter, L. N. D., Helman, R. G., Greene, W., Breider, M. A., Thurber, E. T., and Peetz, R. H. (1988). Experimental bovine respiratory tract disease with *Haemophilus somnus*. *Vet. Pathol.* **25**, 124–130.

Pruett, J. H., Fisher, W. F., and Deloach, J. R. (1987). Effects of dexamethasone on selected parameters of the bovine immune system. *Vet. Res. Commun.* **11**, 305–323.

Reyero, C., Stockl, W., and Thalhammer, J. G. (1979). Stimulation of the antibody response to sheep red blood cells in piglets and young pigs by levamisole. *Br. Vet. J.* **135**, 17–24.

Roney, C. S., Rossi, C. R., Smith, P. C., Laverman, L. C., Spano, J. S., Hanrahan, L. A., and William, J. C. (1985). Effect of human leukocyte A interferon on prevention of infectious bovine rhinotracheitis virus infection of cattle. *Am. J. Vet. Res.* **46**, 1251–1255.

Roth, J. A. (1984). Immunosuppression and immunomodulation in bovine respiratory disease. In "Bovine Respiratory Disease" (R. W. Loan, ed.), pp. 143–192. Texas A&M Univ. Press, College Station.

Roth, J. A. (1985). Cortisol as a mediator of stress-associated immunosuppression in cattle. In "Animal Stress" (G. P. Moberg, ed.), pp. 225–243. Am. Physiol. Soc., Bethesda, Maryland.

Roth, J. A., and Frank, D. E. (1989). Recombinant bovine interferon gamma as an immunomodulator in dexamethasone-treated and nontreated cattle. *J. Interferon Res.* **9**, 143–151.

Roth, J. A., and Kaeberle, M. L. (1981). Effects of *in vivo* dexamethasone administration on *in vitro* bovine polymorphonuclear leukocyte function. *Infect. Immun.* **33**, 434–441.

Roth, J. A., and Kaeberle, M. L. (1982). Effects of glucocorticoids on the bovine immune system. *J. Am. Vet. Med. Assoc.* **180**, 894–901.

Roth, J. A., and Kaeberle, M. L. (1984). Effect of levamisole on lymphocyte blastogenesis and neutrophil function in dexamethasone-treated cattle. *Am. J. Vet. Res.* **45**, 1781–1784.

Roth, J. A., and Kaeberle, M. L. (1985a). Enhancement of lymphocyte blastogenesis and neutrophil function by avridine in dexamethasone-treated and nontreated cattle. *Am. J. Vet. Res.* **46**, 53–57.

Roth, J. A., and Kaeberle, M. L. (1985b). *In vivo* effect of ascorbic acid on neutrophil function in healthy and dexamethasone-treated cattle. *Am. J. Vet. Res.* **46**, 2434–2436.

Roth, J. A., Kaeberle, M. L., and Griffith, R. W. (1981). Effects of bovine viral diarrhea virus infection on bovine polymorphonuclear leukocyte function. *Am. J. Vet. Res.* **42**, 244–250.

Roth, J. A., Kaeberle, M. L., and Hubbard, R. D. (1984). Attempts to use thiabendazole to improve the immune response in dexamethasone-treated or stressed cattle. *Immunopharmacology* **8**, 121–128.

Roth, J. A., Bolin, S. R., and Frank, D. E. (1986). Lymphocyte blastogenesis and neutrophil function in cattle persistently infected with bovine viral diarrhea virus. *Am. J. Vet. Res.* **47,** 1139–1141.

Roth, J. A., Jarvinen, J. A., Frank, D. E., and Fox, D. E. (1989). Alteration of neutrophil function associated with coccidiosis in cattle: Influence of decoquinate and dexamethasone. *Am. J. Vet. Res.* **50,** 1250–1253.

Roth, J. A., Abruzzini, A. F., and Frank, D. E. (1990). Influence of recombinant human interleukin 2 administration on lymphocyte and neutrophil function in clinically normal and dexamethasone-treated cattle. *Am. J. Vet. Res.* **51,** 546–549.

Saperstein, G., Mohanty, S. B., Rockemann, D. D., and Russek, E. (1983). Effect of levamisole on induced bovine viral diarrhea. *J. Am. Vet. Med. Assoc.* **183,** 425–427.

Siegel, H. S. (1985). Immunological responses as indicators of stress. *World's Poult. Sci. J.* **41,** 36–44.

Slauson, D. O., Clifford, C. B., and Holden-Stauffer, W. (1987). Alterations in membrane deformability and superoxide anion generation by neonatal calf neutrophils. *J. Leukocyte Biol.* **42,** 342 (abstr.).

Steinbeck, M. J., Roth, J. A., and Kaeberle, M. L. (1986). Activation of bovine neutrophils by bovine recombinant interferon-gamma. *Cell. Immunol.* **98,** 137–144.

Stevenson, R. D. (1977). Mechanism of anti-inflammatory action of glucocortoicoids. *Lancet* **1,** 225–226.

Valone, F. H. (1984). Regulation of human leukocyte function by lipoxygenase products of arachidonic acid. *Contemp. Top. Immunobiol.* **14,** 115–170.

Van Der Maaten, J. J., Schmerr, M. J. F., Miller, J. M., and Sacks, J. M. (1983). Levamisole does not affect the virological and serological responses of bovine leukemia virus-infected cattle and sheep. *Can. J. Comp. Med.* **47,** 474–479.

Waldman, R. H., and Ganguly, R. (1978). Effect of CP-20,961, an interferon inducer, on upper respiratory tract infections due to rhinovirus type 21 in volunteers. *J. Infect. Dis.* **138,** 531–535.

Webb, D. S. A., and Roth, J. A. (1987). Relationship of glucocorticoid suppression of arachidonic acid metabolism to alteration of neutrophil function. *J. Leukocyte Biol.* **41,** 156–164.

Woodard, L. F., Jasman, R. L., Farrington, D. O., and Jensen, K. E. (1983). Enhanced antibody-dependent bactericidal activity of neutrophils from calves treated with a lipid amine immunopotentiator. *Am. J. Vet. Res.* **44,** 389–394.

Yen, J. T., and Pond, W. G. (1987). Effect of dietary supplementation with vitamin C or carbadox on weanling pigs subjected to crowding stress. *J. Anim. Sci.* **64,** 1672–1681.

Ziv, G., Storper, M., and Saran, A. (1981). The effect of levamisole therapy during the dry period on clinical and subclinical bovine mastitis. *Refu. Vet.* **38,** 108–113.

Mechanisms of Action of Some Immunomodulators Used in Veterinary Medicine

P. J. QUINN

Department of Veterinary Microbiology and Parasitology, University College Dublin, Ballsbridge, Dublin, 4, Ireland

I. Introduction
II. Structure and Function of the Immune System
    A. B Lymphocytes
    B. T Lymphocytes
    C. Monocytes and Macrophages
    D. Immunity to Infectious Diseases
III. Immunomodulation
    A. Historical Aspects of Immunomodulation
    B. Objectives of Immunomodulation
    C. Classification of Immunomodulators
    D. Mechanism of Action of Immunomodulators
IV. Physiologically Important Immunomodulators
    A. Immunomodulation by Neuroendocrine Hormones
    B. Thymic Hormones
    C. Cytokines, Including Interferons
    D. Glucocorticoids
V. Synthetic Compounds with Immunomodulatory Activity
    A. Levamisole
    B. Isoprinosine
    C. Synthetic Polynucleotides
VI. Microbial Products as Immunomodulators
    A. *Proprionibacterium acnes*
    B. Lentinan
VII. Liposomes
    A. Potential Role in Immunomodulation
    B. Mechanism of Action of Liposomes
VIII. Concluding Comments
    References

I. Introduction

The immune system is a highly regulated network of mainly lymphoid cells, which undergo differentiation, activation, and renewal in a structured manner as the body develops full immunological competence postnatally. Two components exist within this network of lymphoid cells, one of which is responsible for humoral immunity, the other for cell-mediated immunity. These cell populations, originally considered distinct, are now clearly demonstrated as interdependent and cooperate in initiating immune responses and in protecting the body. They do this either by the secretion of antibody from plasma cells, derived from the bursa equivalent or B cell series, or through cell-mediated immunity delivered by thymus-derived or T lymphocytes. Nonlymphoid cells also contribute to immunological competence. Soluble factors, some naturally occurring, others induced by antigenic challenge, assist or amplify defense mechanisms of the host. It is the integration of these various components, some specific, others nonspecific, that constitutes a functional immune system.

The immune system has evolved to protect the host from the many potential pathogens that are present in the environment. The functions of the immune system include defense against infectious agents and neoplastic changes, and discrimination of self from nonself. Apart from T and B cells, there is an additional population of lymphoid cells, the natural killer (NK) cells, which are apparently neither T or B cell-derived and probably represent the first line of defense in immune surveillance against malignant or virally transformed cells prior to the development of antigen-specific responses. Cells of the monocyte–macrophage series play a central role in immune reactivity as effector cells capable of destroying invading pathogens and presenting antigen to lymphocytes.

Other cells, such as polymorphonuclear leukocytes and mast cells serve as effectors of inflammation elicited by the immune response. The role of these cells as the first line of defense in innate (nonspecific) immunity is frequently crucial in combating pyogenic infections by initiating acute inflammatory changes at the site of invasion. Together with nonspecific secretions such as complement and lysozyme they provide an immediate, effective barrier to infection while the slower but more efficient, highly specific immune responses are being mobilized.

II. Structure and Function of the Immune System

In postnatal life, the bone marrow is the source of stem cells from which both lymphoid cells and those cells that contribute to nonspecific immunity, through phagocytic activity or other mechanisms, derive

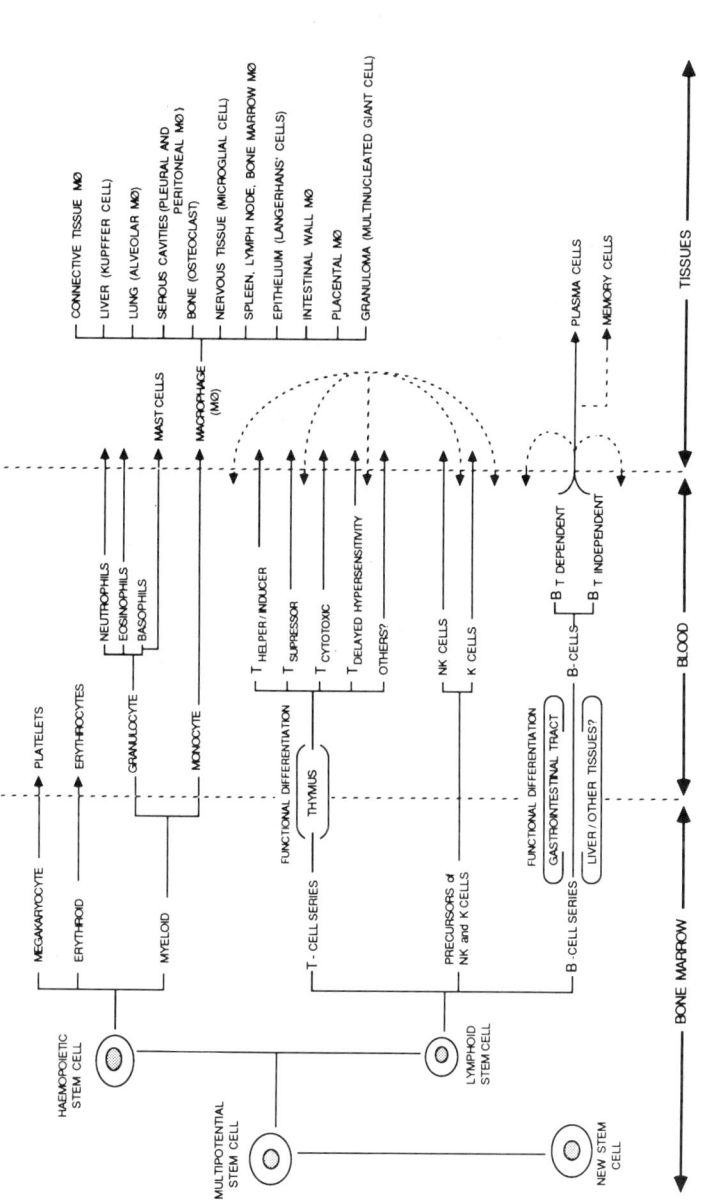

FIG. 1. The origin, development, differentiation, and maturation of cells participating in immune responses in mammals. Associated cell types are also included. The lymphoid cells of avian species destined to become B cells migrate to the bursa where they acquire appropriate characteristics. The counterpart of the bursa has not been conclusively identified in mammals but gut-associated lymphoid tissue such as Peyer's patches and perhaps other structures seeded with lymphoid cells from the bone marrow may have a comparable role to the bursa.

(Fig. 1). There are at least three recognizable subdivisions of lymphoid cells: T lymphocytes, B lymphocytes, and a third subset, referred to as null-cells, distinct from the other two lineages.

A. B Lymphocytes

B cell differentiation commences in the bone marrow and maturation in mammals probably occurs in gut-associated lymphoid tissue or in other lymphoid organs. In birds, pre-B lymphocytes migrate to the bursa of Fabricius where differentiation occurs in close association with epithelial components. The existence of molecules that specifically stimulate B cell development, comparable to thymic hormones for T cells, seems likely, but thus far remains unproved. The development of B cells can be divided into four distinct stages: stem cell, pre-B cell, B cell, and plasma cell. Soon after they are formed, B cells enter the circulation and migrate to special areas of residence in the spleen and other peripheral lymphoid tissues. B cells that encounter antigen complementary to their surface immunoglobulin receptors and receive appropriate T cell cooperation differentiate into antibody-secreting plasma cells or into memory cells ready to make antibodies of high affinity on later encounter with the same antigen (Cooper, 1987; Feldman, 1988).

The principal function of plasma cells in protective immunity is the production of antibodies capable of opsonizing or agglutinating bacteria or other infectious microorganisms, thereby facilitating their engulfment by phagocytes or initiating their destruction through activation of the complement system. Antibodies can also neutralize bacterial toxins and viruses and prevent attachment of bacteria and viruses to cell receptors. They can also facilitate the participation of cells of the lymphoid series (NK or K cells) in the destruction of target cells in antibody-dependent cell-mediated cytotoxicity (ADCC). The passive transfer of antibodies to the newborn animal via colostrum is one of the most effective methods of conferring temporary protection on susceptible neonates who, although potentially immunologically competent, are naive to the vast array of infectious agents that beset them in their early independent existence. The immunoglobulin classes IgM, IgG, and IgA are associated with antibody activity against a wide range of infectious agents, and are bifunctional in that they can react with antigens on infectious agents, and in addition initiate other biological reactions such as attachment to the membranes of phagocytic cells and activation of the complement system. Two other immunoglobulins, IgE and IgD, have unique roles in immune responses; IgE is associated with allergic reactions and IgD functions as an antigen receptor on B cells.

The first antibodies produced in response to antigenic stimulation are IgM. They are highly efficient in agglutination reactions and in complement activation. Being large molecules they are normally confined to the blood vascular system. IgG is the predominant immunoglobulin in serum, interstitial fluid, and colostrum of many species. IgG can bind to receptors on phagocytic cells thereby facilitating phagocytic destruction of invading microorganisms. IgG antibodies neutralize bacterial toxins and viruses, and some IgG subclasses fix complement. IgA, although present in serum, is selectively transported across mucous membranes and is the principal immunoglobulin in body secretions. Antibodies of the IgA class play an important part in protecting mucosal surfaces, particularly in the respiratory and intestinal tracts.

Although IgE is present in low concentrations in serum, it binds with high affinity to mast cells, and sometimes other cells, via a site in the Fc region. When cross-linked by allergens, IgE antibodies cause mast cells to degranulate and release vasoactive substances that lead to local or systemic anaphylactic reactions. Apart from triggering acute local inflammatory reactions, such events may also result in increased intestinal motility and contribute to the elimination of intestinal parasites. The role of IgD is not well defined at present in domestic animals. In man, together with IgM, it is the predominant immunoglobulin on the surface of B lymphocytes where it acts as a receptor for antigen. When cross-linked by antigen, IgD induces the resting B cell to enlarge, preparatory to cell division.

B. T Lymphocytes

Following migration to the thymus, lymphoid cells destined to become T lymphocytes acquire special characteristics that equip them to fulfill their role in cell-mediated reactions (Male et al., 1987; Roitt, 1988). During differentiation within the thymus, T cells learn to recognize self-Major Histocompatibility Complex (MHC) gene products. Unlike B cells, T cells usually do not recognize antigen in its native state. Only when antigen is displayed on the surface of a macrophage in physical association with Class II histocompatibility molecules will recognition by T cells occur. This "dual" recognition for both antigen and MHC is necessary for activation of cytotoxic and immunoregulatory T cells, and is augmented by macrophage-secreted interleukin-1

(IL-1). The antigen receptor on the T cell is a heterodimer, which although bearing some structural and functional similarities to immunoglobulin molecules is distinctly different in many important respects (Royer and Reinherz, 1987). Following interaction with antigen and MHC, the number of surface antigen receptors rapidly decreases and induction of surface interleukin-2 (IL-2) receptors, not previously present on the resting T cell, quickly occurs. This is accompanied by endogenous induction and secretion of IL-2 and subsequent binding of it to IL-2 receptors on the same cell. When a critical number of IL-2 receptors have bound IL-2, DNA synthesis and cell mitosis occurs. IL-2, therefore, acts as an autacoid as it expands that particular T cell clone (Stobo, 1987). In addition, for successful activation of T cells, macrophage-derived IL-1 is required. Sustained exposure of activated T cells to IL-2 results in a diminished response so that continuous replication and the potential for malignant transformation does not occur. In the absence of continued antigenic stimulation, there is reexpression of the surface antigen receptor complex and a reciprocal reduction of IL-2 receptors.

The number of T cells specific for a single antigenic determinant is believed to be exceedingly small. Reactivity of T cells to an infectious agent with multiple antigenic determinants does not result in substantial immune reactivity unless these cells are capable of augmenting their numbers and activity. This is achieved by the liberation from activated T lymphocytes of lymphokines such as IL-2, polypeptide products that participate in a variety of cellular responses, including regulation of the immune system (Dinarello and Mier, 1987). Individual lymphokines amplify the immune response to antigen in a nonspecific manner. In addition to IL-2, activated T cells produce an array of lymphokines, including IL-3, IL-4, IL-5, IL-6, and interferon gamma (IFNγ). IL-3 promotes the development of multipotential bone marrow stem cells. IL-4 is a growth factor for activated B cells and for resting T cells. It also enhances the cytolytic activity of cytotoxic T cells. IL-5 supports induction of the IgA response, while IL-6 exerts antiviral activity and promotes proliferation and differentiation of thymocytes and B cells. Recently, another lymphokine, IL-7, has been isolated and characterized (Henney, 1989). IL-7 provides direct proliferative signals only to T and B precursor cells. Resting T cells respond only in the presence of secondary stimuli such as antigen or mitogen, while mature B cells are unresponsive to IL-7. IFNγ induces Class I and Class II histocompatibility molecules and other surface antigens on a variety of cells. In addition, it is a potent activator of macrophage function, an activity previously attributed to macrophage-activating factor (MAF);

it augments B cell stimulatory lymphokines and increases antibody production (De Maeyer and De Maeyer-Guignard, 1988). It also enhances NK cells and exerts antiviral activity.

Apart from their direct involvement in cell-mediated responses, T cells play a central role in regulating immunological development. B cell maturation is directly influenced by T cell maturation and each in turn responds to stimuli and secretions from macrophages and occasionally other accessory cells.

C. Monocytes and Macrophages

Cells of the monocyte—macrophage series originate in the bone marrow from a multipotential stem cell common to all of the haemopoietic cells and myeloid cells (Fig. 1). Monocytes in the circulation are heterogeneous with regard to cell density, size, morphology, and surface antigens. In the absence of localized inflammation, migration of monocytes into different tissues appears to be a random phenomenon (Johnston, 1988). Once in tissues, monocytes probably do not reenter the circulation. Tissue macrophages arise by maturation of monocytes that have emigrated from the blood. They undergo "transformation" and exhibit morphological and functional properties that are characteristic of the tissue in which they reside. Mature macrophages have a limited capacity for division but some macrophages may be produced locally by this means (Nelson, 1984). Although precise data are not available, individual macrophages in tissue are believed to have a life span of several months. One terminal stage of development in the mononuclear-phagocyte line is the multinucleated giant cell, which characterizes some granulomatous inflammatory diseases. Macrophages play an essential part in nonspecific immunity by ingesting and killing invading microorganisms and by releasing many soluble factors that contribute to host defense and to inflammation. They also have a central role in initiating immune responses by presenting antigen to lymphocytes during the development of specific immunity and by regulating the proliferation of T cells through release of IL-1 (Dinarello and Mier, 1987). Secreted products of macrophages include a wide range of enzymes, complement components, prostaglandins, and a number of monokines with regulatory functions, such as IFNγ (Werb, 1987). A feature of macrophages, unusual in phagocytic cells, is their ability to become activated (Ezekowitz and Gordon, 1984). Activation occurs during infection through the release of macrophage-activating lymphokines from T lymphocytes specifically sensitized to antigens from invading microorganisms, and it constitutes the basis of cell-mediated immunity to infectious disease. IFNγ appears to be an important lymphokine in this process (Johnston, 1988), but other substances such as muramyl dipeptide can also induce activation. Activated macrophages migrate more vigorously in response to chemotactic factors and deal more efficiently with intracellular parasites than normal macrophages. They also show enhanced antimicrobial and anticellular activity and express markedly different surface properties (Ezekowitz and Gordon, 1984; Griffin, 1984).

D. Immunity to Infectious Diseases

The body's ability to maintain itself free of infectious disease derives, not only from highly specialized and adaptable cells capable of responding specifically to invading pathogens and their products, but also from natural barriers in the structure and function of tissues. The various elements that participate in innate immunity do not exhibit specificity against invading agents, while acquired immunity always exhibits specificity. Table I lists innate immune and other mechanisms that limit colonization, multiplication, and penetration of tissues by pathogenic microorgnisms. Although these are essentially nonspecific mechanisms, their role in combating pathogens is often central to the development of a specific immune response through involvement of phagocytic cells and subsequent interaction with lymphocytes which, in turn, generate cell-mediated immunity or humoral immunity. Specific immune responses also rely heavily on elements of nonspecific immunity such as the complement system for amplification through the generation of chemotactic factors, promotion of phagocytosis and the development of ultrastructural lesions on target membranes.

In most animals the combination of natural resistance and stimulation of adaptive responses to infectious agents is usually adequate for disease prevention (Fig. 2). Specific infectious agents capable of overcoming body defenses and producing disease require special consideration. The options for the control and prevention of such diseases include quarantine and isolation, chemoprophylaxis, chemotherapy, vaccination, and disinfection.

The choice of methods for the control and prevention of infectious diseases in domestic animals ranges from relatively simple isolation procedures to refined vaccination regimes and chemoprophylactic measures that either strengthen body defenses in a specific manner or prevent the establishment of infectious agents in susceptible animals. Where the specific causal agent has been identified and where it can be attenuated by culture *in vitro* or otherwise rendered less virulent,

TABLE I
NON-SPECIFIC ANTIMICROBIAL MECHANISMS IN VERTEBRATE ANIMALS

Physical barriers, design features, and mechanical activity	Cellular elements	Secreted products	Competitive microbial mechanisms	Other factors
Skin: desquamation of epithelial cells at body surfaces	Polymorphonuclear leukocytes	Mucus	Commensal microorganisms in the intestine, female urogenital tract, and on the skin	Species vary widely in their susceptibility and resistance to infectious agents, e.g., horses are resistant to foot-and-mouth disease virus
Mucous membranes: turbinate "baffles"; mucociliary clearance; coughing and sneezing	Mononuclear phagocytes (i) circulating monocytes (ii) fixed or tissue-associated macrophages	Lysozyme Complement Interferons Fatty acids (skin) Gastric acid Intestinal enzymes		
Peristalsis		Bile		Body temperature may render some species resistant to particular pathogens, e.g., poultry
Flushing activity of tears		Lacrimal secretions Sebaceous secretions Lactoperoxidase		
Flushing activity of urine		Spermine Waxy secretions (ears)		

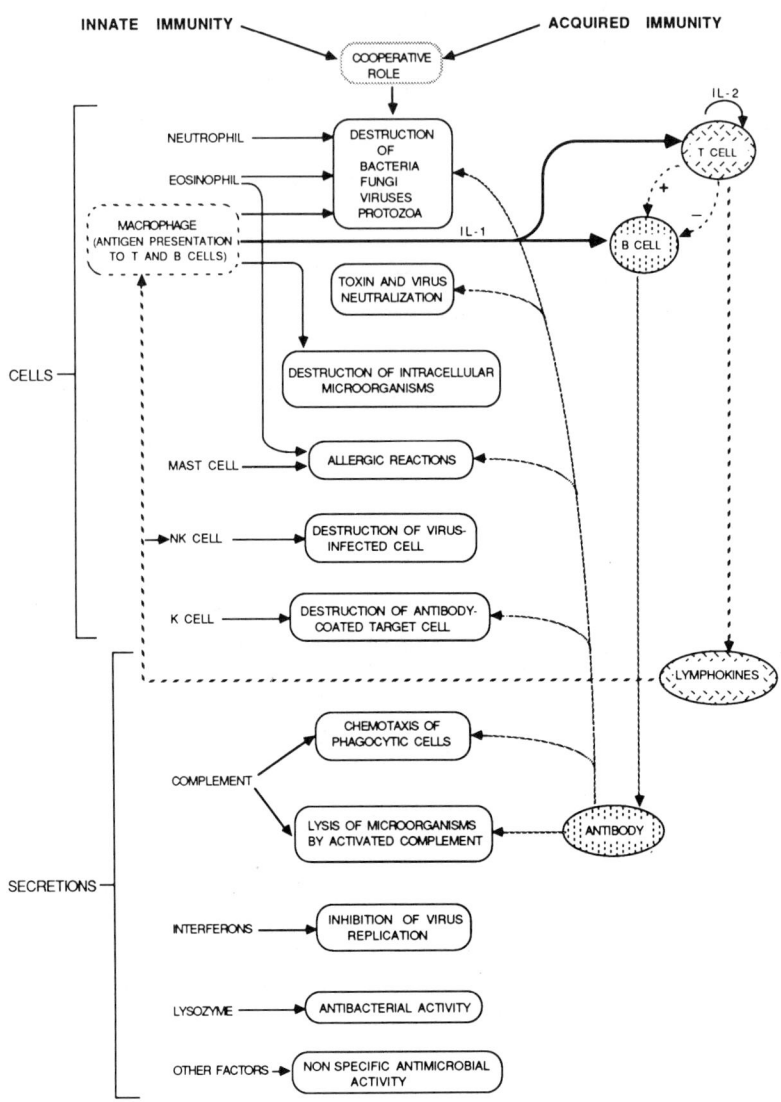

FIG. 2. Cells and secretions that contribute to innate (nonspecific) and acquired immunity against infectious agents. A more complete list of nonspecific antimicrobial secretions is given in Table I. The helper/suppressor role of T cells is indicated by + or − signs. IL-1, Interleukin-1; IL-2, interleukin-2.

vaccination production is a feasible and sometimes effective step in disease prevention. A substantial number of infectious agents, however, do not provoke a protective immune response either following natural infection or vaccination. Thus, although most clostridial diseases of domestic animals can be prevented by vaccination, there remains a large number of bacterial and viral diseases for which vaccination is thus far unsuccessful. African swine fever and staphylococcal mastitis are but two examples of such economically important diseases. Protozoal infections in poultry have eluded control through immunological means and coccidiostats are still the principal method of control.

With intensification of husbandry methods for food producing animals, "complex" diseases have emerged. These frequently occur with recognizable clinical signs and affect a high proportion of susceptible animals in the group. Laboratory investigations, however, often fail to identify the primary agent, if there is one. In these complex disease situations, vaccination and chemotherapy have obvious limitations. For vaccination to succeed the primary agents must be identified for incorporation into the vaccine. In addition, the target organs or tissues should have levels of local protective antibody, cell-mediated immunity or nonspecific protective factors sufficient to withstand attack. Few vaccines administered by conventional means are fully effective. Chemotherapy, although beneficial in defined bacterial infections, is of little value in a primary viral attack beyond controlling secondary bacterial invasion.

III. Immunomodulation

Vaccines, if effective, are the preferred method of disease control of specific infectious diseases. When, however, a variety of infectious agents contribute to the pathogenesis of a particular disease or when the impact of the agents is apparently determined by stressful environmental conditions, nonspecific stimulators of cell-mediated and humoral immunity offer several advantages over current prophylactic and therapeutic approaches. Chemical modification of the immune response has become an increasing possibility as an alternative to conventional disease control measures and may be an attractive alternative to routine measures such as isolation or segregation, vaccination, and disinfection.

During the early years of immunological research it was generally accepted that the only factors that influenced the initiation and maintenance of the immune response were specific antigens. Indeed, the very concept of vaccination was aimed at conferring protection against specific infectious diseases or specific agents capable of infecting animals or humans. With the advent of vaccines, antibiotics, and other antimicrobial agents, the serious recurring losses from epizootics in food animals were halted. Only those infections that were resistant to either chemotherapy or immunoprophylaxis remained as serious obstacles to increased animal production.

Developments in clinical and experimental immunology strongly suggest that many infectious diseases in mature animals arise because of stressful environmental conditions associated with suppression of the immune system. A substantial amount of circumstantial evidence supports the concept that certain types of stress evoke physiological changes that influence susceptibility to infection and malignancy (Griffin, 1989). Intensification, transportation over long distances, and a variety of inappropriate management systems have contributed to conditions that favor transmission of infectious agents and militate against defense mechanisms. It is in such circumstances that immunomodulation may be of benefit in food animals.

The ability to modify the immune responses of animals and humans evolved from a desire to confer greater protection against infectious agents through a more complete understanding of the functioning of the immune system, and of the ways in which nonspecific and specific immune mechanisms developed. Naturally occurring or synthetic compounds capable of altering those mechanisms offered further possibilities for modulating immune responses.

This chapter will consider the mode of action of immunomodulators used in domestic food animals and other potentially useful compounds currently being developed or undergoing field evaluation.

A. Historical Aspects of Immunomodulation

The idea of immunomodulation can be traced back to observations recorded by workers more than a century ago (Sedlacek et al., 1986). Attempts had been made to influence tumors with living bacteria as early as 1850 (Latour, 1850) and subsequently other investigators used extracts of bacteria for tumor therapy. In the early part of this century, it was demonstrated that exposure to certain types of bacteria rendered an animal more resistant to subsequent infections by unrelated organisms. It was quickly realized that either suppression or enhancement of immunological activity could be produced by immunoactive substances and that dosage and timing of administration were crucial to the final outcome. With improved experimental techniques and a greater understanding of the functioning of the immune system, it is now possible to classify a large number of physiological, microbial, and synthetic substances as immunomodulators.

One of the surprising features of research on immunomodulation was its partial eclipse by the successes of chemotherapy and vaccination. The gradual realization that vaccines and chemotherapy have important but defined roles in disease prevention and control, together with knowledge of the limited chemotherapy available for viral diseases, have again focused attention on immunostimulants as a means of minimizing the impact of disease in domestic food animals.

B. Objectives of Immunomodulation

The term immunomodulation is generally used to describe the pharmacological manipulation of the immune system. This may involve an increase in the magnitude of the immune response, immunostimulation, or a decrease in the magnitude, immunosuppression. Specific immunomodulation implies a change in the response of the immune system to a particular antigenic stimulus, as achieved by vaccination, whereas nonspecific immunomodulation implies a more fundamental change whereby the "state of alertness" of the immune system is altered to a wide range of antigenic stimuli. The principal components of the immune system targeted for immunomodulation include T and B lymphocytes, the monocyte–macrophage series, and the granulocyte series. NK and K cells are also selected for pharmacological manipulation in some infectious diseases and in virus-associated neoplasms. Complement levels, cytokines, and other antimicrobial secretions are also amenable to immunomodulatory strategies. As many of the current immunomodulatory drugs act on more than one immunologically active cell type, the final effect will depend on the relative susceptibility of those cell types to the agent used and the contribution they make to nonspecific or specific immune responses (Fig. 2). Generally it appears easier to suppress rather than to stimulate the immune response.

The objectives of immunostimulation in domestic food animals include the following:

1. Promoting a greater and more effective, sustained immune response to those infectious agents producing subclinical or clinical disease, without the risks of toxicity, teratogenicity, carcinogenicity, or tissue residues.
2. Hastening the maturation of nonspecific and specific immunity in neonatal and young susceptible animals.
3. Achieving a high level of reactivity at the local tissue or organ level to invading microorganisms, and thereby enhancing local

protective immune reactions at vulnerable sites such as the mammary gland in dairy cattle or the gastrointestinal tract in neonatal ruminants.
4. Enhancing the level and duration of specific immune responses, both cell-mediated and humoral, following vaccination.
5. Overcoming the immunosuppressive effects of stress and of those infectious agents that damage or interfere with the functioning of cells of the immune system, or that produce a persistent infection.
6. Selectively stimulating the relevant components of the immune system or nonspecific immune mechanisms that preferentially confer protection against replicating microorganisms, for example, via interferon release, especially for those infectious agents for which no vaccines currently exist.
7. Maintaining immune surveillance at a heightened level to ensure early recognition and elimination of incipient neoplastic changes in tissues.

The characteristics of an ideal immunomodulator with immunostimulatory activity are listed in Table II.

TABLE II

CHARACTERISTICS OF AN IDEAL IMMUNOMODULATOR WITH IMMUNOSTIMULATORY ACTIVITY FOR DOMESTIC FOOD ANIMALS

1. It should be nontoxic, even at high dosage rates, for animals and humans.
2. It should not be teratogenic, carcinogenic, or have long-term side effects in animals or humans.
3. At therapeutic levels, it should have a short withdrawal period with low tissue residues.
4. If administered with vaccines it should exert an adjuvant effect.
5. It should stimulate a wide range of nonspecific immune responses against bacteria, viruses, fungi, protozoa, and helminths.
6. Primary and secondary immune responses to infectious agents should be amplified.
7. Breakdown products of the compound should be either inactive or readily biodegradable in the environment.
8. It should be nonantigenic, nonpyrogenic, and of defined chemical composition or biological activity.
9. It should be active by the oral route and should be stable both in its native state and after incorporation into food and water.
10. It should be compatible with a wide range of drugs including antibiotics and anthelmintics.
11. It should not be excreted in milk or eggs.
12. It should be inexpensive and either tasteless or palatable.

C. Classification of Immunomodulators

Various substances extracted from animal sources, bacteria, viruses, parasites, and plants are capable of modifying the immune response. A wide range of synthetic compounds also have immunomodulating activity (Sedlacek et al., 1986). The mechanisms whereby this diverse group of substances achieve immune modification are not well known and classification of these compounds according to their activity is often unreliable. Immunomodulators have been classified by Poli (1984) as either biological or chemical in origin. Others have grouped them into those of biological origin and those synthetically derived (Reizenstein and Mathé, 1984), with each group subdivided according to the source of each compound. Immunoactive compounds have also been divided into three categories: (1) physiological products; (2) substances of microbial origin; and (3) synthetic compounds (Mulcahy and Quinn, 1986). Although strict classification of these agents is not always possible, the latter classification will be used in this chapter.

D. Mechanism of Action of Immunomodulators

In terms of modifying the immune response in animals, the changes induced can be conveniently described as: immunorestoration of immunosuppressed animals; immunostimulation of normal animals; and immunosuppression of normal animals. These altered states of responsiveness can be achieved in many different ways and, at the cellular level, the precise mechanisms operating are diverse and not completely understood. What is evident, however, is that it is often possible to relate changes induced by drugs in immunologically active cells to alteration of intracellular nucleotide levels (Coffey and Hadden, 1985). It is known that many *in vitro* functions can be inhibited by high levels of intracellular cAMP in lymphocytes. Many substances that act to increase cAMP, such as glucocorticoids, are immunosuppressive and inhibit the effector function of lymphocytes. In contrast, agents that increase cyclic cGMP levels promote or augment lymphocyte activity and thus have immunopotentiating properties. Plant lectins, lipopolysaccharide, and IL-1 are included in this group of cGMP agonists.

The effects of cyclic nucleotides on lymphocytes, therefore, indicate that cGMP stimulates effector functions of mature lymphocytes, while cAMP inhibits these functions (Coffey and Hadden, 1985). The action of many immunomodulators affecting lymphocytes can probably be related to the cAMP : cGMP balance established in individual cells. Cells of the monocyte–macrophage series often respond to immunomodulation by exhibiting altered surface properties (Ezekowitz and Gordon, 1984) and different metabolic activity (Murray, 1984; Meltzer *et al.*, 1987), while the response of neutrophils can be assessed by their generation of superoxide anion, prostaglandin E, and lysosomal enzyme release (Abramson *et al.*, 1984).

Desirable characteristics of immunotherapeutic drugs have been proposed by Renoux (1986) who also recommended testing regimes for determining their pharmacological activity and safety.

IV. Physiologically Important Immunomodulators

A. IMMUNOMODULATION BY NEUROENDOCRINE HORMONES

In recent years there has been much interest in endogenous opioid peptides—small peptides with morphinelike actions. Three distinct families of endogenous opioid peptides have been identified: the enkephalins, the endorphins, and the dynorphins (Jaffe and Martin, 1985). Each family is derived from a genetically distinct precursor polypeptide and has a characteristic anatomical distribution. Reports of lymphocyte receptors for opioid substances and the various effects of endorphins and enkephalins on immunological phenomena led to the realization that endorphins released from the neurohypophysis and enkephalins from the adrenal glands had immunomodulatory activity (Plotnikoff *et al.*, 1985).

The central nervous system (CNS) and the immune system share many common characteristics. Both systems have evolved specialized tissue that can respond to external stimuli in a discriminating manner and often with unique responses, including a memory component. Although a direct communication between the CNS and organs of the immune system is indicated by innervation of lymphoid organs, including the spleen and thymus, the existence of other links such as neuroendocrine hormones and neurotransmitters has only become apparent in recent years (Coffey and Hadden, 1985; Wybran, 1985; Blalock and Smith, 1985). Currently, it is believed that the immune and neuroendocrine systems interact with each other through common signal molecules and receptors (Smith *et al.*, 1985; Sternberg and Parker, 1988).

Lymphocytes bear receptors for a wide variety of endogenous substances including neurotransmitters, autacoids, hormones, and other mediators that influence cellular functions (Coffey and Hadden, 1985; Wybran, 1985). It is suggested by many workers that the nervous system is capable of altering the course of immune responses via autonomic and neuroendocrine pathways and, reciprocally, products of the activated immune system are capable of transmitting information not only to lymphocytes and macrophages but also to neurons that may regulate the course of the immune response. The term "immunotransmitter" has been proposed to describe molecules produced predominantly by cells of the immune system that transmit specific signals to neurons and other cell types (Hall et al., 1985).

All immune responses involve cell-to-cell communication. Many distinct functional types of lymphocytes are known and each appears to communicate with its target by means of distinct molecules. Unlike the nervous system, the immune system generally lacks a fixed anatomical relationship between its cells. Lymphocytes and macrophages migrate throughout the body and are responsible for immune surveillance of tissues and organs. In this way, infectious agents or their products are promptly detected and likewise the immune system can confront incipient neoplastic cells bearing tumor-specific antigens.

The detection of adrenocorticotrophic hormone (ACTH) and endorphinlike substances from Newcastle disease virus (NDV)-infected lymphocytes was the first demonstration that the immune system is capable of producing peptides that can transmit signals to the neuroendocrine system (Blalock and Smith, 1985). Many soluble products capable of transmitting information from the immune system to the CNS are currently recognized. They include thymosins, lymphokines, opioid peptides, ACTH, and thyroid stimulating hormone (Hall et al., 1985).

Evidence for the existence of a bidirectional circuit between the CNS and the immune system comes from many different sources (Smith et al., 1985; Plotnikoff et al., 1985; Blalock et al., 1985). Up to 100% of lymphocytes infected with NDV synthesize endorphins, immunoreactive ACTH, and IFNα (Smith et al., 1985). Spleen cells from NDV-infected hypophysectomized or normal mice contain γ endorphins, whereas control mice spleens do not. In addition, orally administered dexamethasone blocks the induction of both immunoreactive endorphins and ACTH in infected mouse spleen cells. The immunoreactive hormones, therefore, seem structurally identical and sensitive to the same negative feedback as pituitary products. Data from many sources indicate that leukocyte immunoreactive endorphins are structurally, antigenically, and biologically identical to pituitary endorphins. Two factors seem to determine the type of hormone that is produced by leukocytes: the stimulus and the cell type. NDV leads to ACTH and endorphin production by all of the cells, while lipopolysaccharide elicits this response in about 25% of cells (Blalock et al., 1985). Although T cells have the potential to produce ACTH and endorphins, they produce thyroid stimulating hormone in response to the T cell mitogen, staphylococcal enterotoxin A. Culture supernatant fluid from NDV-infected, endorphin-positive lymphocytes, blocks specific binding of dihydromorphine to mouse brain homogenate, a source of opiate receptors, in a dose-dependent manner, and approximately 10% of this activity is associated with human IFNα (Smith et al., 1985). When two types of human interferon α and γ were applied locally into various regions of the rat brain, only IFNα altered single cell activity in all brain structures in a dose-dependent manner (Dafny et al., 1985). Following systemic administration, IFNα altered naloxone-induced abstinence syndrome in morphine-dependent rats. The data from these experiments indicate that human IFNα is capable of modifying CNS activity as assessed by electrophysiological and behavioral experiments, indicating that this cytokine may serve as a messenger between the immune system and the CNS.

Leukocyte-derived peptide hormones seem to function both in a neuroendocrine capacity and in an immunomodulatory capacity. Immune responses are affected by neuropeptides, such as leu- and met-enkephalins, which enhance proliferation of peripheral blood lymphocytes when stimulated with phytohemagglutinin (Plotnikoff et al., 1985). Both met- and leu-enkephalins were capable of increasing the number of survivors in mice injected with murine leukemia cells (Plotnikoff and Miller, 1983).

Opium addicts show a number of alterations in immune function including impaired mitogenic response to phytohemagglutinin (PHA) and Con A, and decreased total lymphocytes. A direct relationship exists between both the frequency and dosage of morphine administration and the severity of infections. In a study of morphine addicts, there was marked immunosuppression with impairment of phagocytosis and intracellular killing by polymorphonuclear leukocytes and monocytes (Tubaro et al., 1985). In mice, morphine pellet administration resulted in a depression of T and B lymphocyte proliferation, with marked atrophy of the spleen and thymus accompanied by reduced splenocyte proliferation (Bryant et al., 1988). Adrenal hypertrophy was also noted in chronically "morphinized" mice, suggesting the possibility that sustained morphine administration mimicked behavioral stress. Synthetic human β-endorphin shows a biphasic effect on the production of specific antibodies and NK cells in vitro (Williamson et al., 1988). At higher concentrations antibody production is reduced and at lower concentrations it is enhanced.

The pineal gland is recognized as an important neuroendocrine organ, and synthesis and secretion of melatonin, a neurohormone, by this gland is dependent on activation of pineal β-adrenergic receptors by photo stimuli (the length and intensity of light and the duration of darkness). Consequently, pineal and serum concentrations of melatonin show a circadian, as well as a seasonal periodicity in most species (Deguchi and Axelrod, 1973). Pharmacological inhibition of melatonin synthesis in mice by the β-adrenergic antagonist propranolol, in the evening, and by daily injections of p-chlorophenylalanine resulted in significant depression of the primary antibody response to sheep red blood cells, and spleen cells from these mice showed reduced reactivity against antigens in the autologous mixed lymphocyte reaction (Maestroni et al., 1986). Restoration of the nighttime level of plasma melatonin reversed the immune suppression. Melatonin administration antagonized the depression of antibody production induced by corticosterone and also increased the total number of nucleated spleen cells without affecting the ratio of plaque-forming cells as a proportion of spleen cells.

The cooperative interaction of the CNS and the immune system may be considered as an integration of two highly specialized systems, each equipped with its own methods of recognizing hostile environmental alteration or invasive threats from infectious agents. Thymic factors, glucocorticoids, opioid peptides and selected cytokines may be seen as true hormonal influences on the immune system, as they are secreted from one site and transported by the bloodstream to another where they exert their effects. Physiological modulation of the immune system also involves local mediators and the ability of the two systems to function through similar signal molecules and common receptors confirms their interdependence. Of particular relevance with respect to domestic food animals, is the recognition that acute stress may enhance the immune response whereas chronic stress may suppress the immune system (Riley, 1981).

B. Thymic Hormones

The central role of the thymus gland in the development and maintenance of the immune system has been recognized for many years (Good et al., 1962). Involution of the thymus is associated with aging, and a corresponding decline in immune reactivity, particularly of T cells. The incidence of age-related diseases increases in inverse proportion to the involution of the thymus and to the decrease in thymic-dependent immunity (Low and Goldstein, 1984).

The thymic endocrine tissue produces many factors known as "thymic hormones." These peptides are, apparently, not true hormones, as they are incapable of functionally replacing the thymus. They are believed to act at different sites and on different subsets of T cells and contribute to the normal maintenance of immune function and balance. More than twenty thymic factors have been described. Several of these circulate in the blood and their levels decline rapidly following removal of the thymus or slowly with thymic involution. Among the best characterized factors are thymosin fraction 5, thymosin α_1, thymosin $\beta 4$, thymopoietin, thymulin, and thymic humoral factor (THF) (Low and Goldstein, 1984). A phylogenetic association of the thymus with the humoral immune system is suggested by the fact that thymopoietin has some structural similarities to immunoglobulins, suggesting a common ancestral gene (Hahn and Hamburger, 1983). On isoelectric focusing, thymosin fraction 5 consists of more than 30 individual polypeptide components (Low and Goldstein, 1984). Activities attributed to it include the induction of T cell markers on bone marrow cells, enhancement of Migration Inhibitory Factor (MIF) production, induction of suppressor cells, enhanced antibody production, and increased interferon production following viral challenge. Thymosin α_1 increases mitogenic responsiveness of murine lymphocytes and interferon production. Thymopoietin, which is composed of two related peptides, induces T cell differentiation and has a modulating influence on mature lymphocytes. Among the biological activities ascribed to thymic humoral factor are increased cytotoxic reactivity of lymphoid cells against syngeneic tumors, *in vivo* and *in vitro*, and restoration of some thymus-dependent responses in neonatal thymectomized mice. Originally identified in serum and referred to as Facteur Thymique Serique (FTS), thymulin disappears from serum shortly after thymectomy. It enhances the generation of effector cytotoxic T cells both *in vivo* and *in vitro*. Secretions of the thymus may regulate the adrenal cortex and also influence the functioning of the central nervous system; hormones under CNS control are affected by neonatal thymectomy or by genetic absence of the thymus (Hall and Goldstein, 1984).

Both thymopoietin and thymosin fraction 5 increase cGMP (Coffey and Hadden, 1985), which is consistent with their immunostimulatory activity, especially in animals with reduced T cell levels. Overall, thymic hormones seem to exert their effects primarily on developing cells of the prothymocyte/thymocyte lineage and not on mature T cells. They have immunopotentiating properties and can restore some immunological responses in animals lacking thymic function. Perhaps one of the more important roles of thymic hormones is the maintenance of an active population of circulating precursor lymphocytes that can divide throughout the animal's life.

The identity and characteristics of avian thymic hormones are not as well defined as in mammals. A factor designated T_1 was identified in extracts of chicken thymus, which has characteristics resembling mammalian thymic hormones (Murthy and Ragland, 1984).

A number of thymic hormones have been synthesized chemically or produced by recombinant DNA procedures. Thymosin α_1 has been synthesized by several laboratories and its biological activities were similar to natural α_1 (Low and Goldstein, 1984). In a murine model, thymosin fraction 5 and thymosin α_1, used as a synthetic polypeptide, had similar modulatory properties on an equidose basis (Talmadge, 1984). The therapeutic activity appeared to be due to the maturation-stimulating activity on T cells. Thymopentin, a synthesized pentapeptide that contains the active site of the thymopoietin molecule, was found to improve both neutrophil and macrophage function in a *Pseudomonas aeruginosa*-burn-wound sepsis model in guinea pigs (Waymack *et al.*, 1985). The immunomodulatory activities of two synthetic thymopoietin derivatives, TP4 and TP3, were compared with a biologically active pentapeptide, TP5, in inbred mice (Rajnavölgyi *et al.*, 1986). All three synthetic compounds increased primary and secondary antibody responses but delayed-type hypersensitivity responses were decreased. Synthetic FTS (thymulin) at low concentrations increased NK cell activity in human cancer patients, whereas at high levels it had the opposite effect (Dokhelar *et al.*, 1983). It was concluded that at high doses, FTS stimulated suppressor cell function while effector cells were more readily stimulated at lower doses. It was also suggested that the differences might be due to FTS receptor numbers on various NK cell subsets. High doses of synthetic thymosin α_1 increased the number and *in vitro* resistance of murine polymorphonuclear leukocytes to *Candida albicans* (Bistoni *et al.*, 1985). Whether the immunomodulatory effect of thymosin α_1 on polymorphonuclear (PMN) leukocytes was due to a direct effect on PMN precursor cells or was mediated indirectly by other cells of the immune system was not determined.

C. Cytokines, Including Interferons

In vertebrates, cells, tissues, and organs are in constant communication with each other. The channel of communication may be via the nervous system or chemical messengers produced in specialized cells. Cytokines represent a third method of intercellular communication, transmitting to cells of the immune system "messages" that regulate and coordinate immune responses. These cytokines act as hormonelike mediators that function as intercellular signals that regulate local and, at times, systemic responses in inflammation. They include lymphokines, produced by T and B lymphocytes, and monokines secreted by monocytes or macrophages. Cytokines may interact in various ways either synergistically or as antagonists, thereby enhancing or suppressing their own production and, in some instances, receptor expression. Several cytokines were originally named according to their first observed biological effect. It is now clear that they exert pleotropic effects and the earlier terminology is being replaced.

1. Interleukin-1

Interleukin-1 is the term used for two polypeptides (IL-1α and IL-1β) that possess a wide spectrum of immunological and physiological activity (Dinarello, 1989). Their production is stimulated by interferons α, β, and γ, and conversely, IL-1 itself is an inducer of IFNβ in fibroblasts, and a stimulator of IFNγ synthesis by T cells (De Maeyer and De Maeyer-Guignard, 1988). Although both forms of IL-1 are distinct gene products, they recognize the same receptor and share the same biological properties (Dinarello, 1989). Originally called endogenous pyrogen and found in inflammatory exudates and extracted from granulocytes, monocytes, and macrophages (Wood, 1970), IL-1 is now known to be produced by many cell types, including monocytes and macrophages, neutrophils, T and B cells, endothelial cells, fibroblasts, and platelets (De Maeyer and De Maeyer-Guignard, 1988). Cells produce IL-1 in response to infection, microbial toxins, inflammatory agents, and products of activated lymphocytes. IL-1 is biologically similar to tumor necrosis factor (TNF) and shares with it multiple overlapping biological activities, including T cell activation, cytotoxic action on tumor cells, osteoclast activation, mitogenic action on fibroblasts, and induction of IFNβ and other cytokines (Gilman and Mochan, 1988). Unlike interferons, IL-1 cytokines do not display species specificity and IL-1 from one mammalian species can act on cells of another mammalian species (De Maeyer and De Maeyer-Guignard, 1988). Both forms of IL-1 induce sleep, fever, hepatic acute-phase protein synthesis, neutrophilia, and increased levels of hormones (Dinarello, 1989). T, B, and NK cell responses are augmented by IL-1. Interleukin-1 acts on target cells via specific plasma membrane receptor proteins. Receptors for IL-1 are found on many cell types, including neutrophils, T and B cells, monocytes, fibroblasts, and epithelial cells. There is evidence that the highest number of high-affinity receptors for IL-1 exist on T cell lines (Dinarello, 1989). The effect of IL-1 on T cells indicates that there is synergism between IL-1, antigens, mitogens, and ionophores for the induction of IL-2 by these cells. In B cell activation, IL-1 seems to function as helper or cofactor together with IL-4. Murine IL-1 stimulates the growth and maturation of murine B cells into immunoglobulin-secreting cells (De Maeyer and De Maeyer-Guignard, 1988). Interleukin-1 also binds to NK cells and since IL-1 induces interferon, which in turn enhances NK cell tumoricidal activity, both cytokines have a synergistic antitumor effect. Recombinant IL-1 has been used to confirm the role of IL-1 in T and B cell activation, eliminating previous doubts about the purity of IL-1 preparations and confirming its ability to participate in immune responses (Dinarello, 1989).

2. *Interleukin-2*

Interleukin-2 is an inducible glycoprotein made by T cells following activation by mitogens or antigens in the presence of IL-1 (De Maeyer and De Maeyer-Guignard, 1988). In addition to promoting the proliferation of cytotoxic T effector cells and acting as a T-helper factor, IL-2 induces the release of a number of cytokines, such as IFNγ and B cell growth factor from activated T lymphocytes (Kimball and Grob, 1988). Additional activities that have been attributed to IL-2 include supporting growth of thymocytes and activated T cells in culture, increasing NK cell activity, enhancing the activity of lymphokine-activated killer cells, and stimulating the generation of cytotoxic T lymphocytes. The specific high-affinity membrane receptors for IL-2 are absent on resting T cells but are rapidly synthesized following the interaction of mitogens or antigens with the T cell antigen receptor. Thus, production of both IL-2 and its receptor are prerequisites for the T cell immune response (De Maeyer and De Maeyer-Guignard, 1988). IL-2 is also a B cell growth factor. B cells activated with lipopolysaccharide or by anti-immunoglobulin treatment express IL-2 receptors. Production of this lymphokine by human mononuclear cells is suppressed by histamine, but this inhibition can be reversed by the addition of exogenous IL-2 (Dohlsten *et al.*, 1986). The availability of recombinant IL-2 facilitates detailed investigation of its regulatory role in immune responses.

The comparatively recent discovery that the activity of IL-2 may be modulated by neuropeptides and that lymphocytes have surface receptors for endorphins and enkephalins confirms the close communication that exists beween the immune system and the central nervous system (Blalock and Smith, 1985; Coffey and Hadden, 1985; Wybran, 1985).

3. *Interleukin-3*

Interleukin-3 stimulates the proliferation of a broad range of hemopoietic cell types. It is normally produced by antigen- or mitogen-stimulated T cells. Mice receiving recombinant murine IL-3 show a marked increase in many white blood cells and their spleens increase in weight by 50% (De Maeyer and De Maeyer-Guignard, 1988).

Lymphocytes possess receptors for a large number of endogenous substances and apparently respond to these compounds via the same intracellular mechanisms that operate in other cells. Substances for which lymphocytes bear receptors include neurotransmitters, hormones, and other mediators that influence cellular functions, in part through cyclic nucleotide metabolism (Coffey and Hadden, 1985). Receptors for other endogenous compounds, such as transferrin, low-density lipoproteins, and prostaglandins, are also found on lymphocytes. Metabolites of the essential fatty acid, arachidonic acid, are of undoubted importance in regulating inflammatory and immunological reactions. Cellular activation by IL-1 is often accompanied by cyclooxygenation as well as lipoxygenation of arachidonic acid. The major cyclooxygenase metabolites are the prostaglandins PGE_2 and $PGF_2\alpha$ (Kimball and Grob, 1988). While PGE increases cAMP levels in lymphocytes and inhibits their activation, leukotrienes, products of the lipoxygenase enzymatic pathway, decrease cAMP and contribute to activation (Coffey and Hadden, 1985). There is evidence that the activity of IL-1 on thymocytes is directly controlled via lipoxygenase metabolism of arachidonic acid (Dinarello *et al.*, 1983). The lipoxygenase pathway may also be required for IL-2 production and IL-2-induced proliferation of T cells (Goodwin *et al.*, 1977).

4. Interferons

Interferons are a heterogeneous family of inducible secretory proteins originally identified by their ability to prevent viral replication. They can be classified according to their cells of origin and divided into antigenically distinct types. Interferons classified as IFNα, IFNβ, and IFNγ are produced by leukocytes, fibroblasts or epithelial cells, and T cells or NK cells, respectively. Apart from their antiviral activity they have a number of immunoregulatory effects. IFNγ is functionally similar in some respects to IFNα and IFNβ, but it also has several distinct effects on cells of the immune system. The availability of recombinant IFNγ and antibodies specific for IFNα subtypes and for IFNβ and IFNγ has allowed their regulatory role to be thoroughly investigated. Overall, the effect of interferons on cells is inhibitory, although they do have stimulatory effects on some aspects of immune cell function. All three types enhance NK cell activity (Herberman *et al.*, 1979). Interferons α and β depress antigenic, mitogenic, and allogeneic cell-stimulated lymphocyte proliferation (Sternberg and Parker, 1988). The fact that interferons sometimes stimulate and at other times inhibit T suppressor cell function depends on many factors including antigen dose, genetic factors, and their interaction with other cytokines (De Maeyer and De Maeyer-Guignard, 1988). The immunomodulatory effect of IFNγ on the monocyte–macrophage series includes an increase in Fc receptors for IgG, macrophage activation, and expression of Class I and II MHC antigens (Schultz and Kleinschmidt, 1983; Varesio et al., 1984). Endotoxin-induced IL-1 secretion by monocytes is enhanced also. Interferons α, β, and γ have been reported to both increase and decrease synthesis and secretion of multiple proteolytic enzymes by macrophages.

Interferons also affect humoral immunity and produce time- and dose-dependent alterations in antibody responses. Low-dose IFN α, β, and γ may inhibit antibody production *in vitro* (Johnson et al., 1975). Recombinant IFNγ has a stimulatory effect on late antibody production (Leibson et al., 1984) and it seems likely that IFNγ is one of the major components of T cell-derived helper factors for late B cell responses.

All three types of interferon exert their effect after binding to cell surface receptors. The mechanism by which they induce changes in immune cell function and antiviral activity has been investigated through an analysis of the effects of interferons on the regulation of gene transcription. Interferons not only rapidly induce transcription of unique genes, but they also inhibit transcription of genes induced by other growth factors (Sternberg and Parker, 1988). It is clear that interferons exert effects on the expression of a variety of cell surface molecules essential to a wide spectrum of immune responses. Whether modulation of all these surface molecules is the primary mechanism through which interferons alter immune cell function, or whether these molecules are simply markers of a stage of cell differentiation induced by interferons remains to be determined.

5. Therapeutic Applications of Cytokines

For many years the prophylactic and therapeutic use of cytokines was limited because of difficulties with their production and purification. The recent availability of recombinant cytokines has overcome some of these difficulties and many are undergoing clinical evaluation, not only in rodents and humans, but also in domestic food animals.

Polyinosinic-polycytiditic acid (Poly I:C) used as an interferon inducer in mice, restored a large amount of NK activity lost during treatment with immunosuppressive agents (Djeu and Ramsey, 1984). Both murine recombinant IFNγ and human recombinant IFNα induced high levels of NK cell activity against target cells and the gamma interferon was also a potent activator of peritoneal macrophages (Pinto et al., 1988). Recombinant IFNα also protected mice against challenge with a togavirus, a flavivirus, and a herpes virus, whereas recombinant IFNγ had less antiviral activity.

The immunomodulatory and therapeutic activities of recombinant murine IFNγ and poly I:C were evaluated in treating metastatic disease in mice (Black et al., 1988). Both compounds had immunomodulatory activity when NK cell, lymphokine-activated killer cells, and cytolytic T lymphocyte functions were assessed. With the knowledge that anti-IL-2 receptor monoclonal antibodies were immunosuppressive (Kelley et al., 1986), Murphy et al. (1988) used "protein engineering" to synthesize diphtheria toxin, with IL-2 replacing the receptor binding domain of the toxin. This IL-2-toxin inhibited protein synthesis in both human and murine T cell lines bearing high affinity IL-2 receptors, whereas the hybrid toxin was not active against cells lacking this receptor. In murine delayed-type hypersensitivity, the IL-2-toxin treatment induced marked immunosuppression.

The administration of recombinant bovine IL-2 to calves vaccinated and then challenged with bovine herpesvirus-1 (BHV1) resulted in clinical benefit (Blecha, 1988). Neutralizing antibody levels increased sixfold following treatment with IL-2 and there was induction of lymphokine-activated killer cells. An undesirable effect of IL-2 treatment was illness attributed to the recombinant lymphokine, which ceased when treatment was terminated. Calves treated with recombinant bovine interferon α_1, prior to challenge with BHV1 had an enhanced ability to withstand subsequent *Pasteurella haemolytica* challenge (Babiuk and Ohmann, 1984). Treatment with interferon reduced temperature responses, clinical signs of disease, lung pathology, and mortality.

Recombinant human IFNα_2 conferred protection in calves against challenge with vaccinia virus and also protected bovine cells *in vitro* (Schwers et al., 1984). Although IFNγ is often considered species-specific, recombinant porcine IFNγ protected homologous cells as well as heterologous cells of bovine origin against the cytopathic effects of vesicular stomatitis virus (Charley et al., 1988). This recombinant lymphokine also protected porcine epithelial cells and pulmonary alveolar macrophages against transmissible gastroenteritis virus.

D. GLUCOCORTICOIDS

The adrenal cortex synthesizes two classes of steroids: the corticosteroids (glucocorticoids and mineralocorticoids) and androgens. Glucocorticoids are considered to have a homeostatic role in relation to inflammatory and immune responses in addition to their pronounced effect on carbohydrate and protein metabolism (Dale, 1984). Mineralocorticoids act on the distal tubules of the kidney enhancing the reabsorption of sodium ions and increasing urinary excretion of both potassium and hydrogen ions (Haynes and Murad, 1985). Glucocorticoids have a broad range of effects on cells involved in the induction of immune responses. Cortisol and corticosterone are the principal naturally-occurring glucocorticoids, the former being the more potent. They are released when cells of the adrenal cortex are stimulated by ACTH (corticotrophin), the peptide hormone elaborated by the adenohypophysis (anterior pituitary). Adrenocortical steroids and their synthetic analogues have antiinflammatory and immunosuppressive effects apart from their negative feedback action on the hypothalamus and adenohypophysis (Dale, 1984).

Glucocorticoids inhibit not only the early phenomena associated with the inflammatory process (edema, capillary dilation, and migration of leukocytes into the inflamed area and phagocytic activity) but also the later stages, characterized by capillary proliferation, fibroblast proliferation, and deposition of collagen. Circulating white blood cells are also affected. Species differences in the responses of immunoactive cells to glucocorticoids exist; those with relatively high lymphocyte numbers respond with a lymphopenia and neutrophilia (Griffin, 1989). The subpopulations of lymphocytes are differently affected by steroids; T cells are decreased proportionately more than B cells (Cupps and Fauci, 1982).

1. Mechanism of Action at the Cellular Level

Endogenous glucocorticoids probably have a major role in regulating immune function, particularly the expression of immunological reactivity. The effects of exogenous corticosteroids on immunological reactivity are complicated by many variables including the potency and concentration of steroid, treatment schedules, species and age of animals, and assay systems. Species can be grouped as steroid sensitive (hamster, mouse, rat, and rabbit), in which steroids produce lymphocytolysis, or steroid resistant (human, guinea pig, monkey, and ferret), in which there is lymphopenia without lymphocytolysis (Sternberg and Parker, 1988).

These drugs also inhibit the synthesis of various inflammatory mediators including prostaglandins, thromboxanes, and leukotrienes. The suppression of mediator synthesis is attributed to the ability of the steroids to induce synthesis of regulatory antiphospolipase proteins, collectively called lipocortins. Lipocortins suppress mediator biosynthesis by inhibiting the release of arachidonate from membrane phospholipids, thereby limiting the amount of substrate available for mediator production (Hirata and Iwata, 1983; Flower, 1984; Becker and Grasso, 1988).

In general, a decrease in the absolute number of circulating lymphocytes follows oral or parenteral administration of glucocorticoids

(Tsokos, 1987; Katz and Fauci, 1988). Following pharmacological doses, there is a sharp decrease in absolute and relative numbers of eosinophils, basophils, monocytes, and lymphocytes (Tsokos, 1987). Neutrophils, however, increase both in absolute numbers and relative proportions. This neutrophilia, which may last up to 8 hours, may result from (1) an increase in circulatory half-life; (2) accelerated release from the bone marrow; or (3) decreased transfer from the circulation to sites of inflammation (Katz and Fauci, 1988). It has been suggested that glucocorticoid-induced changes in neutrophil surface charge and other membrane effects lessen their attachment to blood vessel endothelium (MacGregor et al., 1974). This effect, in association with alterations in vascular permeability, may account in part for decreased neutrophil migration to extravascular sites and the antiinflammatory activity of these substances. The *in vitro* influence of glucocorticoids on bovine polymorphonuclear leukocyte chemotaxis appears to be minimal (Jayappa and Loken, 1983).

Glucocorticoid-induced lymphocytopenia may involve different mechanisms in different species ranging from lymphocytolysis to redistribution of these cells to extravascular spaces (Katz and Fauci, 1988). In humans, T cells are more affected than B cells, and among T cells, helper populations are more susceptible than the suppressor subpopulation (Tsokos, 1987). Some lymphocyte functions are sensitive to steroids, particularly effector functions dependent on early stages of activation, proliferation, and differentiation. Glucocortocoids generally depress the blastogenic response of lymphocytes to mitogens (Langhoff et al., 1987; Ghio et al., 1988). Dogs, although often regarded as steroid resistant, showed transient lymphocytopenia and a prolonged inhibition of peripheral blood lymphocyte–phytomitogen response following oral prednisolone treatment, but their antibody response to canine distemper virus vaccination was normal (Nara et al., 1979). The effects of steroids on B cell function are unclear. In humans, primary antibody responses were reduced, while secondary responses were unaffected (Tsokos, 1987).

A decrease in circulating eosinophils, apparently due to redistribution of these cells in other body compartments, is a consistent feature of glucocorticoid administration (Kaeberle, 1984). Presumably this effect may account for some of the benefits of steroid treatment in eosinophil-mediated allergic states. In rats, pretreatment of peritoneal mast cells with dexamethasone prevented IgE-Fc receptor-dependent stimulation of histamine release by Con A or antigen, whereas histamine release by a nonimmunological stimulus was unaffected (Walajtys-Rode et al., 1988).

NK cells are reported by some workers to be refractory to glucocorticoids (Katz and Fauci, 1988) but by others to be suppressed by these drugs (Nair and Schwartz, 1984; Fuggetta et al., 1988; Goldstein et al., 1988). Prednisolone inhibited NK and ADCC activities of purified human lymphocytes and the reaction was reversible with interferon or IL-2 (Nair and Schwartz, 1984). The mechanism of steroid suppression of NK activity is unclear but the induction of an inhibitor of phospolipase by these drugs is suggested (Goldstein et al., 1988).

Depletion of monocytes, probably by redistribution, occurs in several species following the administration of glucocorticoids (Kaeberle, 1984). Horses and cattle appear to be exceptions while monocytosis has been reported in dogs and cattle receiving steroid therapy. Steroids have multiple effects on human monocytes. They interfere with their ability to present antigen, to produce lymphokines, to differentiate into macrophages, and to phagocytoze (Tsokos, 1987). They also seem to increase the Immune Response-Associated Antigen (Ia) expression by monocytes while inhibiting production of IL-1, response to migration inhibitory factor, and macrophage mitogenic factor production (Duncan et al., 1982).

In mice, glucocorticoids inhibit expression of Ia antigens by peritoneal macrophages, both *in vivo* and *in vitro*, reduce production of IL-1, and inhibit antigen presentation for T cell proliferation by macrophages (Snyder and Unanue, 1982). Dexamethasone inhibition of yeast phagocytosis by murine macrophages is mediated by a factor present in homogenates of steroid-treated macrophages. This factor appears to belong to the lipocortin family of phospholipase inhibitory proteins (Becker and Grasso, 1988). It also inhibits accumulation of macrophages and the generation of macrophage chemotactic activity in peritonitis in mice (Nagaoka et al., 1988).

Dexamethasone inhibits IL-2 production but it does not block responsiveness to IL-2 to prevent this lymphokine from interacting with its receptor (Lillehoj and Shevach, 1985). Cortisol decreases the levels of bovine IL-2 *in vivo* and *in vitro* (Blecha and Baker, 1986).

Complement levels and metabolism seem to be relatively resistant to glucocorticoids. High dose glucocorticoid therapy depresses complement levels in guinea pigs and normal levels were not reached for two weeks after discontinuation of therapy (Atkinson and Frank, 1973).

2. Mechanism of Action at the Subcellular Level

The means whereby steroids exert their effect on cells of the immune system are not completely understood. It seems likely that glucocorticoids first bind to specific receptors. The drug–receptor complex migrates to the cell nucleus where it attaches to the cell genome, inducing nuclear DNA to transcribe a specific messenger RNA. This mRNA affects the intracytoplasmic synthesis of proteins, which presumably direct the drug's final action (Baxter and Funder, 1979; Katz and Fauci, 1988; Sternberg and Parker, 1988). Glucocorticoid receptors have been identified on lymphocytes, monocytes, neutrophils, and eosinophils. In the case of the B cell, the immunomodulatory activity of glucocorticoids seems to be exerted by binding to its nuclear receptor, thereby preventing the generation of second messengers required for cell activation after agonist–receptor interaction (Dennis *et al.*, 1987).

The method whereby glucocorticoids induce lymphocytolysis seems to be via receptor-mediated endonuclease activation. Thymocyte death is related to activation of a calcium- and magnesium-dependent endonuclease (Cohen and Duke, 1984). It appears that glucocorticoids may induce cell death via an endonuclease-activating protein, possibly a cytoplasm-to-nucleus calcium-transporting protein, present in thymocytes but not mature T cells. The lack of glucocorticoid-inducible endonuclease-activating protein in mature lymphocytes may explain their glucocorticoid resistance compared with immature thymocytes.

Glucocorticoid sensitivity is probably influenced by many factors apart from receptor number or binding affinity. The state of maturation and activation of cells, the ratio and susceptibility of mixed cell populations, together with the subtypes present are likely to determine the outcome of a treatment regime.

V. Synthetic Compounds with Immunomodulatory Activity

A. LEVAMISOLE

Levamisole, the levoisomer of tetramisole, was originally introduced as an anthelmintic for use in animals and humans more than 20 years ago and is now widely recognized and employed for its immunomodulatory activity (Webster, 1985). The observation by Renoux and Renoux (1971) that *Brucella*-vaccinated mice had an increased immunity against *Brucella* infection following levamisole medication led to active research not only on this imidazole derivative but also on many other potentially useful immunomodulatory compounds.

Apart from its anthelmintic activity in domestic food animals, the pharmacology, pharmacokinetics, and toxicology of this compound have received much attention (Assem, 1984; Fudenberg and Whitten,

1984). Likewise, its effect on the immune system has been the subject of numerous investigations and reports (Irwin et al., 1976; Kaneene et al., 1981; Babiuk and Misra, 1982; Rogers et al., 1985; Mulcahy, 1988). Despite the substantial body of information accumulated from in vivo and in vitro experiments with this compound, its effect on the immune system is not well understood and, indeed, much of the published data seems, on primary examination, to be contradictory. In common with many other immunomodulatory compounds, the dosage used, the frequency of administration, and the immune status of the animal have a major influence on the effects observed. Thus, levamisole treatment of immunosuppressed or stressed animals generally proves beneficial (Babiuk and Misra, 1982; Flesh et al., 1982), whereas in normal animals its effect on the immune response is minimal and sometimes even slightly immunosuppressive (Irwin et al., 1976). The somewhat unpredictable nature of its efficacy combined with its unpleasant side effects, which may include nausea, malaise, and severe granulocytopenia, have diminished its popularity as an immunostimulant in human medicine (Fudenberg and Whitten, 1984; Bardana, 1985).

Levamisole has a wide and sometimes confusing spectrum of biological effects. It has been reported to act primarily on cellular rather than humoral immune responses and to restore the immune response of normal animals. It enhances the chemotactic response of bovine polymorphonuclear leukocytes in vitro without enhancing phagocytosis or intracellular killing in vivo or in vitro (Jayappa and Loken, 1982). No differences in the severity of infection or rate of recovery was noted between levamisole-treated and control calves experimentally infected with bovine viral diarrhea (BVD) virus (Sapertstein et al., 1983). The only difference observed was that leukopenia associated with BVD infection was prevented; the mean white blood cell counts were consistently higher in the levamisole-treated group than in the control group. The application of levamisole in the prevention and treatment of bovine mastitis has been reviewed from published sources by Anderson (1984), who concluded that it offered limited benefit for treatment but might have a role in prevention.

When used in vitro with peripheral blood lymphocytes, levamisole significantly potentiated the Brucella abortus-induced lymphocyte blastogenesis from unresponsive cattle (Kaneene et al., 1981). Potentiation was achieved only when levamisole was added to lymphocyte cultures 24 hours prior to the addition of the Brucella antigen. The authors concluded that levamisole appeared to "prime" the lymphocytes and macrophages for interaction with antigen. The effect of levamisole on the immune response of cattle to infectious bovine rhinotracheitis vaccine (IBRV) was assessed under controlled and commercial feed lot conditions by Babiuk and Misra (1982). In all instances, regardless of when levamisole was administered, there was an enhanced immune response to vaccination. A previous report by Irwin et al. (1976) concluded that the simultaneous administration of levamisole and IBRV suppressed the primary immune response in calves. Van Der Maaten et al. (1983) evaluated the effect of levamisole on the virological and serological responses of bovine leukemia virus-infected cattle and sheep and concluded that neither recommended anthelmintic doses, nor repeated doses of the drug, produced significant changes in antibody titer or in bovine leukemia virus replication in persistently infected sheep and cattle. Levamisole treatment increased PHA responsiveness of peripheral blood lymphocytes of normal chickens and initially enhanced PHA stimulation in Marek's disease virus-inoculated chickens compared to untreated virus-inoculated chickens (Confer and Adldinger, 1981).

A report on the immunopotentiating effect of levamisole in the prevention of bovine mastitis, fetal death, and endometritis in dairy cattle, based largely on clinical parameters, claimed that there was a substantial improvement in the health status of treated animals over the control group (Flesh et al., 1982). Mulcahy (1988) failed to demonstrate any clinical benefit from levamisole treatment in calves with enzootic pneumonia, and pulmonary alveolar macrophages recovered by bronchopulmonary lavage from treated and control animals had similar distribution patterns of Fc and C3 receptors. Using a luminol-amplified chemiluminescence assay to evaluate the effect of levamisole on the metabolic activity of pulmonary alveolar macrophages from parainfluenza-3 and IBR virus-infected calves, Ogunbiyi et al. (1988) concluded that treatment of calves with levamisole partially reversed the virus-induced impairment of pulmomary alveolar macrophage β_1-adrenoreceptor function without influencing β_2-adrenoreceptor activity.

The immunomodulatory activity of levamisole in artificially reared neonatal pigs was assessed using lymphocyte proliferative responses to mitogens by Hennessy et al. (1987), who concluded that it enhanced the responses of artificially reared pigs to values comparable to those of sow-reared controls. The addition of levamisole to cultures of normal mouse spleen cells in vitro in the presence of staphylococcal enterotoxin B (which activates antigen nonspecific suppressor T cells) resulted in increased suppressor cell activity as judged by antibody production in a plaque-forming cell assay (Rogers et al., 1985).

1. Mechanism of Action

The imidazole structure is found in several synthesized chemicals that have been reported to regulate one or more of the cellular components of the immune system. Imidazole elevates cGMP levels in lymphocytes *in vitro* and enhances their proliferative response to mitogens or foreign cells (Chirigos, 1984). The imidazole ring seems to be one of the active moieties of levamisole responsible for the functional increase of peripheral T cells and macrophages (Amery and Hörig, 1984). Levamisole or its products appear to have thymomimetic properties and one of its metabolites dl-2-oxo-3-[2-mercapto-ethyl]-5-phenylimidazolidine (OMPI) is believed to have a direct effect on the immune system through its oxygen radical scavenging properties, which may limit oxidative destruction of β-adrenoreceptors (Van Ginckel and De Brabender, 1979; Fudenberg and Whitten, 1984; Engels *et al.*, 1985).

Levamisole and OMPI restore cell functions by inhibition of peroxide formation, and accordingly it is proposed that either levamisole or OMPI exert an antioxidant effect by preventing accumulation of peroxides and free radicals that limit the metabolism of immunocytes (Amery and Hörig, 1984).

2. Comments

The apparent contradictory results arising from levamisole treatment reported by various workers probably reflect the many variables present in their experimental designs. In general, clinical trials with levamisole both in human and veterinary medicine have demonstrated a marked effect on cellular immunological variables but equivocal effects on antibody production. Beneficial results are most likely to be achieved when the drug is given to animals whose immune system is functioning suboptimally, but even then, a positive response is not always obtained. Irrespective of its mode of action at the cellular level, the outcome of a treatment regime should include consideration of the initial immune status of the animals under test. Most other results seem to be time and dose dependent.

B. Isoprinosine

Isoprinosine is a synthetic immunomodulator with antiviral activity, formed from the p-acetamidobenzoate salt of n-n-dimethylamino-2-propanol and inosine in a 3:1 molar ratio. Activities attributed to it include enhanced lymphocyte proliferative responses, augmented lymphokine production, and increased NK cell cytotoxicity. *In vitro* experiments have demonstrated that isoprinosine inhibits the replication of both DNA and RNA viruses in tissue culture (Fudenberg and Whitten, 1984) and *in vivo* it promotes resistance against a wide range of viruses (Tsang et al., 1984). In immunosuppressive conditions, unrelated to virus infections, it increases various immune responses both *in vivo* and *in vitro*. Isoprinosine seems to be remarkably free of side effects. Following oral or intravenous administration in humans it is rapidly metabolized. The half-life of the inosine moiety is 50 minutes following an oral dose and only 3 minutes following an intravenous dose (Campoli-Richards et al., 1986), the major excretion product being uric acid. An important feature of isoprinosine's activity is its thymic hormonelike properties (Tsang et al., 1984; Hadden, 1987). This feature has been demonstrated *in vitro* by the induction of differentiation in both human and murine prothymocytes. Interleukin-1 and -2 production, and neutrophil, monocyte, and macrophage chemotaxis and phagocytosis are also potentiated by this inosine-containing complex (Campoli-Richards et al., 1986). The capacity of mitogens to induce lymphocyte DNA synthesis is substantially increased by isoprinosine (O'Neill et al., 1984).

As is the case with levamisole, the immunostimulatory effects of isoprinosine are most easily demonstrated where there is a preexisting impairment of the immune system. The effects of isoprinosine treatment on the lymphocyte stimulation response to PHA, NK cytotoxicity, and monocyte chemotaxis in aging hamsters were studied in three age groups by continuous weekly intraperitoneal injection (Tsang et al., 1984). This compound restored depressed immune functions in aging hamsters and produced a significant prolongation of life span in that species.

Immunosuppression due to viral infection has traditionally been a target for isoprinosine treatment, and its protective effects in hamsters and mice against DNA and RNA viruses have been investigated by Ohnishi et al. (1983). A broad spectrum of antiviral activity was evident; treatment with isoprinosine resulted in a statistically significant increase in survival of treated hamsters and mice. The same workers reported an enhanced primary immune response to sheep red blood cells as determined by plaque assay. The drug also enhanced delayed-type hypersensitivity reactions; macrophage activity increased but there was no effect on NK cells. *In vitro*, IFNγ production was increased by isoprinosine treatment. Adminstration of isoprinosine to humans had variable effects on NK cell activity, but three days after cessation of treatment there was a significant increase in activity (Hersey and

Edwards, 1984). Isoprinosine restored the *in vitro* T lymphocyte functions of cyclophosphamide immunosuppressed mice but no effect was observed on B cell proliferation by lipopolysaccharide (Barasoain *et al.*, 1987).

The immunomodulatory activity of isoprinosine against three avian viruses, Newcastle disease, avian influenza, and avian infectious bronchitis was evaluated by Moya *et al.* (1984). Isoprinosine delayed the mean death day in chickens infected with Newcastle disease or avian influenza, provided the drug was given before and after virus infection. The antiviral effect of treatment appeared to be due mainly to interferon production. In artificially reared neonatal pigs, isoprinosine enhanced the lymphocyte proliferative responses to mitogens to values comparable to those of sow-reared controls (Hennessy *et al.*, 1987). Isoprinosine did not affect shedding of virus from calves infected with BHV1 (Blecha *et al.*, 1987). It did not appear to reverse BHV1 suppression of lymphocyte proliferation and it tended to decrease the bacteriocidal activity of alveolar macrophages. Mulcahy (1988) reported an increase *in vitro* expression of Fc and C3 receptors on pulmonary alveolar macrophages following isoprinosine treatment. Alveolar macrophages from isoprinosine-treated calves had greater numbers of Fc and C3 receptors than control animals, but no associated increase in phagocytic activity was evident. Following naturally occurring respiratory disease, treated calves had significantly less neutrophil infiltration into the lower respiratory tract.

Mode of Action

Since it contains the imidazole structure, the immunomodulatory effects of isoprinosine are consistent with its proposed action of affecting enzymes controlling cyclic nucleotide levels in immunocytes by increasing the availability of precursor substances, thereby raising intracellular cGMP and the activity of effector cells (Chirigos, 1984; Barasoain *et al.*, 1987). The thymomimetic activity of isoprinosine and substances with similar molecular structures, such as NPT 15392, is believed to contribute substantially to their immunomodulatory role (Tsang *et al.*, 1984; Hadden, 1987). In a comprehensive review of isoprinosine Campoli-Richards *et al.* (1986) have assembled data on its activity on individual cells of the immune system. They concluded that mitogen- or antigen-stimulated T lymphocyte differentiation and proliferation are accelerated by concurrent exposure to isoprinosine, and production of IL-2 from blood lymphocytes of healthy persons is potentiated. When human monocytes and alveolar macrophages are incubated *in vitro* with isoprinosine, production of IL-1 is stimulated and they have increased levels of lysosomal enzymes. Although its effect on NK cell function is disputed, in general it seems to increase NK cell activity. The *in vitro* effect on neutrophils and eosinophils is beneficial, especially if immunosuppression is present, with enhanced chemotaxis and phagocytosis by neutrophils and increased Fc and C3 receptors on eosinophils.

The *in vivo* antiviral activity of isoprinosine in an avian model has been attributed to enhancement of interferon production or to a synergistic interferon–isoprinosine interaction (Moya *et al.*, 1984). From their studies on hamsters and mice treated with isoprinosine and challenged with DNA and RNA viruses, Ohnishi *et al.* (1983) concluded that the compound acts on T lymphocytes with release of lymphokines, thus altering macrophage activity; alternatively it may act directly on macrophages. The total protection conferred on treated mice against secondary influenza infection may be due to a direct antiviral effect and a general elevation of the immune status. The *in vivo* antiviral activity is believed to result from enhancement of immunological processes once lymphocytes have been triggered by viral antigens or mitogens. Resting lymphocytes are usually not stimulated by isoprinosine. The clinical efficacy of this compound for the treatment of viral infections may be attributed to its direct effect on viral replication combined with its ability to augment the host's immune responses (Ruszala-Mallon *et al.*, 1988). The enhancement of immunological responses by isoprinosine may be explained in part by its effect on cAMP and cGMP levels or by lymphokine release from T cells, especially IFNγ.

The biochemical activity of isoprinosine at the cellular level is uncertain. One theory proposed to explain its antiviral activity is that the drug links to the ribosomes of the infected cells, which through steric modification offers advantage to cellular RNA over viral RNA in the competition for linkage with the ribosomal sites (Campoli-Richards *et al.*, 1986). A second theory attributes the immunostimulatory activity of isoprinosine to lymphokine production, which leads to enhanced expression of immune functions. It is probable that the immunostimulatory activity of this compound derives from its diverse activity at the cellular level, including enhancement of mitogen-induced proliferation of T cells with associated lymphokine release and, in addition, its thymomimetic properties.

C. Synthetic Polynucleotides

The realization that interferons represented a major defense system of animals against viral diseases stimulated much interest in the development of interferon inducers. In 1967, Field *et al.* demonstrated that protected RNAs, such as polyinosinic-polycytidylic acid (poly I:C), were excellent stimulators of interferon synthesis. Subsequently, it was demonstrated that they were effective, both prophylactically and therapeutically in experimental viral infections in animals and that they were also active against experimental tumors in animals (Levy, 1970). In recent years, much attention has been directed to determine the efficacy of polyribonucleotide complexes in inducing nonspecific resistance in many species to infectious agents.

Polyribonucleotide complexes are formed through mixing of the polymerized single strands of synthetic mononucleotide with another complementary base pair. Poly I:C, a double-stranded RNA, is a potent IFN inducer in rodents but has weak IFN-inducing activity in primates and humans because of rapid hydrolysis by serum nucleases (Hartmann et al., 1987). A stabilized poly I:C complex has been prepared, which appears to resist hydrolysis by serum nucleases and is an effective IFN inducer in subhuman primates and rodents (Chirigos, 1984).

The stabilized product is a complex of high molecular weight poly I:C and low molecular weight poly-L-lysine with carboxymethylcellulose as a stabilizer. This stabilized preparation, referred to as poly ICLC, is reported to protect rhesus monkeys against otherwise lethal viral infections, augment natural killer cell activity, activate macrophage tumoricidal activity, stimulate lymphocytes to PHA, and enhance delayed-type hypersensitivity responses to sheep red blood cells (Chirigos, 1984).

Because of toxicity problems with poly I:C other polyribonucleotide complexes were formed such as polyadenylic acid mixed with polyuridilic acid (poly A·poly U). Many of these synthetic polyribonucleotides have well-defined immunomodulatory properties, apart from interferon induction. These include stimulation of many cell types, without increased cell division, including nonimmunocompetent cells. Polyribonucleotides appear to stimulate both macrophages and T cells (Johnson, 1985). Poly A·poly U-exposed macrophages show heightened nonspecific cytotoxicity against tumor cells in culture and there is increasd production of IL-1. Poly ICLC is a potent enhancer of liver-associated NK activity (Wiltrout et al., 1985). Polyribonucleotides, generally, appear to have a dual effect on antibody production. If antigen is administered within hours of polyribonucleotide administration, helper cells tend to dominate the response, whereas if antigen administration is delayed for 24 hours a suppressive effect is reported (Johnson, 1985). Nonspecific suppressor activity in mice is enhanced by poly A·poly U, either *in vivo* or *in vitro*, when used 2 days prior to antigen.

The prophylactic and therapeutic efficacy of poly ICLC in mice against Rift Valley fever virus indicates its potential use as an antiviral agent (Kende, 1985). Its ability to protect rabbits against challenge with rabies street virus confirms its potent antiviral activity (Fenje and Postic, 1970).

The immunomodulatory role of polyribonucleotides is not confined to viral infections. They can also induce protection against Gram-positive and Gram-negative bacteria. The survival patterns of neonatal and young mice were substantially improved by treatment with poly A·poly U 1 day before challenge with *Pseudomonas aeruginosa* and *Streptococcus pneumoniae* (Johnson, 1987).

The inherent toxicity of polyribonucleotides, however, tends to limit their usefulness as therapeutic immunomodulators in some domestic food animals. Poly I:C caused several transient toxic manifestations in young pigs including elevated blood urea nitrogen and marked leukopenia (Gainer and Guarnieri, 1985). In mice, the injection of toxic doses of poly ICLC significantly reduced body weight and induced serological and histological abnormalities, including pulmonary thrombosis and hepatic necrosis (Hartmann et al., 1987).

Mechanism of Action

Poly I:C, and Poly A·poly U have been reported to be potent IFN inducers in rodents but not in primates, while poly ICLC is reported to be a potent interferon inducer in rodents and primates (Chirigos, 1984; Hartmann et al., 1987). It is suggested that synthetic polyribonucleotides are capable of inducing interferon production by lymphocytes because they may simulate viral genetic material. The generalized cell stimulation associated with this group of compounds is believed to operate via a common membrane component, possibly adenyl or guanyl cyclase, or by interaction with the cell nucleus (Johnson, 1985).

Poly A·poly U induces release of some T helper lymphokines, including, presumably, IL-2. Nonspecific polyclonal activation of cytotoxic T cells is also induced by poly A·poly U. Poly ICLC is a potent stimulator of NK cell activity both *in vivo* and *in vitro* (Talmadge et al., 1985a). The activation of NK cells appears to be systemic, and peak IFN levels seem to parallel peak stimulation of NK cell activity. Poly ICLC can also be used to induce colony-stimulating factor-mediated myelopoiesis (Schlick et al., 1984).

VI. Microbial Products as Immunomodulators

Crude preparations of selected microorganisms, such as dead mycobacteria in Freund's complete adjuvant, have long been used to increase immune responsiveness in a nonspecific manner. A great variety of taxonomically different bacteria have been used in the immunotherapy of experimental animal tumors and also in patients with neoplasia. A common finding in treatments with microbial products is nonspecific activation of macrophages and stimulation of NK cell activity. It is now possible to identify particular components of bacteria and fungi that have immunostimulatory activity.

A. PROPIONIBACTERIUM ACNES

This organism, well established in immunological literature for many years under its former name, *Corynebacterium parvum*, has long been associated with immunostimulatory activity in humans and domestic animals. Recently reclassified as *Propionibacterium spp.*, most strains are now classed as *P. acnes*, but strain differences in terms of immunopharmacological effects have been noted (Cummins, 1984). Despite the fact that they have a longer history than do chemical immunomodulators, the mechanisms of action of immunoactive substances of microbial origin are generally less well defined than those of synthetic compounds, and *P. acnes* is no exception. Heat-killed or formaldehyde-treated suspensions of *P. acnes* are used for immunotherapy.

Several studies have indicated that *P. acnes* is effective in increasing host resistance to bacterial, viral, and protozoal infections (Adlam *et al.*, 1972; Glasgow *et al.*, 1977; Manickam *et al.*, 1983). The ability of *P. acnes* to induce tumor regression has been extensively investigated and reported (Ghaffar *et al.*, 1981; North, 1984; Mastroeni *et al.*, 1985). The principal effects of *P. acnes* on experimental animals are:

1. Macrophage activation, increased particle clearance, and development of hepatosplenomegaly.
2. Modulation of both humoral and cellular aspects of the immune response.
3. Alteration of liver enzyme levels (Cummins, 1984).

Suppression of macrophage-mediated antibacterial resistance in mice to *Listeria monocytogenes*, induced by fibrosarcoma cells, was not observed if mice were pretreated with *P. acnes* (Miyata *et al.*, 1981). Treatment with P40, a fraction of *P. acnes* (*Corynebacterium granulosum*), restored peritoneal macrophage activity from a depressed level to the normal chemotactic level in tumor-bearing rats, and phagocytic values observed in untreated normal animals (Mastroeni *et al.*, 1985). The ability of *P. acnes* to induce tumor regression has been attributed to greatly enhanced cytolytic T cell responses, coinciding with the onset of tumor regression (North, 1984). Ghaffar *et al.* (1981) have suggested that *P. acnes* can either inhibit or promote the growth of tumors, depending on the tumor model system and the immunogenicity of the tumor.

Although alterations in bone marrow activity and associated hematological alterations have been reported following *P. acnes* administration, Al-Izzi and Maxie (1982) found no significant enhancement of the macrophage colony-forming potential in calves. There were, however, increases in macrophage numbers in the spleen, lungs, liver, and lymph nodes and an accompanying lymphoid hyperplasia in the thymus, lymph nodes, and pulmonary-associated lymphoid tissue following intravenous administration of *P. acnes*.

P. acnes has been used to enhance resistance to a range of protozoa, including *Plasmodium* and *Babesia* spp. (Clark et al., 1977), *Toxoplasma gondii* (Swartzberg et al., 1975), and *Theileria annulata* (Manickam et al., 1983).

An increase in bacterial clearance was observed in the liver, spleen, and blood of mice injected intravenously with *Salmonella enteritidis*, previously treated with *P. acnes* (Collins and Scott, 1974). The enhanced clearance of the salmonellae was attributed to increased phagocytosis by activated macrophages. The immunomodulatory activity of killed *P. acnes* in guinea pigs simultaneously vaccinated with *Brucella abortus* strain-19 vaccine and later challenged with a virulent *B. abortus* strain was investigated by Panangala et al. (1986). The mean splenic colony-forming units of *Brucella* in the group immunopotentiated with *P. acnes* and vaccinated was significantly decreased when compared to guinea pigs vaccinated with *B. abortus* alone. The immunomodulation was attributed to either activated macrophages, T cell-mediated cytolytic mechanisms, or both combined. The pulmonary clearance of *Pasteurella haemolytica* in calves given *P. acnes* and infected with parainfluenza-3 virus was investigated by Al-Izzi et al. (1982). *P. acnes* appeared to enhance bacterial clearance. The alveolar macrophages were generally larger in *P. acnes*-treated calves and bacterial clearance was enhanced in those calves that had larger macrophages. Subcutaneous administration of *P. acnes* to calves resulted in increased intracellular killing of bacteria by alveolar macrophages, but this was not accompanied by increased Fc of C3 receptor expression (Mulcahy, 1988). An increased responsiveness to skin sensitization with Dinitrochlorobenzene (DNCB) also followed *P. acnes* administration.

The oral administration of P40, a fraction of *P. acnes*, to mice prior to challenge with herpes and influenza viruses resulted in some protection, but not when used subcutaneously for treatment after challenge (Fattal-German and Bizzini, 1988).

Mechanism of Action

In general it appears that *P. acnes* and its fractions are not as efficient in stimulating antibody production as other microbial products, such as killed mycobacteria. Among the prominent immunomodulating properties of *P. acnes* are its nonspecific tumor effects. Apart from enhancing tumor resistance, this organism modulates phagocytic and cytotoxic functions of macrophages, their lysosomal enzyme contents, and their histochemical characteristics (Ghaffar et al., 1981). The antitumor activity following systemic administration of *P. acnes* appears to be largely due to generalized and nonspecific activation of macrophages in the reticuloendothelial system. The increase in macrophage numbers in the spleen, lungs, liver, and lymph nodes of calves, following intravenous administration of *P. acnes*, together with lymphoid hyperplasia evident in many lymphoid organs, clearly indicate the stimulatory effect this organism exerts on the reticuloendothelial system (Al-Izzi and Maxie, 1982). The restoration of impaired macrophage functions in tumor-bearing rats (Mastroeni et al., 1985) and in tumor-bearing mice confirms the immunostimulatory role of this organism in tumor-induced immunosuppression. Stimulation of cytotoxic T cells has also been reported in tumor-bearing mice (North, 1984). A generalized stimulation of most cells of the immune system, including T and B cells, NK cells, and macrophages, appears to be the method whereby *P. acnes* exerts its immunostimulatory effect in most animals (Cummins, 1984). The immunopotentiation of the immune response to protozoal and bacterial infections is attributed to macrophage activation, probably in association with enhanced T cell-mediated responses.

B. Lentinan

A number of fungal-derived immunomodulators have received much attention from research workers in recent years. These include protein-bound polysaccharides and pure polysaccharides extracted from fungi, often by simple methods. Lentinan is one such substance, a neutral polysaccharide, isolated from the hot-water extract of mycelia of *Lentinus edodes*, an edible mushroom prevalent in Japan.

Lentinan is a β-1,3-glucan with a high molecular weight, and its repeating unit is composed of five β-1,3-glucopyranoside linkages with two β-1,6-glucopyranoside-linked branches. Thus, it is composed only of glucose with no other sugar component (Hamuro and Chihara, 1984). It has a triple-helix structure, is water soluble, and is heat and acid stable but alkalilabile (Aoki, 1984). Lentinan has been studied extensively for its potency as an antitumor immunotherapeutic agent and also for its immunostimulatory activity against bacteria, viruses, and parasites (Hamuro and Chihara, 1984). It has low toxicity and does not induce hypersensitivity reactions in guinea pigs.

Lentinan stimulates pinocytosis of murine peritoneal macrophages *in vitro* and it is suggested that this stimulation occurs via polysaccharide receptors on macrophages (Ábel *et al.*, 1986). Interferon production is stimulated *in vivo*, but apparently not *in vitro*. Interleukin-1 production is augmented and T cell-dependent immune responses are enhanced (Hamuro and Chihara, 1984). Lentinan not only augments antigen-specific cellular immune responses, but it is also capable of triggering antigen-nonspecific immune responses against neoplastic cells.

In *Mesocestoides corti*-infected mice treated with lentinan, there was a marked reduction in the number of parasites in the peritoneal cavity (White *et al.*, 1988). Giant cells and macrophages appeared to be the effector cells mediating parasite damage. Although the effect of lentinan on humoral immunity is not as well documented as on cell-mediated immunity, it has been shown to enhance the number of plaque-forming cells in mice against sheep red blood cells, both *in vivo* and *in vitro* (Aoki, 1984). In the murine system, activation of the complement pathway, via the classical and alternate pathway, has also been documented.

Mode of Action of Lentinan

Lentinan is believed to augment the reactivity of precursor effector cells that respond to some of the major lymphokines, with subsequent amplification of the responses of cytotoxic T lymphocytes, NK cells, and activated macrophages, and with increased antibody production. Lentinan has also been shown to affect macrophage function independent of specific immune responses, to increase chemiluminescence (Sipka *et al.*, 1985), to regulate the production of acute-phase protein (Suga *et al.*, 1986), to interact with the alternate complement pathway (Hamuro *et al.*, 1978), and to induce macrophage cytotoxicity (Hamuro *et al.*, 1980). This fungal polysaccharide increases IL-1 production by direct interaction with macrophages or indirectly, via augmented colony-stimulating factor produced by lentinan-stimulated alveolar macrophages. The increased production of IL-1 results in augmented maturation of immature lymphoid cells into mature cells capable of responding to lymphokines, and in turn these mature cells differentiate into effector cytotoxic T cells, NK cells, and plasma cells in the presence of IL-2 (Hamuro and Chihara, 1984). The augmentation and modulation of lentinan-induced responses appears to be T cell-dependent, as this drug fails to induce the strong inflammatory responses to *Mesocestoides corti* in athymic mice that are seen in normal mice following lentinan treatment (White *et al.*, 1983, 1988).

VII. Liposomes

A. Potential Role in Immunomodulation

Liposomes are membranous vesicles of naturally occurring phospholipids, separated by aqueous compartments. Various types of biologically active substances can be incorporated into liposomes by encapsulation, surface absorption, or covalent linkage (Swenson *et al.*, 1988). They consist of one or more closed concentric phospholipid bilayers that are formed when phospholipids are suspended in aqueous solution, and depending on the method of preparation, multilamellar vesicles or unilamellar vesicles are formed (Swenson *et al.*, 1988). Their composition and properties can be varied at will and they can be safely administered parenterally as drug carriers. In addition to phospholipids, liposomes may contain cholesterol, which improves their *in vivo* and *in vitro* stability, and other compounds that impart a positive or negative surface charge (Emmen and Storm, 1987). The adjuvant effect of liposomes in terms of increased antibody titers has been demonstrated both *in vivo* and *in vitro* for protein antigens, toxoid, a number of viral antigens, and also a malarial peptide vaccine (Richards *et al.*, 1987). The immunogenic potency of liposomes can be further increased by the inclusion of immunostimulators, such as muramyldipeptide (MDP), lymphokines, lipopolysaccharide, and lipid A.

Incorporation of immunostimulatory substances in liposomes enhances the therapeutic effect, reduces the toxicity, and substantially increases the therapeutic index of these substances (Emmen and Storm, 1987). Advantages of liposomal encapsulation of immunomodulators include the possibility of direct delivery to phagocytic cells, with the potential for higher drug concentrations at the sites of infection without the risk of toxicity (Koff and Fidler, 1985). The encapsulation of lymphokines and MDP within the same liposome induces synergistic activation of tumoricidal properties in rat alveolar macrophages (Sone and Fidler, 1980). Liposome-encapsulated lymphokines can activate murine macrophages to lyse virus-infected cells, and human peripheral blood monocytes incubated with human IFNγ encapsulated in liposomes behave similarly (Swenson *et al.*, 1988). Some technical difficulties remain to be resolved, however, before this method can be given unqualified approval, as entrapment of murine recombinant IFNγ prevented the interaction of this interferon with its specific receptor on the cell surface (Eppstein *et al.*, 1985).

B. Mechanism of Action of Liposomes

Following intravenous administration, liposomes are engulfed by macrophages, especially in the liver and spleen (Poste *et al.*, 1982). The rate of endocytotic uptake, intralysosomal degradation, and resulting intracellular release of the drug is influenced by the physiochemical characteristics of the liposome, particularly its size, composition, surface charge, and stability. Immunomodulators liberated from the liposomes during intralysosomal degradation are believed to exert their effect locally. Where lymphokines or biologically active molecules are presented in a liposomal form, it is necessary for them to be released before or after phagocytosis to ensure interaction with the cell receptor (Swenson *et al.*, 1988). Encapsulation of immunomodulators in liposomes may trigger other mechanisms of antimicrobial resistance, such as increased NK cell activity in the lung and liver, probably through release of monokines from activated macrophages (Talmadge *et al.*, 1985b).

VIII. Concluding Comments

For several decades antibiotics, sulphonamides and other antimicrobial compounds, coccidiostats, and anthelmintics have been employed, often in a routine manner, to limit the impact of infectious disease on domestic food animals. A wide range of vaccines, many of increased potency, have found a ready market with those who recognize the limitations of antimicrobial strategies in this ongoing struggle between intensively reared animals and recurring infectious diseases. It could be said that the impact of chemotherapy and vaccination on the many complex diseases in cattle, pigs, and poultry has reached a plateau, and if further progress is to be made different strategies will have to be considered. Immunomodulation offers many worthwhile alternatives to current standard practices in disease control with the additional potential advantage of amplifying specific responses to vaccines administered routinely. Immunomodulatory compounds also offer the prospect of reversing stress- or virus-induced immunosuppression, believed by many to be one of the fundamental problems in overcoming recurring infectious diseases, particularly those affecting the respiratory tract.

The delicate balance that exists in the regulatory mechanisms that maintain the body in a state of health is capable of rapid alteration in response to infectious agents, inflammatory changes, hormonal alteration, or through other indirect means. By deliberate intervention, it is now possible to pharmacologically modulate the immune response in a manner appropriate to the perceived clinical state of the animal, or in anticipation of imminent change in the animal's environmental condition which may predispose it to attack from respiratory, enteric, or other pathogens.

A distinct limitation to the interpretation and application of the extensive data that have accumulated on the use of immunomodulatory compounds is the widespread use of laboratory animal models, *in vitro* test systems, and the variety of dosage regimes employed. Extrapolation of these results to food animals is unlikely to be reliable due to differences in dosage regimes, diets, life span, and rate and type of tissue metabolism of immunomodulatory drugs in different species. The unique attributes of some species, such as ruminants, renders comparison with rodents very tenuous. Of even greater importance, perhaps, is the rate of maturation and functioning of the immune system in different species. This has been closely investigated in small rodents, such as the mouse, but less thoroughly investigated in ruminants. Models for infectious disease appropriate for laboratory animals frequently have little relevance to the major respiratory and enteric problems encountered in food animals. Consequently, there is an obvious need to conduct appropriate experiments in those species for which immunomodulatory drugs are intended. Some of the paradoxical results reported with immunomodulators may be due to dosage regimes, species differences, or to variation in experimental design.

A wide gulf exists between the detailed information available on the structure of immunomodulators, particularly those of synthetic origin, and their site and mode of action. Safety for the consumer is another aspect of immunomodulation in food animals worthy of attention so that mistakes made with antimicrobial therapy will not be repeated with different immunomodulatory compounds used for similar purposes. Developments with some immunomodulatory drugs, therefore, may shortly require careful monitoring and evaluation in a manner analogous to antibiotics, to ensure compliance with regulatory controls and to establish consumer confidence in these therapeutic substances. The long-term effects of many immunomodulators are still uncertain, and as the therapeutic benefits of many compounds frequently obscure their side effects, it is essential for producers and consumers (and also in the interest of environmental safety), that these compounds be regulated in an appropriate manner for domestic food animals.

Many of the immunomodulators currently available were discovered fortuitously, and some share characteristics that limit their prophylactic or therapeutic application. Thus far, no drug has been shown to have absolute selectivity at all levels of the immune response. Even drugs that appear to alter specifically the immune response at a particular level are known to exert their effects at several biochemical subcellular sites, not only on cells of the immune system but also on a wide variety of cell types, thereby decreasing further the specificity of their effects.

A common mechanism of action could hardly be expected for such a large and diverse collection of substances with few common characteristics apart from their ability to modulate immune responses. A few generalizations can be made, however. The action of many of these compounds is usually not specific to particular cell subsets or even cell types. Although macrophage activation is not a universal mechanism of action among these substances, it is, nevertheless, common to many of them. The timing of drug administration is often critical, as the efficacy of immunomodulators varies with the growth cycle of target cells. Inappropriate dosages can produce equivocal or even undesirable reactions. Beneficial results from immunomodulators are most likely to be achieved when an animal's immune system is functioning suboptimally. Although altered states of responsiveness, following administration of immunomodulators, can be associated with few changes at the cellular level, substances that increase lymphocyte intracellular cAMP are frequently immunosuppressive, whereas agents that increase cGMP levels usually have immunopotentiating properties. Other indices of cellular stimulation that correlate positively with immunostimulation include release of cytokines, increased numbers of membrane receptors, and, for phagocytic cells, increased phagocytic activity and enhanced intracellular killing of ingested microorganisms.

Appropriate delivery systems may soon be available, in the form of liposomes or comparable structures, for the accurate delivery of biologically active substances to organs or tissues requiring immune modulation. Unlike vaccines, which stimulate specific responses to their antigenic components and are used to stimulate immunity against specific infectious agents, immunomodulators may find wider application in domestic food animals as a means of counteracting many emerging complex diseases because of their broad, nonspecific immunopotentiating effects. Apart from their ability to alter the host's response in a nonspecific manner, immunomodulators are likely to find useful applications in stimulating specific immune responses, especially for weakly immunogenic vaccines, for enhancing the immune responses of immunosuppressed animals, and in hastening the development of the immune response in young immature animals.

The fact that the mode of action of many immunomodulators is uncertain or as yet unknown does not detract from their actual or potential importance as agents with diverse applications in the prevention or control of infectious diseases in intensively reared domestic food animals. Compounds fulfilling the criteria of ideal immunomodulators have yet to be discovered, developed, or synthesized. A more complete understanding of the activation and suppression of the immune response would point the way towards the development of specific compounds with known and predictable activity, for either augmenting immune responsiveness at a particular stage in the development of cell-mediated and humoral immunity, or ablating undesirable and deleterious immune reactions in particular organs or tissues. There is an obvious need for drugs that can safely and selectively enhance or suppress one specific class or subclass of immunocyte in domestic food animals. Such compounds will have to conform to defined criteria to ensure safety for the consumer, compatibility with the environment, and minimal deleterious effects on the animals in which they are used. The success of immunomodulatory therapy will depend on continued research into the mechanisms of physiological immunoregulation and the application of this knowledge to develop immunomodulators that combine *in vivo* efficiency with consumer acceptability.

Acknowledgments

I wish to thank L. Doggett for typing the manuscript, D. Maguire for preparing the illustrations, the library staff for assistance with data base searches, and my colleagues for constructive criticism.

References

Ábel, G., Szöllösi, J., Chihara, G., and Fachet, J. (1986). Effect of lentinan on pinocytosis in mouse peritoneal macrophages and the murine macrophage cell line C4Mø *in vitro*. *Int. J. Immunopharmacol.* **8,** 919–924.

Abramson, S., Edelson, H., Kaplan, H., Ludewig, R., and Weissman, G. (1984). Inhibition of neutrophil activity by nonsteroidal anti-inflammatory drugs. *Am. J. Med.* **77,** 3–6.

Adlam, C., Broughton, E. S., and Scott, M. T. (1972). Enhanced resistance of mice to infection with bacteria following pre-treatment with *Corynebacterium parvum*. *Nature (London), New Biol.* **235,** 219–220.

Al-Izzi, S. A., and Maxie, M. G. (1982). Effect of *C. parvum* on bone marrow macrophage colony production, peripheral blood leucocytes and histologic changes of tissue in calves. *Am. J. Vet. Res.* **43**, 2244–2247.

Al-Izzi, S. A., Maxie, M. G., and Savan, M. (1982). The pulmonary clearance of *Pasteurella haemolytica* in calves given *C. parvum* and infected with PI-3 virus. *Can. J. Comp. Med.* **46**, 85–90.

Amery, W. K., and Hörig, C. (1984). Levamisole. In "Immune Modulation Agents and Their Mechanisms" (R. L. Fenichel and M. A. Chirigos, eds.), pp. 383–408. Dekker, New York.

Anderson, J. C. (1984). Levamisole and bovine mastitis. *Vet. Rec.* **114**, 138–140.

Aoki, T. (1984). Lentinan. In "Immune Modulation Agents and Their Mechanisms" (R. L. Fenichel and M. A. Chirigos, eds.), pp. 63–77. Dekker, New York.

Assem, E. S. K. (1984). Levamisole. In "Textbook of Immunopharmacology" (M. M. Dale and J. C. Foreman, eds.), pp. 333–339. Blackwell, Oxford.

Atkinson, J. P., and Frank, M. M. (1973). Effect of cortisone therapy on serum complement components. *J. Immunol.* **111**, 1061–1066.

Babiuk, L. A., and Misra, V. (1982). Effect of levamisole in immune responses to bovine herpesvirus-1. *Am. J. Vet. Res.* **43**, 1349–1354.

Babiuk, L. A., and Ohmann, H. B. (1984). Effect of levamisole and bovine interferon α_1 on bovine immune responses and susceptibility to bovine herpesvirus-1. In "Chemical Regulation of Immunity in Veterinary Medicine" (M. Kende, J. Gainer, and M. Chirigos, eds.), pp. 433–442. Alan R. Liss, New York.

Barasoain, I., Rejas, M. T., Portoles, M. P., Ojeda, G., and Rojo, J. M. (1987). Isoprinosine restores *in vitro* T lymphocyte functions of cyclophosphamide immunosuppressed mice. *Int. J. Immunopharmacol.* **9**, 489–496.

Bardana, E. J. (1985). Recent developments in immunomodulatory therapy. *J. Allergy Clin. Immunol.* **75**, 423–436.

Baxter, J. D., and Funder, J. W. (1979). Hormone receptors. *N. Engl. J. Med.* **301**, 1149–1161.

Becker, J., and Grasso, R. J. (1988). Suppression of yeast ingestion by dexamethasone in macrophage cultures: Evidence for a steroid-induced phagocytosis inhibitory protein. *Int. J. Immunopharmacol.* **10**, 325–338.

Bistoni, F., Baccarini, M., Blasi, E., Riccardi, C., Marconi, P., and Garaci, E. (1985). Modulation of polymorphonucleate-mediated cytotoxicity against *Candida albicans* by thymosin α_1. *Thymus* **7**, 69–84.

Black, P. L., Phillips, H., Tribble, H. R., Pennington, R., Schneider, M., and Talmadge, J. E. (1988). Correlation of immunomodulatory and therapeutic activities of interferon and interferon inducers in metastatic disease. *J. Cell. Biochem.* **36**, 377–392.

Blalock, J. E., and Smith, E. M. (1985). A complete regulatory loop between the immune and neuroendocrine systems. *Fed. Proc.* **44**, 108–111.

Blalock, J. E., Harbour-McMenamin, D., and Smith, E. M. (1985). Peptide hormones shared by the neuroendocrine and immunologic systems. *J. Immunol.* **135**, Suppl., 858S–861S..

Blecha, F. (1988). Immunomodulation: A means of disease prevention in stressed livestock. *J. Anim. Sci.* **66**, 2084–2090.

Blecha, F., and Baker, P. E. (1986). Effect of cortisol *in vitro* and *in vivo* on production of bovine interleukin 2. *Am. J. Vet. Res.* **47**, 841–845.

Blecha, F., Anderson, G. A., Osorio, F., Chapes. S. K., and Baker, P. E. (1987). Influence of isoprinosine on bovine herpesvirus type-1 infection in cattle. *Vet. Immunol. Immunopathol.* **15**, 253–265.

Bryant, H. U., Bernton, E. W., and Holaday, J. W. (1988). Morphine pellet-induced immunomodulation in mice: Temporal relationships. *J. Pharmacol. Exp. Ther.* **245**, 913–920.

Campoli-Richards, D. M., Sorkin, E. M., and Heel, R. C. (1986). Inosine Pranobex. A preliminary review of its pharmacodynamic and pharmacokinetic properties, and therapeutic efficacy. *Drugs* **32**, 383–424.

Charley, B., McCullough, K., and Martinod, S. (1988). Antiviral and antigenic properties of recombinant porcine interferon gamma. *Vet. Immunol. Immunopathol.* **19**, 95–103.

Chirigos, M. A. (1984). Overview of chemicals and biologicals capable of regulating immunity. *In* "Chemical Regulation of Immunity in Veterinary Medicine" (M. Kende, J. Gainer, and M. Chirigos, eds.), pp. 423–432. Alan R. Liss, New York.

Clark, I. A., Cox, R. E. G., and Allison, A. C. (1977). Protection of mice against *Babesia* spp. and *Plasmodium* spp. with killed *Corynebacterium parvum*. *Parasitology* **74**, 9–18.

Coffey, R. G., and Hadden, J. W. (1985). Neurotransmitters, hormones, and cyclic nucleotides in lymphocyte regulation. *Fed. Proc.* **44**, 112–117.

Cohen, J. J., and Duke, R. C. (1984). Glucocorticoid activation of a calcium-dependent endonuclease in thymocyte nuclei leads to cell death. *J. Immunol.* **132**, 38–42.

Collins, F. M., and Scott, M. T. (1974). Effect of *Corynebacterium parvum* treatment on the growth of *Salmonella enteritidis* in mice. *Infect. Immun.* **9**, 863–869.

Confer, A. W., and Adldinger, H. K. (1981). The *in vivo* effect of levamisole on PHA stimulation in normal and Marek's disease virus inoculated chickens. *Res. Vet. Sci.* **30**, 243–245.

Cooper, M. D. (1987). B lymphocytes. Normal development and function. *N. Engl. J. Med.* **317**, 1452–1456.

Cummins, C. S. (1984). *Corynebacterium parvum* and its fractions. *In* "Immune Modulation Agents and Their Mechanisms" (R. L. Fenichel and M. A. Chirigos, eds), pp. 163–190. Dekker, New York.

Cupps, T. R., and Fauci, A. S. (1982). Corticosteroid-mediated immunoregulation in man. *Immunol. Rev.* **65**, 133–150.

Dafny, N., Prieto-Gomez, B., and Reyes-Vazquez, C. (1985). Does the immune system communicate with the central nervous system? *J. Neuroimmunol.* **9**, 1–12.

Dale, M. M. (1984). Corticosteroids and their anti-inflammatory effects. *In* "Textbook of Immunopharmacology" (M. M. Dale and J. C. Foreman, eds.), pp. 283–288. Blackwell, Oxford.

Deguchi, T., and Axelrod, J. (1973). Control of circadian change of serotonin N-acetyltransferase in the pineal organ by beta-adrenergic receptor. *Proc. Natl. Acad. Sci. U.S.A.* **70**, 2411–2414.

De Maeyer, E., and De Maeyer-Guignard, J., eds. (1988). Production of IFN-y by T cells and modulation of T cell, B cell and NK cell activity by interferons. *In* "Interferons and Other Regulatory Cytokines," pp. 221–273. Wiley, New York.

Dennis, G., June, C. H., Mizuguchi, J., Ohara, J., Witherspoon, K., Finkelman, F. D., McMillan, V., and Mond, J. J. (1987). Glucocorticoids suppress calcium mobilization and phospholipid hydrolysis in anti-Ig antibody-stimulated B cells. *J. Immunol.* **139**, 2516–2523.

Dinarello, C. A. (1989). Interleukin-1 and its biologically related cytokines. *Adv. Immunol.* **44**, 153–205.

Dinarello, C. A., and Mier, J. W. (1987). Lymphokines. *N. Engl. J. Med.* **317**, 940–945.

Dinarello, C. A., Marnoy, S. O., and Rosenwasser, L. J. (1983). Role of arachidonate metabolism in the immunoregulatory function of human leukocytic pyrogen/lymphocyte activating factor/IL1. *J. Immunol.* **130**, 890–895.

Djeu, J. Y., and Ramsey, K. M. (1984). Interaction of interferon and chemotherapeutic agents in modulation of natural killer cell activity. In "Immune Modulation Agents and Their Mechanisms" (R. L. Fenichel and M. A. Chirigos, eds.), pp. 489–498. Dekker, New York.

Dohlsten, M., Sjögren, H. O., and Carlsson, R. (1986). Histamine inhibits interferon-γ production via suppression of interleukin 2 synthesis. *Cell. Immunol.* **101,** 493–501.

Dokhelar, M.-C., Tursz, T., Dardenne, M., and Bach, J.-F. (1983). Effect of a synthetic thymic factor (Facteur Thymique Serique) on natural killer cell activity in humans. *Int. J. Immunopharmacol.* **5,** 277–282.

Duncan, M. R., Salik, J. R., and Hadden, J. W. (1982). Glucocorticoid modulation of lymphokine-induced macrophage proliferation. *Cell. Immunol.* **67,** 23–36.

Emmen, F., and Storm, G. (1987). Liposomes in treatment of infectious diseases. *Pharm. Weekbl.* **9,** 162–171.

Engels, F., Oosting, R. S., and Nijkamp, F. P. (1985). Pulmonary macrophages induce deterioration of guinea pig tracheal β-adrenergic function through release of oxygen radicals. *Eur. J. Pharmacol.* **111,** 143–144.

Eppstein, D. A., Marsh, Y. V., Vander Pas, M., Felgner, P. L., and Schreiber, A. B. (1985). Biological activity of liposome-encapsulated murine interferon gamma is mediated by a cell receptor. *Proc. Natl. Acad. Sci. U.S.A.* **82,** 3688–3692.

Ezekowitz, R. A. B., and Gordon, S. (1984). Alterations of surface properties by macrophage activation: Expression of receptors for Fc and mannose-terminal glycoproteins and differentiation antigens. In "Macrophage Activation" (D. O. Adams and M. G. Hanna, eds.), pp. 33–56. Plenum, New York.

Fattal-German, M., and Bizzini, B. (1988). The *Corynebacterium granulosum*-derived P40 immunomodulator exerts a synergistic effect on the activity of antiviral drugs in the treatment of experimental viral infections. *Biomed. Pharmacother.* **42,** 217–220.

Feldman, M. (1988). Lymphocyte interactions and their mediators. In "The Lymphocyte" (J. J. Marchalonis, ed.), pp. 121–142. Dekker, New York.

Fenje, P., and Postic, B. (1970). Protection of rabbits against experimental rabies by poly (I:C). *Nature (London)* **226,** 171–172.

Field, A. K., Tytell, A. A., Lampson, G. P., and Hilleman, M. R. (1967). Inducers of interferon and host resistance. II. Multi-stranded synthetic polynucleotide complexes. *Proc. Natl. Acad. Sci. U.S.A.* **58,** 1004–1010.

Flesh, J., Harel, W., and Nelken, D. (1982). Immunopotentiating effect of levamisole in the prevention of bovine mastitis, fetal death and endometritis. *Vet. Rec.* **111,** 56–57.

Flower, R. J. (1984). The inhibition of prostaglandin synthesis by the glucocorticoids. In "Textbook of Immunopharmacology" (M. M. Dale and J. C. Foreman, eds.), pp. 289–304. Blackwell, Oxford.

Fudenberg, H. H., and Whitten, H. D. (1984). Immunostimulation: Synthetic and biological modulators of immunity. *Annu. Rev. Pharmacol. Toxicol.* **24,** 147–174.

Fuggetta, M. P., Graziani, G., Aquino, A., D'Atri, S., and Bonmassar, E. (1988). Effect of hydrocortisone on human natural killer activity and its modulation by beta interferon. *Int. J. Immunopharmacol.* **10,** 687–694.

Gainer, J. H., and Guarnieri, J. (1985). Effects of Poly I:C in porcine iron deficient neutropenia. *Cornell Vet.* **75,** 454–465.

Ghaffar, A., Paul, R. D., Sigel, M. M., Lichter, W., and Wellham, L. L. (1981). Immunomodulation by *Corynebacterium parvum*. In "Immunomodulation by Bacteria and Their Products" (H. Friedman, T. W. Klein, and A. Szentiuanyi, eds.), pp. 135–149. Plenum, New York.

Ghio, R., Pistoia, V., Romagnoli, M., D'Elia, P., and Boccaccio, G. P. (1988). Inhibition of phytohaemagglutinin (PHA) induced human T-cell colonies by methylprednisolone. *Int. J. Immunopharmacol.* **10,** 237–245.

Gilman, S. C., and Mochan, E. (1988). Cytokines and their antagonists as therapeutic agents. *Agents Actions* **25,** 57–59.

Glasgow, L. A., Fischbach, S. M., Bryant, S. M., and Kern, E. R. (1977). Immunomodulation of host resistance to experimental viral infection in mice: Effect of *Corynebacterium acnes, Corynebacterium parvum* and *Bacille Calmette-Guérin. J. Infect. Dis.* **135,** 763–770.

Goldstein, D., Dawson, J., and Laszlo, J. (1988). Suppression of natural killer cell activity by hydrocortisone. *J. Biol. Regul. Homeostatic Agents* **2,** 25–30.

Good, R. A., Dalmasso, A. P., Martinez, C., Archer, O. K., Pierce, J. C., and Papermaster, B. W. (1962). The role of thymus in the development of immunological capacity in rabbits and mice. *J. Exp. Med.* **116,** 773–796.

Goodwin, J. S., Bankhurst, A. D., and Messner, R. P. (1977). Suppression of T-cell mitogenesis by prostaglandin. *J. Exp. Med.* **146,** 1719–1734.

Griffin, F. M. (1984). Activation of macrophage complement receptors for phagocytosis. In "Macrophage Activation" (D. O. Adams and M. G. Hanna, eds.), pp. 57–70. Plenum, New York.

Griffin, J. F. T. (1989). Stress and immunity: A unifying concept. *Vet. Immunol. Immunopathol.* **20,** 263–312.

Hadden, J. W. (1987). Immunotherapy in the treatment of infectious diseases. In "Immunopharmacology of Infectious Diseases" (J. A. Majde, ed.), pp. 337–349. Alan R. Liss, New York.

Hahn, G. S., and Hamburger, R. N. (1983). Revolutionary relationship of thymopoietin to immunoglobulins and cellular recognition molecules. *J. Immunol.* **126,** 459–462.

Hall, N. R., and Goldstein, A. L. (1984). Endocrine regulation of host immunity. In "Immune Modulation Agents and Their Mechanisms" (R. L. Fenichel and M. A. Chirigos, eds.), pp. 533–563. Dekker, New York.

Hall, N. R., McGillis, J. P., Spangelo, B. L., and Goldstein, A. L. (1985). Evidence that thymosins and other biologic response modifiers can function as neuroactive immunotransmitters. *J. Immunol.* **135,** Suppl., 806S–811S.

Hamuro, J., and Chihara, G. (1984). Lentinan, a T-cell-oriented immunopotentiator. In "Immune Modulation Agents and Their Mechanisms" (R. L. Fenichel and M. A. Chirigos, eds.), pp. 409–436. Dekker, New York.

Hamuro, J., Hadding, U., and Bitter-Suerman, D. (1978). Solid phase activation of alternative pathway of complement by beta 1-3 glucans and its possible role for tumour regressing activity. *Immunology* **34,** 695–705.

Hamuro, J., Rollinghoff, M., and Wagner, H. (1980). Induction of cytotoxic peritoneal exudate cells by T-cell immune adjuvants of the beta (1-3) glucan-type lentinan and its analogues. *Immunology* **39,** 551–559.

Hartmann, D., Schneider, M. A., Lenz, B. F., and Talmadge, J. E. (1987). Toxicity of polyinosinic-polycytidilic acid admixed with poly-L-lysine and solubilized with carboxymethylcellulose in mice. *Pathol. Immunopathol. Res.* **6,** 37–50.

Haynes, R. C., and Murad, F. (1985). Adrenocorticotropic hormone; adrenocortical steroids and their synthetic analogs; inhibitors of adrenocortical steroid biosynthesis. In "The Pharmacological Basis of Therapeutics" (A. G. Gilman, L. S. Goodman, T. W. Rall, and F. Murad, eds.), 7th ed., pp. 1459–1489. Macmillan, New York.

Hennessy, K. J., Blecha, F., Pollmann, D. S., and Kluber, E. F. (1987). Isoprinosine and levamisole immunomodulation in artificially reared neonatal pigs. *Am. J. Vet. Res.* **48**, 477–480.

Henney, C. S. (1989). Interleukin 7: Effects on early events in lymphopoiesis. *Immunol. Today* **10**, 170–173.

Herberman, R. R., Ortald, J. R., and Bonnard, G. D. (1979). Augmentation by interferon of human natural and antibody-dependent cell-mediated cytotoxicity. *Nature (London)* **277**, 221–223.

Hersey, P., and Edwards, A. (1984). Effect of isoprinosine on natural killer cell activity of blood mononuclear cells *in vitro* and *in vivo*. *Int. J. Immunopharmacol.* **6**, 315–320.

Hirata, F., and Iwata, N. (1983). Role of lipomodulin, a phospholipase inhibitory protein, in immunoregulation of thymocytes. *J. Immunol.* **130**, 1930–1936.

Irwin, M. R., Holmberg, C. A., Knight, H. D., and Hjerpe, C. A. (1976). Effect of vaccination against infectious bovine rhinotracheitis and simultaneous administration of levamisole on primary humoral responses in calves. *Am. J. Vet. Res.* **37**, 223–226.

Jaffe, J. H., and Martin, W. R. (1985). Opioid analgesics and antagonists. *In* "The Pharmacological Basis of Therapeutics" (A. G. Gilman, L. S. Goodman, T. W. Rall, and F. Murad, eds.), 7th ed., pp. 491–531. Macmillan, New York.

Jayappa, H. G., and Loken, K. I. (1982). Enhancement of the chemotactic response of bovine polymorphonuclear leukocytes by levamisole. *Am. J. Vet. Res.* **43**, 2138–2142.

Jayappa, H. G., and Loken, K. I. (1983). Effect of antimicrobial agents and corticosteroids on bovine polymorphonuclear leukocyte chemotaxis. *Am. J. Vet. Res.* **44**, 2155–2159.

Johnson, A. G. (1985). Immunomodulating effects of synthetic polyribonucleotides. *J. Biol. Response Modif.* **4**, 481–483.

Johnson, A. G. (1987). Non-specific resistance against microbial infections induced by polyribonucleotide complexes. *In* "Immunopharmacology of Infectious Diseases" (J. A. Majde, ed.), pp. 291–301. Alan R. Liss, New York.

Johnson, H. M., Smith, B. G., and Barron, S. (1975). Inhibition of the primary *in vitro* antibody response by interferon preparations. *J. Immunol.* **114**, 403–409.

Johnston, R. B. (1988). Monocytes and macrophages. *N. Engl. J. Med.* **318**, 747–752.

Kaeberle, M. L. (1984). Effect of steroids of immunologic function. *In* "Chemical Regulation of Immunity in Veterinary Medicine" (M. Kende, J. Gainer, and M. Chirigos, eds.), pp. 325–335. Alan R. Liss, New York.

Kaneene, J. M. B., Okino, F. C., Anderson, R. K., Muscoplat, C. C., and Johnson, D. W. (1981). Levamisole potentiation of antigen specific lymphocyte blastogenic response in *Brucella abortus* exposed but unresponsive cattle. *Vet. Immunol. Immunopathol.* **2**, 75–85.

Katz, P., and Fauci, A. S. (1988). Immunosuppressives and adjuvants. *In* "Immunological Diseases" (M. Samter, D. W. Talmage, M. M. Frank, K. F. Austen, and H. N. Claman, eds.), 4th ed., pp. 675–698. Little, Brown, Boston, Massachusetts.

Kelley, V. E., Naor, D., Tarcic, N., Gaulton, G. N., and Strom, T. B. (1986). Anti-interleukin 2 receptor antibody suppresses delayed type hypersensitivity to foreign and syngeneic antigens. *J. Immunol.* **137**, 2122–2124.

Kende, M. (1985). Prophylactic and therapeutic efficacy of poly (I,C)-LC against Rift Valley Fever virus infection in mice. *J. Biol. Response Modif.* **4**, 503–511.

Kimball, E. S., and Grob, P. M. (1988). Molecular biology and mechanisms of action of Interleukins 1 and 2. *In* "The Lymphocyte" (J. J. Marchalonis, ed.), pp. 71–94. Dekker, New York.

Koff, W. C. and Fidler, I. J. (1985). The potential use of liposome-mediated antiviral therapy. *Antiviral Res.* **5**, 179–190.

Langhoff, E., Olgaard, K., and Ladefoged, J. (1987). The immunosuppressive potency *in vitro* of physiological and synthetic steroids on lymphocyte cultures. *Int. J. Immunopharmacol.* **9,** 469–473.

Latour, A. (1850). Le traitement des affections cancéreuses et tuberculeuses. Union méd. de Paris. *Gaz. Méd. de Paris,* p. 8.

Leibson, H. J., Gefter, A., Zlotnik, A., Marrack, P., and Kappler, J. W. (1984). Role of γ-interferon in antibody-producing responses. *Nature (London)* **309,** 799–801.

Levy, H. B. (1970). Genome function and disease. *In* "Resistance to Infectious Disease" (R. H. Dunlop and H. W. Moon, eds.), pp. 13–24. Saskatoon Modern Press, Saskatoon, Saskatchewan, Canada.

Lillehoj, H., and Shevach, F. M. (1985). A comparison of the effects of cyclosporin A, dexamethasone and oubain on the interleukin-2 cascade. *J. Immunopharmacol.* **7,** 267–284.

Low, T. L., and Goldstein, A. L. (1984). Thymosin, peptidic moieties, and related agents. *In* "Immune Modulation Agents and Their Mechanisms" (R. L. Fenichel and M. A. Chirigos, eds.), pp. 135–162. Dekker, New York.

Maestroni, G. J. M., Conti, A., and Pierpaoli, W. (1986). Role of pineal gland in immunity. *J. Neuroimmunol.* **13,** 19–30.

Male, D., Champion, B., and Cooke, A. (1987). The basis of immunity. *In* "Advanced Immunology," pp. 1.1–1.12. Lippincott, Philadelphia, Pennsylvania.

Manickam, R., Dhar, S., and Singh, R. P. (1983). Non-specific immunization against bovine tropical theilerosis (*Theileria annulata*) using killed *Corynebacterium parvum*. *Vet. Parasitol.* **13,** 115–119.

Mastroeni, P., Bizzini, B., Bonina, L., Iannello, D., Merendino, R. A., Delfino, D., Berlinghieri, M. C. Leonardi, M. S., Arena, A., Liberto, M. C., and Gazzara, D. (1985). The restoration of impaired macrophage functions using as immunomodulator the *Corynebacterium granulosum*-derived P40 fraction. *Immunopharmacology* **10,** 27–34.

MacGregor R. R., Spagnuolo, P. J., and Lentnek, A. L. (1974). Inhibition of granulocyte adherence by ethanol, prednisone, and aspirin, measured with an assay system. *N. Engl. J. Med.* **291,** 642–646.

Meltzer, M. S., Crawford, R. M., Gilbreath, M. J., Finbloom, D. S., Davis, C. E., Fortier, A. H., Schreiber, D., and Nacy, C. A. (1987). Lymphokine regulation of nonspecific macrophage cytotoxicity against neoplastic and microbial targets. *In* "Immunopharmacology of Infectious Diseases" (J. A. Majde, ed.), pp. 27–39. Alan R. Liss, New York.

Miyata, H., Himeno, K., Miake, S., and Nomoto, K. (1981). Alterations of host resistance to *Listeria monocytogenes* in tumour-bearing mice and in those given *C. parvum*. *Immunology.* **44,** 305–310.

Moya, P., Alonso, M. L., Baixeras, E., and Ronda, E. (1984). Immunomodulatory activity of isoprinosine on experimental viral infections in avian models. *Int. J. Immunopharmacol.* **6,** 339–343.

Mulcahy, G. (1988). The effect of immunomodulators on the lower respiratory tract of the calf. Ph.D. Thesis, National University of Ireland.

Mulcahy, G., and Quinn, P. J. (1986). A review of immunomodulators and their application in veterinary medicine. *J. Vet. Pharmacol. Ther.* **9,** 119–139.

Murphy, J. R., Kelley, V. E., and Strom, T. B. (1988). Interleukin 2 toxin: A step toward selective immunomodulation. *Am. J. Kidney Dis.* **11,** 159–162.

Murray, H. W. (1984). Macrophage activation: Enhanced oxidative and antiprotozoal activity. *In* "Macrophage Activation" (D. O. Adams and M. G. Hanna, eds.), pp. 97–115. Plenum, New York.

Murthy, K. K., and Ragland, W. L. (1984). Immunomodulation by thymic hormones: studies with an avian thymic hormone. In "Chemical Regulation of Immunity in Veterinary Medicine" (M. Kende, J. Gainer, and M. Chirigos, eds.), pp. 481–491. Alan R. Liss, New York.

Nagaoka, I., Kaneko, H., and Yamashita, T. (1988). Inhibition of the accumulation of macrophages and the generation of macrophage chemotactic activity by dexamethasone in concanavilin A-induced peritonitis in mice. Agents Actions 25, 156–163.

Nair, M. P. N., and Schwartz, S. A. (1984). Immunomodulatory effects of corticosteroids on natural killer and antibody-dependent cellular cytotoxic activities of human lymphocytes. J. Immunol. 132, 2876–2882.

Nara, P. L., Krakowka, S., and Powers, T. E. (1979). Effect of prednisolone on the development of immune responses to canine distemper virus in beagle pups. Am. J. Vet. Res. 40, 1742–1747.

Nelson, D. S. (1984). Macrophages. In "Cell-mediated Immunity" (P. J. Quinn, ed.), pp. 8–25. Commission of the European Communities, Luxembourg.

North, R. J. (1984). Models of adoptive T-cell-mediated regression of established tumours. In "Macrophage Activation" (D. O. Adams and M. G. Hanna, eds.), pp. 243–257. Plenum, New York.

Ogunbiyi, P. O., Conlon, P. D., Black, W. D., and Eyre, P. (1988). Levamisole-induced attenuation of alveolar macrophage dysfunction in respiratory virus-infected calves. Int. J. Immunopharmacol. 10, 377–385.

Ohnishi, H., Kosuzume, H., Inaba, H., Ohkura, M., Shimada, S., and Suzuki, Y. (1983). The immunomodulatory action of inosiplex in relation to its effects in experimental viral infections. Int. J. Immunopharmacol. 5, 181–196.

O'Neill, B. B., Ginsberg, T., and Hadden, J. (1984). Immunopharmacology of the hypoxanthine containing compounds isoprinosine and NPT 15392. In "Chemical Regulation of Immunity in Veterinary Medicine" (M. Kende, J. Gainer, and M. Chirigos, eds.), pp. 525–541. Alan R. Liss, New York.

Panangala, V. S., Haynes, T. B., Schultz, R. D., and Mitra, A. (1986). Immunomodulation with killed *Propionibacterium acnes* in guinea pigs simultaneously vaccinated with *Brucella abortus* strain 19. Vet. Immunol. Immunopathol. 13, 71–84.

Pinto, A. J., Morahan, P. S., and Brinton, M. A. (1988). Comparative study of various immunomodulators for macrophage and natural killer cell activation and antiviral efficacy against exotic RNA viruses. Int. J. Immunopharmacol. 10, 197–209.

Plotnikoff, N. P., and Miller, G. C. (1983). Enkephalins as immunomodulators. Int. J. Immunopharmacol. 5, 437–441.

Plotnikoff, N. P., Murgo, A. J., Miller, G. C., Corder, C. N., and Faith, R. E. (1985). Enkephalins: Immunomodulators. Fed. Proc., Fed. Am. Soc. Exp. Biol. 44, 118–122.

Poli, G. (1984). Immunomodulators. In "Adjuvants, Interferon and Nonspecific Immunity" (F. M. Cancellotti and D. Galassi, eds.), pp. 111–126. Commission of the European Communities, Luxembourg.

Poste, G., Bucana, C., Raz, A., Bugelski, P., Kirsh, R., and Fidler, I. J. (1982). Analysis of systemically administered liposomes and implications for their use in drug delivery. Cancer Res. 42, 1412–1422.

Rajnavölgyi, E., Kulics, J., Szilágyvári, M., Kisfaludy, L., Nyéki, O., Schön, I., and Gergely, J. (1986). The influence of new thymopoietin derivatives on the immune response of inbred mice. Int. J. Immunopharmacol. 8, 167–177.

Reizenstein, P., and Mathé, G. (1984). Immunomodulating agents. In "Immune Modulation Agents and Their Mechanisms" (R. L. Fenichel and M. A. Chirigos, eds.), pp. 347–361. Dekker, New York.

Renoux, G. (1986). The ten commandments for immunotherapeutic drugs at the example of sulfur-containing agents. *Comp. Immunol. Microbiol. Infect. Dis.* **9,** 121–129.

Renoux, G., and Renoux, M. (1971). Effet immunostimulant d'un imidothiazole dans l'immunisation des souris contre l'infection par *Brucella abortus. C. R. Hebd. Seances Acad. Sci., Ser. D.* **272,** 349–350.

Richards, R. L., Wirtz, R. A., Hockmeyer, W. T., and Alving, C. R. (1987). Liposomes as carriers for a malaria peptide vaccine: Developmental aspects. *In* "Immunopharmacology of Infectious Diseases" (J. A. Majde, ed.), pp. 171–180. Alan R. Liss, New York.

Riley, V. (1981). Psychoneuroendocrine influences on immunocompetence and neoplasia. *Science* **212,** 1100–1109.

Rogers, C. M., Rogers, T. J., and Gilman, S. C. (1985). Effect of WY-18,251 (3-(P-chlorophenyl) thiazolo[3, 2-a] benzimidazole-2-acetic acid), levamisole and indomethacin on the generation of murine T suppressor cells *in vitro. J. Immunopharmacol.* **7,** 479–488.

Roitt, I. M. (1988). The acquired immune response. *In* "Essential Immunology," pp. 134–153. Blackwell, Oxford.

Royer, H. D., and Reinherz, E. L. (1987). T lymphocytes: Ontogeny, function, and relevance to clinical disorders. *N. Engl. J. Med.* **317,** 1136–1142.

Ruszala-Mallon, V., Lin, Y., Durr, F. E., and Wang, B. S. (1988). Low molecular weight immunopotentiators. *Int. J. Immunopharmacol.* **10,** 497–510.

Saperstein, G., Mohanty, S. B., Rockemann, D. D., and Russek, E. (1983). Effect of levamisole on induced bovine viral diarrhea. *J. Am. Vet. Med. Assoc.* **183,** 425–427.

Schlick, E., Hartung, K., and Chirigos, M. A. (1984). Comparison of *in vitro* and *in vivo* modulation of myelopoiesis by biological response modifiers. *Cancer Immunol. Immunother.* **18,** 226–232.

Schultz, R. M., and Kleinschmidt, N. J. (1983). Functional identity between murine γ interferon and macrophage activating factor. *Nature (London)* **305,** 239–240.

Schwers, A., Goossens, A., Vandenbroecke, C., Maenhout, M., Bugyaki, L., Pastoret, P. P., and Wérenne, J. (1984). Antiviral efficiency of bacterially produced human interferon in the bovine species. *In* "Adjuvants, Interferon and Non-specific Immunity" (F. M. Cancellotti and D. Galassi, eds.), pp. 51–58. Commission of the European Communities, Luxembourg.

Sedlacek, H. H., Dickneite, G., and Schorlemmer, H. U. (1986). Chemotherapeutics: A questionable or promising project. *Comp. Immunol. Microbiol. Infect. Dis.* **9,** 99–119.

Sipka, S., Abel, G., Csongor, J., Chihara, G., and Fachet, J. (1985). Effect of lentinan on the chemiluminescence produced by human neutrophils and the murine macrophage cell line C4Mø. *Int. J. Immunopharmacol.* **7,** 747–751.

Smith, E. M., Harbour-McMenamin, D., and Blalock, J. E. (1985). Lymphocyte production of endorphins and endorphin-mediated immunoregulatory activity. *J. Immunol.* **135,** Suppl., 779S–782S.

Snyder, D. S., and Unanue, E. R. (1982). Corticosteroids inhibit murine macrophage Ia expression and interleukin 1 production. *J. Immunol.* **129,** 1803–1805.

Sone, S., and Fidler, I. J. (1980). Synergistic activation by lymphokines and muramyl dipeptide of tumoricidal properties in rat alveolar macrophages. *J. Immunol.* **125,** 2454–2460.

Sternberg, E. M., and Parker, C. W. (1988). Pharmacologic aspects of lymphocyte regulation. *In* "The Lymphocyte" (J. J. Marchalonis, ed.), pp. 1–54. Dekker, New York.

Stobo, J. D. (1987). Lymphocytes. *In* "Basic and Clinical Immunology" (D. P. Stites, J. D. Stobo, and J. V. Wells, eds.), pp. 65–81. Appleton & Lange, Norwalk, Connecticut.

Suga, T., Macda, Y. Y., Uchida, H., Rokutanda, M., and Chihara, G. (1986). Macrophage-mediated acute-phage transport protein production induced by lentinan. *Int. J. Immunopharmacol.* **8**, 691–699.

Swartzberg, J. E., Krahenbuhl, J. L., and Remington, J. S. (1975). Dichotomy between macrophage activation and degree of protection against *Listeria monocytogenes* and *Toxoplasma gondii* in mice stimulated with *Corynebacterium parvum*. *Infect. Immun.* **12**, 1037–1043.

Swenson, C. E., Popescu, M. C., and Ginsberg, R. S. (1988). Preparation and use of liposomes in the treatment of microbial infections. *CRC Crit. Rev. Microbiol.* **15**, Suppl. 1, S1–S31.

Talmadge, J. E. (1984). Thymosin: Immunomodulatory and therapeutic characteristics. *In* "Chemical Regulation of Immunity in Veterinary Medicine" (M. Kende, J. Gainer, and M. Chirigos, eds.), pp. 457–465. Alan R. Liss, New York.

Talmadge, J. E., Adams, J., Phillips, H., Collins, M., Lenz, B., Schneider, M., Schlick, E., Ruffmann, R., Wiltrout, R. H., and Chirigos, M. A. (1985a). Immunomodulatory effects in mice of polyinosinic-polycytidylic acid complexed with poly-L-lysine and carboxymethylcellulose. *Cancer Res.* **45**, 1058–1065.

Talmadge, J. E., Schneider, M., Collins, M., Phillips, H., Heberman, R. B., and Wiltrout, R. H. (1985b). Augmentation of NK cell activity in tissue specific sites by liposomes incorporating MTP-PE. *J. Immunol.* **135**, 1477–1483.

Tsang, K. Y., Fudenberg, H. H., and Koehler, F. K. (1984). Immunostimulating compounds isoprinosine and NPT 15396. *In* "Immune Modulation Agents and Their Products" (R. L. Fenichel and M. A. Chirigos, eds.), pp. 79–95. Dekker, New York.

Tsokos, G. C. (1987). Immunomodulatory treatment in patients with rheumatic diseases: Mechanisms of action. *Semin. Arthritis Rheum.* **17**, 24–38.

Tubaro, E., Avico, U., Santiangeli, C., Zuccaro, P., Cavallo, G., Pacifici, R., Croce, C., and Borelli, G. (1985). Morphine and methadone impact on human phagocytic physiology. *Int. J. Immunopharmacol.* **7**, 865–874.

Van Der Maaten, M. J., Schmerr, M. J. F., Miller, J. M., and Sacks, J. M. (1983). Levamisole does not affect the virological and serological responses of bovine leukemia virus-infected cattle and sheep. *Can. J. Comp. Med.* **47**, 474–479.

Van Ginckel, R., and De Brabander, M. (1979). The influence of a levamisole metabolite (DL-2-oxo-3-[2-mercaptoethyl]-5-phenylimidazolidine) on carbon clearance in mice. *J. Reticuloendothel. Soc.* **25**, 125–131.

Varesio, L., Blasi, E., Thurman, G. B., Talmadge, J. E., Wiltrout, R. H., and Heberman, R. B. (1984). Potent activation of mouse macrophages by recombinant interferon-γ. *Cancer Res.* **44**, 4465–4469.

Walajtys-Rode, E., Dabrowski, A., Grubek-Jaworska, H., Machnicka, B., and Droszcz, W. (1988). Binding of dexamethasone and its effect on histamine release from rat mast cells. *Int. J. Immunopharmacol.* **10**, 925–930.

Waymack, J. P., Gonce, S., Miskell, P., and Alexander, J. W. (1985). Mechanism of action of two new immunomodulators. *Arch. Surg. (Chicago)* **120**, 43–48.

Webster, L. T. (1985). Drugs used in the chemotherapy of helminthiasis. *In* "The Pharmacological Basis of Therapeutics" (A. G. Gilman, L. S. Goodman, T. W. Rall, and F. Murad, eds.), 7th ed., pp. 1009–1028. Macmillan, New York.

Werb, Z. (1987). Phagocytic cells: Chemotaxis and effector functions of macrophages and granulocytes. *In* "Basic and Clinical Immunology" (D. P. Stites, J. D. Stobo, and J. V. Wells, eds.), pp. 96–113. Appleton & Lange, Norwalk, Connecticut.

White, T. R., Thompson, R. C. A., and Penhale, W. J. (1983). The effects of selective immunosuppression on resistance to *Mesocestoides corti* in strains of mice showing high and low initial susceptibility. *Z. Parasitenkd.* **69**, 91–104.

White, T. R., Thompson, R. C. A., Penhale, W. J., and Chihara, G. (1988). The effect of lentinan on the resistance of mice to *Mesocestoides corti*. *Parasitol. Res.* **74,** 563–568.

Williamson, S. A., Knight, R. A., Lightman, S. L., and Hobbs, J. R. (1988). Effects of beta endorphin on specific immune responses in man. *Immunology* **65,** 47–51.

Wiltrout, R. H., Salup, R. S., Twilley, T. A., and Talmadge, J. E. (1985). Immunomodulation of natural killer activity by polyribonucleotides. *J. Biol. Response Modif.* **4,** 512–517.

Wood, W. B. (1970). The pathogenesis of fever. *In* "Infectious Agents and Host Reactions" (S. Mudd, ed.), pp. 146–162. Saunders, Philadelphia, Pennsylvania.

Wybran, J. (1985). Enkephalins and endorphins as modifiers of the immune system: Present and future. *Fed. Proc.* **44,** 92–94.

Part II
Chemical Immunomodulation

Chemically Induced Immunomodulation in Domestic Food Animals

MARCUS E. KEHRLI, JR.* AND JAMES A. ROTH[†]

* Metabolic Diseases and Immunology Research Unit, National Animal Disease Center, USDA-Agricultural Research Service, Ames, Iowa, and
[†] Department of Veterinary Microbiology and Preventive Medicine, Iowa State University, Ames, Iowa

I. Introduction
II. Chemical Immunomodulation in Domestic Food Animal Species
   A. Levamisole
   B. Thiabendazole
   C. Imuthiol
   D. Avridine
   E. Isoprinosine
   F. Glucan
   G. Indomethacin
   H. Ascorbic Acid Derivatives
   I. RU 41470 (Biostim®)
   J. Dihydroheptaprenol
III. Chemical Immunomodulators Which Have Apparently Not Been Evaluated in Domestic Food Animals
IV. Summary
   References

I. Introduction

Enhancing the specific and nonspecific defense mechanisms against infectious diseases is of interest to clinicians in both human and veterinary medicine. Advances in immunomodulation have been the subject of three recent international symposia (Majde, 1987; Masihi and Lange, 1988; Bizzini and Bonmassar, 1988) and of recent reviews focusing on immunomodulators in domestic animals (Mulcahy and Quinn, 1986;

Blecha, 1988; Brunner and Muscoplat, 1980; Roth, 1988). This review will focus on chemicals that nonspecifically augment immune responses in contrast to the action of adjuvants that augment the specific immune response to a coadministered antigen. It will emphasize immunomodulating chemicals (not nutrients or cytokines, which are the topics of other chapters in this book), which have been evaluated in domestic food animals (poultry, swine, sheep, and cattle). We will also present information on some promising immunomodulators being developed and evaluated for use in humans that may have value in domestic food animals.

Immunomodulation may have its rudimentary beginnings in the use of herbs and teas that were taken as preventatives or administered for the treatment of various maladies in oriental cultures. Ancient Chinese medicine used ginseng tea, which has been found to contain unusually high amounts of the trace element germanium, which has immunomodulating activity (Goodman, 1988).

The specific mechanisms by which immunomodulators act in the body are undoubtedly diverse and currently are ill defined. Much of the mechanism of action data is based on indirect evidence of alterations in immune cell activity without any direct knowledge of the specific signal transduction mechanisms that may change gene expression, mRNA processing, protein synthesis, posttranslational protein modification, intracellular protein transport, and protein secretion or its expression on the surface of a cell. All of these cellular processes are potential targets of immunomodulating chemicals.

The criteria for immunomodulator selection should be based on knowledge about the nature of immunosuppression experienced by the host. Having specific information on the immunologic profile of a compromised host is, therefore, necessary for the rational selection of an immunomodulator. Careful and complete characterization of the syndromes whose pathogenesis involves immunosuppression, as well as complete characterization of the pharmacological effects of immunomodulators *in vivo* is necessary for predicting efficacious immunomodulator therapy.

Care must be taken in selecting diseases that are amenable to immunomodulation. Much of human research emphasizes immunomodulation in cancer patients and the experimental models used to evaluate compounds reflect this focus. Veterinary medicine has similar interests for companion animal medicine, however, immunomodulating compounds with less dramatic activity may have value in food animal medicine where animals experience transient episodes of immunosuppression leading to increased incidence of infectious diseases. Examples of disease syndromes where immunosuppression has been implicated in the disease pathogenesis include the bovine respiratory disease complex observed in association with transport and management stress factors after weaning, and periparturient clinical bovine mastitis.

Chemical immunomodulation in domestic food animals must meet certain criteria that are not of concern in the human medical field. First, residues in meat, milk, and eggs must be avoided, especially if the chemical immunomodulator has any potential to be carcinogenic. Ease of administration, a reasonably long duration of activity, and low cost are essential if an immunomodulator is to be utilized in a practical livestock production setting. Chemical immunomodulators that are orally active would have an obvious advantage for administration to large herds or flocks of animals.

II. Chemical Immunomodulation in Domestic Food Animal Species

A. LEVAMISOLE

Levamisole was the first chemically defined agent found to have immunomodulatory effects (Renoux, 1986) and has been evaluated in mice, rats, guinea pigs, chickens, turkeys, cattle, sheep, and swine. Levamisole is a phenylimidathiazole anthelmintic, with immunomodulating effects on T cells and macrophages. The effectiveness of levamisole is variable depending upon dose, timing of administration in relation to disease or stress, and host immunocompetence. Enhancement of immune activity by levamisole seems to occur in cells whose function is impaired. Levamisole does not affect primary immune responses to vaccination or prevent infections by bolstering innate immune mechanisms (Brunner and Muscoplat, 1980).

At high doses, levamisole may be immunosuppressive in rodents (Renoux, 1986). The critical nature of the dose of levamisole may represent a general biological phenomenon that has importance for immunomodulation. Many dose–response relationships that impact the reticuloendothelial system are not linear; instead they often involve M- or W-shaped curves (Sampson *et al.*, 1977; Bliznakov and Adler, 1972).

1. Effects of Levamisole in Poultry

At levamisole doses of 1.25 to 5 mg/kg, there is some evidence of immunomodulation against coccidiosis in 3-week-old chicks but not in 6-week-old chicks (Onaga *et al.*, 1984). Subcutaneous administration of levamisole at 2–5 mg/kg enhanced phytohemagglutinin (PHA) stimulation of peripheral blood lymphocytes of normal 5- and 12-week-old chicks but was unable to reserve Marek's disease virus-induced suppression (Confer and Adldinger, 1981). Another study on the immunomodulatory effects of levamisole on the antibody response to Newcastle disease virus in chickens, found a significant increase in the H1 antibody titers in 6-week-old chicks at a dose rate of 2.5 mg/kg. In 1-day-old chicks, however, four doses of levamisole at 1 mg/50 g produced immunosuppression (Sulochana et al., 1984).

In turkeys, levamisole restored the humoral immune responses (determined by vaccination with a killed *Brucella abortus* antigen preparation and a killed Newcastle disease virus preparation) in x-irradiated turkeys and in turkeys immunosuppressed by antibiotics (Panigrahy et al., 1979).

2. Effects of Levamisole in Swine

It has been suggested that levamisole stimulates the development of memory T cells in swine, based on the observation that pretreatment with levamisole has no effect on primary immune response but may enhance the secondary immune response. Increased levels of IgG antibody titers (without an increase in IgM) are seen after booster vaccination in pigs that had been given levamisole at the time of boosting (Reyero et al., 1979). In another study (Hennessy et al., 1987), levamisole was found to ameliorate the suppression of lymphocyte function seen in artificially reared swine.

3. Effects of Levamisole in Cattle

Immunosuppression has been implicated in the pathogenesis of bovine respiratory disease and mastitis. Investigations on the effects of levamisole on these two diseases have not found levamisole to be consistently efficacious for improving resistance to disease. A single treatment with levamisole PO_4 significantly reduced the incidence of shipping fever when compared with the morbidity observed 1 week after cattle had been treated with levamisole HCl or thiabendazole, upon entry into a feedlot (Irwin et al., 1980). Various concentrations of levamisole *in vitro* are known to enhance bovine lymphocyte blastogenesis induced by mitogens (phytohemagglutinin or pokeweed mitogen) or antigens [infectious bovine rhinotracheitis (IBR) virus or purified protein derivative], to increase immune interferon (IFN) production by mononuclear cell cultures, and to increase macrophage Fc receptor activity (Babiuk and Misra, 1981). Mammary gland-derived macrophages are also known to be activated *in vitro* by levamisole as determined by increased Fc receptor activity. *In vivo*, levamisole-treated cattle vaccinated with attenuated IBR virus developed lower serum antibody titers to IBR virus, had lower lymphocyte blastogenic responses to IBR antigen, and lower cytotoxic lymphocyte activity against IBR-infected target cells (Irwin et al., 1976; Babiuk and Misra, 1981). In a subsequent study, an identical dosage of levamisole given at the time of vaccination with attenuated IBR vaccine or 7 days later produced an enhanced antibody response to IBR virus (Babiuk and Misra, 1982). There were no obvious clinical differences between the levamisole-treated groups and controls after challenge exposure, however (Babiuk and Misra, 1982). Another study found a lymphocytosis following levamisole administration to cattle as the only evidence of immunostimulation (Nair and Rajan, 1983).

Repeated levamisole treatments had no effect on bovine leukemia virus replication or the BLV-associated antibody titers in persistently infected sheep or cattle (Van Der Maaten et al., 1983). A double-blind study of effects of levamisole on calves experimentally infected with bovine viral diarrhea virus found no difference in severity of infection, pattern of virus shedding, antibody titers, or speed of recovery between levamisole-treated and placebo control calves (Saperstein et al., 1983). Levamisole had no consistent ability to prevent or reverse the dexamethasone-induced suppression of lymphocyte blastogenesis or neutrophil functions in cattle (Roth and Kaeberle, 1984).

The incidence of bovine mastitis (9.6% vs 3.7%), fetal deaths (24.8% vs 4.8%), and endometritis (24.3% vs 6.4%) all have been reported to be reduced by weekly administration of levamisole for 6 weeks during the dry period with the last injection given at least 2 weeks prepartum (Flesh et al., 1982). This study was conducted in 4 herds with a total of over 4000 cows, with over 1000 cows on treatment. However, not all control cows received placebo injections and were therefore not handled similarly. The reduction in fetal death is difficult to attribute to levamisole since deaths due to all causes (including accidents and dystocias) were included in the analysis. In studies on the effects of levamisole on mammary gland health, levamisole reduced the number of quarters that remained infected 28 days after oral treatment (7.5 mg/kg) and increased the proportion of B lymphocytes in lacteal secretions of normal cows (i.e., without mastitis) (Ishikawa and Shimizu, 1983) and increased the immunoglobulin levels in normal milk (Ishikawa et al., 1982), but had little effect on whey protein content of mastitic milk. Therefore, if levamisole reduces the incidence of mastitis in dairy cows, it appears that it may do so by increasing the level of potentially opsonic antibody in normal milk, which may facilitate normal defense mechanisms involved with antibody clearance of pathogens in the lacteal secretions. Levamisole does not appear to alter the acute and sometimes severe inflammatory response to the presence of pathogens in lacteal secretions.

B. THIABENDAZOLE

Thiabendazole, another anthelmintic compound, has been shown to have immunomodulatory activity in mice (Lovett and Lundy, 1977). It was evaluated in cattle for its ability to overcome dexamethasone-induced and stress-induced immunosuppression. Thiabendazole failed to consistently prevent dexamethasone-induced suppression of neutrophil functions or antibody production. However, in the dosage range of 1.0–25.0 mg/kg it did significantly enhance lymphocyte blastogenic responsiveness to mitogens in dexamethasone-treated cattle. Higher doses were ineffective (Kaeberle and Roth, 1984). Thiabendazole failed to prevent suppression of lymphocyte blastogenesis or antibody production to various antigens in cattle stressed by weaning, vaccination, and castration (Roth et al., 1984).

C. IMUTHIOL

Sodium diethyldithiocarbamate (DTC, imuthiol) has been found to restore T lymphocyte proliferation, interleukin-2 production, and NK activity in cyclophosphamide-immunosuppressed mice (Rejas et al., 1988). Tests of imuthiol on weanling piglets found that it lacked any consistent, beneficial effects on delayed type hypersensitivity, lymphocyte blastogenesis, or IL-2 production by the piglets (Flaming et al., 1988). At the higher dose tested, imuthiol significantly reduced lymphocyte blastogenesis and IL-2 production. Both dosages of imuthiol tested reduced the growth of the animals. The effects of imuthiol on other domestic food animals are apparently not yet known.

D. AVRIDINE

Avridine (N,N-dioctadecyl-N',N'-bis-[2-hydroxyethyl]-propanediamine) is a lipoidal amine, previously referred to as CP 20,961, which possesses IFN-inducing activity in mice and humans. In cattle, avridine in liposomes produced mild alterations in lymphocyte and neutrophil function in normal animals and almost completely reversed the suppression of neutrophil function (except for inhibition of neutrophil iodination) in dexamethasone-treated cattle (Roth and Kaeberle, 1985a). Neutrophils from avridine-treated cattle had increased bactericidal activity against *Escherichia coli* (Woodard et al., 1983). Injection site irritations, however, preclude its widespread use in the form tested (Roth and Kaeberle, 1985a).

E. ISOPRINOSINE

Inosiplex (Isoprinosine), the 3:1 M complex of N,N-dimethylamino-2-propanol, p-acetamidobenzoate, and inosine, has been under study as an antiviral agent for years. It is hypothesized that its immunomodulation effects are the factors responsible for its clinical effectiveness against viral diseases (Ginsberg and Glasky, 1977). Isoprinosine is known to enhance the PHA- and monoclonal antibody OKT3-induced proliferative response of human peripheral blood mononuclear cells. The mechanism for this is unclear since it had no apparent effect on IL-2 receptor expression or on IL-2 activity in culture supernatants from stimulated mononuclear cells. Isoprinosine is also unable to restore immune responsiveness of mononuclear cells suppressed by cyclosporine A (Lomnitzer, 1988).

Isoprinosine-induced modulation of T helper cell subsets and antigen-presenting monocytes (Leu M_3^+ Ia$^+$) results in improvement of T and B lymphocyte functions *in vitro* in AIDS patients and patients with the AIDS-related complex (ARC) (Tsang et al., 1987). Isoprinosine decreases both the suppressor regulating (Leu3$^+$ Leu8$^+$) helper T subset and the reciprocal (Leu3$^+$ Leu8$^-$) helper T subset responsible for inducing the differentiation of B cells into antibody-forming plasma cells in ARC and AIDS patients. Both subsets are required for generation of suppression of cell-mediated immune responses. *In vitro* coincubation of peripheral blood lymphocytes with isoprinosine (1) induced an increase in both the Leu3$^+$ Leu8$^-$ and the reciprocal Leu3$^-$ Leu8$^+$ subsets of helper T cells; (2) restored the normal ratio of B effector to T-suppression cell precursors; (3) potentiated the expression of HLA-DR antigen on helper cells during the process of activation; and (4) enhanced the number of antigen-presenting monocytes (LeuM$_3^+$ Ia$^+$) in mitogen-driven lymphocyte transformation. Isoprinosine may therefore stimulate the differentiation of precursor helper T cells, suppressor T cells, and monocytes, thereby initiating a cascade of cellular interactions leading to partial restoration of the cell-mediated immune response.

Blecha and colleagues have evaluated isoprinosine in three domestic animal models of immunosuppression: artificially reared piglets, bovine herpesvirus 1 (BHV1) infection in cattle, and pseudorabies virus infection in pigs (Blecha, 1988; Flaming et al., 1989; Blecha et al., 1987; Hennessy et al., 1987). Artificial rearing of piglets results in suppressed lymphocyte blastogenic responses to mitogens and delayed-type hypersensitivity reactions compared to sow-reared controls. Orally administered isoprinosine (or levamisole) enhanced the responses of the artificially reared pigs to values comparable to the controls. Pseudorabies virus infection in pigs and BHV1 infection in calves each cause a suppression of the *in vitro* lymphocyte proliferative response to mitogens. Orally administered isoprinosine failed to ameliorate the suppression of lymphocyte blastogenesis in either of these viral infections. The reasons for the difference in effectiveness of isoprinosine in these models is not known. The mechanism for suppression of lymphocyte blastogenesis in the artificial rearing model is most likely different from the mechanisms of suppression in the virus infection model. This illustrates the need to understand the mechanism of immunosuppression and the mechanism of action of immunomodulators in order to rationally approach immunomodulation therapy.

F. Glucan

Glucan is a β-1,3-polyglucose component isolated from the cell wall of *Saccharomyces cerevisiae*. It has been reported to be a potent macrophage stimulant as well as a modulator of cellular and humoral immunity (Wooles and Di Luzio, 1963; Bugaleta *et al.*, 1978; Morrow and Di Luizio, 1965). In sheep challenged 40 days postpartum intramammarily with 10^3 colony-forming units of *Staphylococcus haemolyticus* per gland, glucan treatments reduced the mean milk bacterial counts when compared to controls. Milk somatic cell counts postchallenge for the glucan-treated ewes rose more quickly (1 day postchallenge vs 3 days postchallenge for the controls), suggesting that glucan may have enhanced the chemotactic response of the neutrophils, thus contributing to the lowering of the milk bacterial counts (Buddle *et al.*, 1988).

G. Indomethacin

Indomethacin is an irreversible inhibitor of the cyclooxygenase pathway, which converts arachidonic acid to various prostacyclin, thromboxane, and prostaglandin metabolites. In pig peripheral blood mononuclear cell cultures containing lymphocytes and monocytes (5–10%) the blastogenic responses to PHA were enhanced by up to 30% by the addition of indomethacin (Kingston *et al.*, 1984). When the cultures were depleted of monocytes the addition of indomethacin inhibited lymphocyte blastogenesis. The authors interpreted this to suggest that arachidonic acid metabolites may have both positive and negative effects on lymphocyte activation. We were unable to find any *in vivo* evidence for immunomodulation by indomethacin in domestic food animals.

H. ASCORBIC ACID DERIVATIVES

High doses of ascorbic acid (20–40 mg/kg) administered subcutaneously to cattle tended to reverse or prevent some of the immunosuppressive effects of dexamethasone on bovine neutrophil function (Roth and Kaeberle, 1985b). New immunomodulating ascorbic acid derivatives have been developed that have varying abilities to amplify immune activities. These compounds have been recently reviewed (Fodor *et al.*, 1987). Briefly, one class of these new synthetic immunopharmaceuticals is referred to as the methylfurylbutyrolactones (MFBLs). The MFBLs prime T lymphocytes to respond to antigenic or polyclonal stimulation in a heightened manner and to produce more lymphokines including IFNs and IL-2. The MFBLs also amplify antibody production to T-dependent antigens (sheep erythrocytes and keyhole limpet hemocyanin). *In vitro* MFBLs also enhance neutrophil adherence, chemotaxis, phagocytosis, and intracellular microbial killing. An *in vivo* mouse model has shown MFBLs have immunomodulating activity that is manifested as increased resistance of mice to infection with *Streptococcus pneumoniae* and *Salmonella typhimurium*. A second class of derivatives of ascorbic acid are the ketone ascorbic acid condensates (KAACs). The KAACs amplify T lymphocyte proliferation, lymphokine production, and antibody production.

I. RU 41470 (BIOSTIM®)

Biostim is an immunomodulator of bacterial origin obtained from the K201 strain of *Klebsiella pneumoniae*. It is composed of two macroglobular subunits, one of which is a capsular glycoprotein. Biostim has broad-spectrum immune activity with predominant effects on B lymphocytes and macrophages of rats. Biostim improves delayed-type hypersensitivity responses of rats experiencing protein deprivation-induced immunosuppression (Christou *et al.*, 1988).

Biostim has been evaluated in 8-week-old piglets for its influence on phagocytic cell production of reactive oxygen species, delayed type hypersensitivity, and resistance to intradermal infection caused by *Erysipelothrix rhusiopathiae*. Pigs were administered oral capsules containing two dosage levels of Biostim (10 or 1 mg/kg/day) for 8 consecutive days. Very little effect of Biostim was seen on delayed-type hypersensitivity reactions in these pigs. However, Biostim appears to be capable of enhancing both the bactericidal activity of circulating phagocytes and nonspecific resistance to intradermal injections of *E. rhusiopathiae* (Laval *et al.*, 1988).

J. DIHYDROHEPTAPRENOL

Dihydroheptaprenol (DHP) is a synthetic polyprenol derivative that has been evaluated in calves and adult cattle as a microemulsion with lecithin. Preliminary studies indicated that mice injected intramuscularly with 100 mg of DHP/kg of body weight 1–4 days prior to a challenge infection showed enhanced resistance to subcutaneous infection with *E. coli* (Araki *et al.*, 1987). In normal 3- to 5-week-old healthy Holstein calves a single intramuscular injection of DHP given at 4, 6, and 8 mg/kg of body weight was reported to increase the number of peripheral blood neutrophils and to enhance their phagocytic killing activity (Yoneyama *et al.*, 1989a). Similar results were found with DHP administration to adult Holstein cows at 1 and 2 mg/kg of body weight (Yoneyama *et al.*, 1989b). Effects of DHP on other bovine leukocyte functions or the value of DHP in immunosuppressed cattle have not been reported.

III. Chemical Immunomodulators Which Have Apparently Not Been Evaluated in Domestic Food Animals

There is currently a great deal of basic and applied research aimed at developing immunomodulators for use in cancer and AIDS patients. Most of this research is conducted in rodents and humans and is generating new knowledge about immunomodulator actions and identifying new immunomodulatory compounds at a rapid rate. Because of the more limited resources available, research aimed at applying this new information to benefit domestic food animals is lagging behind. Many compounds with immunomodulatory activity in rodents and man have apparently not yet been evaluated in domestic food animals. At least we were not able to find reference to their use in the scientific literature. It is possible that pharmaceutical companies have evaluated some of these compounds in domestic food animals and that the information generated is proprietary. We will briefly present here the known activities of a few compounds that show promise, and which, in our opinion, should be evaluated for activity in relevant models in domestic food animals.

Bryostatins are a group of macrocyclic lactones isolated from certain marine organisms (the Bryozoan *Bugula neritina*). Bryostatin 1 is cytotoxic to transformed tumor cell lines *in vitro*, and *in vivo* observations indicate that bryostatins increase the survival rate of tumor-bearing mice. Bryostatins share some properties with the phorbol esters in the activation of protein kinase C. *In vitro*, the bryostatins markedly enhance the synthesis of IL-2 and IFNγ. IL-2 production by lymphocytes treated with bryostatins is enhanced by a factor of 100–200 and that of IFNγ by a factor of 10–20 (Mohr *et al.*, 1987). Bryostatins synergize with recombinant IL-4 (B cell stimulatory factor) to stimulate resting T cells to proliferate and to differentiate into cytotoxic T lymphocytes (Trenn *et al.*, 1988). *In vivo*, bryostatin-primed splenocytes have a dramatically reduced concentration of IL-2 needed for the development of cytotoxic T lymphocytes. This may be explained by byrostatin induction of IL-2 receptor expression on human lymphocytes, which is accompanied by only weak proliferative responses, as opposed to phorbol esters, which have a powerful mitogenic effect (Hess *et al.*, 1988). The bryostatins possess a major advantage over the phorbol esters in that they lack tumor-promoting activity and therefore are a promising group of immunomodulators for evaluation.

Immunopharmacological activities of muramyl dipeptide (MDP) (Chédid, 1983; Werner *et al.*, 1986) include stimulation of the reticuloendothelial system and enhancement of nonspecific resistance to infection and tumors. Lipophilic derivatives of MDP have been synthesized which are generally more active than MDP in stimulation of cell-mediated immunity (as opposed to the adjuvant effects on humoral immunity). Many immunomodulating peptides (pimelautide, bestatin, and the MDP derivative murabutide) are undergoing phase I clinical trials aimed at treating patients with immunodeficiencies, cancer, and rheumatoid arthritis.

The immunomodulator FR-900483 is a substance produced by a fungus *Nectria lucida* F-4490. Addition of this substance *in vitro* is known to restore suppressed Con A-induced lymphocyte blastogenesis (mouse spleen cells). Intraperitoneal administration of FR-900483 to mice (7–500 mg/kg) reversed the suppression of antibody synthesis to sheep erythrocytes in mice treated with mitomycin C (1 mg/kg I.P.) (Shibata *et al.*, 1988).

The immunomodulators aerodin and bronhodin are bacterial derivatives that have been evaluated in rats. Both immunomodulators potentiated NK cell activity, stimulated splenocyte RNA and DNA synthesis, and enhanced intradermal delayed hypersensitivity reactions to protein antigens (Popescu *et al.*, 1985).

Swainsonine is an inhibitor of the Golgi enzyme alpha-mannosidase II and also has antimetastatic effects when administered systemically per os to mice in their drinking water. The primary action of swainsonine is to stimulate proliferation of the T cell population. However, it does have some mitogenic activity in nude mice. Therefore other spleen cell populations may also be stimulated by the drug (White et al., 1988).

Oxamisole is a substituted imidazopridine that is orally active. It is capable of enhancing antibody production against T-dependent antigens in immunosuppressed mice but not in normal mice, suggesting that it may selectively restore depressed T cell function (Radov et al., 1988).

A hypoxanthine analogue, NPT 15392, has been shown to be more potent than isoprinosine in the induction of Thy-1 antigen on the surface of precursor T cells and in the enhancement of mitogen stimulation in mice. Isoprinosine and NPT 15342 have also been shown to increase the killing activity of T cells, NK cells, and macrophages (Ikehara et al., 1987).

N-(4-[(4-Fluorophenyl)sulfonyl]phenyl)acetamide (CL 259,763) is an orally active, synthetic compound with a wide range of immunomodulating activities in mice (activating macrophage release of IL-1 increased lymphocyte responses to mitogens and release of IL-2, and inhibition of *in vitro* tumor growth) (Wang et al., 1988).

Two new fluoro-quinolone derivatives, ciprofloxacin and ofloxacin, enhance IL-2 production *in vitro* in human lymphocytes stimulated with PHA. Ciprofloxacin is a costimulator of IL-2 production in PHA-stimulated peripheral blood lymphocytes, while at the same time it exerts a prominent inhibitory effect on the incorporation of radioactive thymidine and amino acids into these cells. Ciprofloxacin, but not ofloxacin, enhances IFN production in PHA-induced peripheral blood lymphocytes, whereas IgM production in a SKW6 cell line is enhanced only by ofloxacin (Zehavi-Willner and Shalit, 1989). Fluorinated 4-quinolones apparently also prolong the kinetics of IL-2 production in human peripheral blood lymphocyte cultures based on IL-2 supernatant activity (Riesbeck et al., 1989).

γ-Aminobutyric acid (GABA) increases the expression of Thy-1 antigen on murine bone marrow precursor T cells *in vitro*. *In vivo* GABA enhances antibody production to sheep erythrocytes, presumably by stimulation of thymus-dependent immunity (Belokrylov and Mochanova, 1987).

Germanium is an element belonging to the 4th group of the periodic table with carbon, silicon, tin, and lead. Several organo-germanium compounds have been synthesized and shown to be immunomodulators: carboxyethyl germanium sesquioxide (GE-132); lactate-citrate-germanate (sanumgerman); and spirogermanium (an azaspirane compound). GE-132 has antitumor activity in mice explained by its ability to induce T cell production of circulating lymphokines, which activate macrophages, which subsequently inhibit the tumors. In human clinical trials, GE-132 induced interferon release in a dose-dependent manner and had a significant effect on life prolongation in lung cancer patients. Organic germanium compounds induce interferon release, activate macrophages, augment NK cell activity, and restore impaired immunoresponsiveness. In addition to cell-mediated immunity effects, GE-132 increases the number of antibody-producing cells in plaque assays in aged mice. Spirogermanium treatment normalizes IL-1 production by adherent spleen cells in adjuvant arthritic rats. Germanium compounds apparently function as free radical scavengers by virtue of outer shell electrons being available to interact with toxic, unpaired electrons. Germanium in low doses raises glutathione levels, thus affording protection against endogenously arising free radicals (Goodman, 1988).

IV. Summary

There is extensive research underway on development of chemical immunomodulators for use in humans. This research is primarily driven by the need for therapeutic immunomodulators for use in patients with cancer or AIDS. Currently, there are no chemicals approved as immunomodulators by the Food and Drug Administration for use in domestic food animals. There is considerable potential for applying the rapid advances in immunomodulation research to benefit domestic animals. In domestic food animals, immunomodulators have the greatest potential for prevention and perhaps therapy in early stages of infectious diseases associated with immunosuppression. There are many different causes for immunosuppression and many different molecular mechanisms responsible for defective function of immune cells. It is unlikely that any one immunomodulator will be capable of preventing or reversing all of these various causes of immunosuppression. Therefore, research is needed to understand the mechanisms of immunosuppression and the mechanism of action of immunomodulators so that rational approaches can be developed for their prophylactic and therapeutic use. Without this information and information on effective dosages and duration of action, attempts to use immunomodulators clinically are likely to produce discouraging results.

REFERENCES

Araki, S., Kagaya, K., Kitoh, K., Kimura, M., and Fukazawa, Y. (1987). Enhancement of resistance of *Escherichia coli* infection in mice by dihydroheptaprenol, a synthetic polyprenol derivative. *Infect. Immun.* **55**, 2164–2170.

Babiuk, L. A., and Misra, V. (1981). Levamisole and bovine immunity: *In vitro* and *in vivo* effects on immune responses to herpesvirus immunization. *Can. J. Microbiol.* **27**, 1312–1319.

Babiuk, L. A., and Misra, V. (1982). Effect of levamisole in immune responses to bovine herpesvirus-1. *Am. J. Vet. Res.* **43**, 1349–1354.

Belokrylov, G. A., and Mochanova, I. V. (1987). Immunostimulating property of gamma-aminobutyric acid. *Bull. Exp. Biol. Med. (Engl. Transl.)* **104**, 1284–1286.

Bizzini, B., and Bonmassar, E., eds. (1988). "Advances in Immunomodulation." Pythagora Press, Roma-Milan.

Blecha, F. (1988). Immunomodulation: A means of disease prevention in stressed livestock. *J. Anim. Sci.* **66**, 2084–2090.

Blecha, F., Anderson, G. A., Osorio, F., Chapes, S. K., and Baker, P. E. (1987). Influence of isoprinosine on bovine herpesvirus type-1 infection in cattle. *Vet. Immunol. Immunopathol.* **15**, 253–265.

Bliznakov, E. G., and Adler, A. D. (1972). Nonlinear response of the reticuloendothelial system upon stimulation. *Pathol. Microbiol.* **38**, 393–410.

Brunner, C. J., and Muscoplat, C. C. (1980). Immunomodulatory effects of levamisole. *J. Am. Vet. Med. Assoc.* **176**, 1159–1162.

Buddle, B. M., Pulford, H. D., and Ralston, M. (1988). Protective effect of glucan against experimentally induced staphylococcal mastitis in ewes. *Vet. Microbiol.* **16**, 67–76.

Bugaleta, C., Territo, M. C., Quan, S. G., and Golde, D. W. (1978). Glucan-activated macrophages: Functional characteristics and surface morphology. *J. Reticuloendothel. Soc.* **23**, 195–204.

Chédid, L. (1983). Muramyl peptides as possible endogenous immunopharmacological mediators. *Microbiol. Immunol.* **27**, 723–732.

Christou, N. V., Zakaluzny, I., Marshall, J. C., and Nohr, C. W. (1988). The effect of the immunomodulator RU 41740 (Biostim) on the specific and nonspecific immunosuppression induced by thermal injury or protein deprivation. *Arch. Surg. (Chicago)* **123**, 207–211.

Confer, A. W., and Adldinger, H. K. (1981). The *in vivo* effect of levamisole on phytohaemagglutinin stimulation of lymphocytes in normal and Marek's disease virus inoculated chickens. *Res. Vet. Sci.* **30**, 243–245.

Flaming, K. P., Thaler, R. C., Blecha, F., and Nelssen, J. L. (1988). Influence of sodium diethyldithiocarbamate (Imuthiol) on lymphocyte function and growth in weanling pigs. *Comp. Immunol. Microbiol. Infect. Dis.* **11**, 181–187.

Flaming, K. P., Blecha, F., Fedorka-Cray, P. J., and Anderson, G. A. (1989). Influence of isoprinosine on lymphocyte function in virus-infected feeder pigs. *Am. J. Vet. Res.* **50**, 1653–1657.

Flesh, J., Harel, W., and Nelken, D. (1982). Immunopotentiating effect of levamisole in the prevention of bovine mastitis, fetal death and endometritis. *Vet. Rec.* **111**, 56–57.

Fodor, B., Sussangkarn, K., Arnold, R., Mathelier, H., Mohacsi, T., Mujumdar, R., Butterick, J., and Veltri, R. W. (1987). From methylglyoxal to new immunopotentiating ascorbic acid derivatives. *Acta Biochim. Biophys. Hung.* **32**, 165–179.

Ginsberg, T., and Glasky, A. J. (1977). Inosiplex: An immunomodulation model for the treatment of viral disease. *Ann. N.Y. Acad. Sci.* **284**, 128–138.

Goodman, S. (1988). Therapeutic effects of organic germanium. *Med. Hypotheses* **26**, 207–215.

Hennessy, K. J., Blecha, F., Pollmann, D. S., and Kluber, E. F. (1987). Isoprinosine and levamisole immunomodulation in artificially reared neonatal pigs. *Am. J. Vet. Res.* **48**, 477–480.

Hess, A. D., Silanskis, M. K., Esa, A. H., Pettit, G. R., and May, W. S. (1988). Activation of human T lymphocytes by bryostatin. *J. Immunol.* **141**, 3263–3269.

Ikehara, S., Hadden, J. W., Good, R. A., Lunzer, D. G., and Pahwa, R. N. (1987). In vitro effects of two immunopotentiators, isoprinosine and NPT 15392, on murine T-Cell differentiation and function. *Thymus* **3**, 87–95.

Irwin, M. R., Holmberg, C. A., Knight, H. D., and Hjerpe, C. A. (1976). Effects of vaccination against infectious bovine rhinotracheitis and simultaneous administration of levamisole on primary humoral responses in calves. *Am. J. Vet. Res.* **37**, 223–226.

Irwin, M. R., Melendy, D. R., and Hutcheson, D. P. (1980). Reduced morbidity associated with shipping fever pneumonia in levamisole phosphate-treated feedlot cattle. *Southwest. Vet.* **33**, 45–49.

Ishikawa, H., and Shimizu, T. (1983). Depression of B-lymphocytes by mastitis and treatment with levamisole. *J. Dairy Sci.* **66**, 556–561.

Ishikawa, H., Shimizu, T., Hirano, H., Saito, N., and Nakano, T. (1982). Protein composition of whey from subclinical mastitis and effect of treatment with levamisole. *J. Dairy Sci.* **65**, 653–658.

Kaeberle, M. L., and Roth, J. A. (1984). Effects of thiabendazole on dexamethasone-induced suppression of lymphocyte and neutrophil function in cattle. *Immunopharmacology* **8**, 129–136.

Kingston, A. E., Ivanyi, J., and Kay, J. E. (1984). The effects of indomethacin on T lymphocyte stimulation. *Immunol. Lett.* **8**, 301–305.

Laval, A., Rommain, M., Fortier, M., Zalisz, R., Dahan, R., and Smets, P. (1988). Immunomodulating effects of orally administered Ru 41740 (Biostim®) in the swine. *Adv. Biosci.* **68**, 103–109.

Lomnitzer, R. (1988). Isoprinosine potentiation of human peripheral blood mononuclear cell response to mitogens. Kinetics and effect on expression of the IL-2 receptor and the activity of interleukin 2. *J. Clin. Lab. Immunol.* **27**, 91–96.

Lovett, E. J., and Lundy, J. (1977). The effect of thiabendazole in a mixed leukocyte culture. *Transplantation* **24**, 93–97.

Majde, J. A., ed. (1987). "Immunopharmacology of Infectious Diseases: Vaccine Adjuvants and Modulators of Non-Specific Resistance," Prog. Leukocyte Biol. Vol. 6. Alan R. Liss, New York.

Masihi, K. N., and Lange, W., eds. (1988). "Immunomodulators and Nonspecific Host Defense Mechanisms Against Microbial Infections," Adv. Biosci., Vol. 68. Pergamon, New York.

Mohr, H., Pettit, G. R., and Plessing-Menze, A. (1987). Co-induction of lymphokine synthesis by the antineoplastic bryostatins. *Immunobiology* **175**, 420–430.

Morrow, S. H., and Di Luzio, N. R. (1965). The fate of foreign red cells in mice with altered reticuloendothelial function. *Proc. Soc. Exp. Biol. Med.* **119**, 647–652.

Mulcahy, G., and Quinn, P. J. (1986). A review of immunomodulators and their application in veterinary medicine. *J. Vet. Pharmacol. Ther.* **9**, 119–139.

Nair, N. D., and Rajan, A. (1983). Immunostimulatory effect of levamisole in calves. *Kerala J. Vet. Sci.* **14**, 31–34.

Onaga, H., Tajima, M., and Ishii, T. (1984). Effect of levamisole on the immune response of chickens to infection with *Eimeria tenella*. *Zentralbl. Bakteriol., Mikrobiol. Hyg., Abt. 1, Orig. A* **256**, 323–327.

Panigrahy, B., Grumbles, L. C., Millar, D., Nagi, S. A., and Hall, C. F. (1979). Antibiotic-induced immunosuppression and levamisole-induced immunopotentiation in turkeys. *Avian Dis.* **23**, 401–408.

Popescu, C., Pencea, I., Economu, D., Grecu, V., Uliciuc, S., Ghincea, V., and Buzdugan, R. (1985). Enhanced immune response in R inbred rats by chemical and/or bacterial immunostimulation. II. Stimulation of cell-mediated immune response after administration of aerodin and bronhodin associated or not with levamisole. *Arch. Roum. Pathol. Exp. Microbiol.* **44**, 55–61.

Radov, L. A., Kamp, D., Trusso, L. A., Sloane, D., Julien, R. P., Clemens, C. M., and Murray, R. J. (1988). The immunological profile of a new immunomodulatory agent, oxamisole. *Int. J. Immunopharmacol.* **10**, 609–618.

Rejas, M. T., Rojo, J. M., Ojeda, G., and Barasoain, I. (1988). Sodium diethyldithiocarbamate restores T lymphocyte proliferation, IL2 production and NK activity in cyclophosphamide-immunosuppressed animals. *Immunopharmacology* **16**, 191–197.

Renoux, G. (1986). The ten commandments for immunotherapeutic drugs at the example of sulfur-containing agents. *Comp. Immunol. Microbiol. Infect. Dis.* **9**, 121–129.

Reyero, C., Stockl, W., and Thalhammer, J. G. (1979). Stimulation of the antibody response to sheep red blood cells in piglets and young pigs by levamisole. *Br. Vet. J.* **135**, 17–24.

Riesbeck, K., Anderson, J., Gullberg, M., and Forsgren, A. (1989). Fluorinated 4-quinolones induce hyperproduction of interleukin 2. *Proc. Natl. Acad. Sci. U.S.A.* **86**, 2809–2813.

Roth, J. A. (1988). Enhancement of nonspecific resistance to bacterial infection by biologic response modifiers. *In* "Virulence Mechanisms of Bacterial Pathogens" (J. A. Roth, ed.), pp. 329–342. Am. Soc. Microbiol., Washington, D.C.

Roth, J. A., and Kaeberle, M. L. (1984). Effect of levamisole on lymphocyte blastogenesis and neutrophil function in dexamethasone-treated cattle. *Am. J. Vet. Res.* **45**, 1781–1784.

Roth, J. A., and Kaeberle, M. L. (1985a). Enhancement of lymphocyte blastogenesis and neutrophil function by avridine in dexamethasone-treated and nontreated cattle. *Am. J. Vet. Res.* **46**, 53–57.

Roth, J. A., and Kaeberle, M. L. (1985b). In vivo effect of ascorbic acid on neutrophil function in healthy and dexamethasone-treated cattle. *Am. J. Vet. Res.* **46**, 2434–2436.

Roth, J. A., Kaeberle, M. L., and Hubbard, R. D. (1984). Attempts to use thiabendazole to improve the immune response in dexamethasone-treated or stressed cattle. *Immunopharmacology* **8**, 121–128.

Sampson, D., Peters, T. G., Lewis, J. D., Metzig, J., and Kurtz, B. E. (1977). Dose dependence of immunopotentiation and tumor regression induced by levamisole. *Cancer Res.* **37**, 3526–3529.

Saperstein, G., Mohanty, S. B., Rockemann, D. D., and Russek, E. (1983). Effect of levamisole on induced bovine viral diarrhea. *J. Am. Vet. Med. Assoc.* **183**, 425–427.

Shibata, T., Nakayama, O., Tsurumi, Y., Okuhara, M., Terano, H., and Kohsaka, M. (1988). A new immunomodulator, FR-900483. *J. Antibiot.* **41**, 296–301.

Sulochana, S., Pillai, R. M., and Nair, G. K. (1984). Immunomodulatory effect of levamisole on the antibody response to Newcastle Disease Virus in chicken. *Kerala J. Vet. Sci.* **15**, 145–149.

Trenn, G., Pettit, G. R., Takayama, H., Hu-Li, J., and Sitkovsky, M. V. (1988). Immunomodulating properties of a novel series of protein kinase C activators. *J. Immunol.* **140**, 433–439.

Tsang, P. H., Sei, Y., and Bekesi, J. G. (1987). Isoprinosine-induced modulation of T-helper cell subsets and antigen-presenting monocytes (Leu M_3^+ Ia^+) resulted in improvement of T- and B-lymphocyte functions, *in vitro* in ARC and AIDS patients. *Clin. Immunol. Immunopathol.* **45**, 166–176.

Van Der Maaten, M. J., Schmerr, M. J. F., Miller, J. M., and Sacks, J. M. (1983). Levamisole does not affect the virological and serological responses of bovine leukemia virus-infected cattle and sheep. *Can. J. Comp. Med.* **47**, 474–479.

Wang, B. S., Ruszala-Mallon, V. M., Lumanglas, A. L., Silva, J., and Durr, F. E. (1988). Restoration of cytolytic T-lymphocyte response with a new immunopotentiator,N-(4-[(4-Fluorophenyl)sulfonyl]phenyl)acetamide (CL 259,763), in mice. *Cancer Res.* **48**, 2135–2137.

Werner, G. H., Floc'h, F., Migliore-Samour, D., and Jollès, P. (1986). Immunomodulating peptides. *Experientia* **42**, 521–531.

White, S. L., Schweitzer, K., Humphries, M. J., and Olden, K. (1988). Stimulation of DNA synthesis in murine lymphocytes by the drug swainsonine: Immunomodulatory properties. *Biochem. Biophys. Res. Commun.* **150**, 615–625.

Woodard, L. F., Jasman, R. L., Farrington, D. O., and Jensen, K. E. (1983). Enhanced antibody-dependent bactericidal activity of neutrophils from calves treated with a lipid amine immunopotentiator. *Am. J. Vet. Res.* **44**, 389–394.

Wooles, W. R., and Di Luzio, N. R. (1963). Reticuloendothelial function and the immune response. *Science* **142**, 1078–1080.

Yoneyama, O., Osame, S., Ichijo, S., Kimura, M., Araki, S., Susuki, M., and Imamura, E. (1989a). Effects of dihydroheptaprenol on neutrophil functions in calves. *Br. Vet. J.* **145**, 531–537.

Yoneyama, O., Osame, S., Kimura, M., Araki, S., and Ichijo, S. (1989b). Enhancement of neutrophil function by dihydroheptaprenol in adult cows. *Jpn. J. Vet. Sci.* **51**, 1283–1286.

Zehavi-Willner, T., and Shalit, I. (1989). Enhancement of interleukin-2 production in human lymphocytes by two new quinolone derivatives. *Lymphokine Res.* **8**, 35–46.

Classical and New Approaches to Adjuvant Use in Domestic Food Animals

KRISTIAN DALSGAARD,* LUUK HILGERS,† AND GÉRARD TROUVE‡

*Animal Biotechnology Research Center, State Veterinary Institute for Virus Research, Lindholm, DK-4771 Kalvehave, Denmark,
† Duphar B. V., Animal Health Division, Veterinary Vaccines, Weesp, Holland, and
‡ SEPPIC, Lacaze Basse, F-81105 Castres Cedex, France

I. Introduction
II. Aluminum Salts
III. Oil Emulsions
IV. Surface Active Agents
  A. Lipophilic Amines
  B. Nonionic Block Polymers
  C. Sulpholipopolysaccharides
  D. Saponins
V. ISCOMS
VI. Muramyldipeptides
VII. Polymeric Adjuvants
VIII. General Conclusions
  References

I. Introduction

The history of immunological adjuvants is almost as long as immunology itself. Although early experience indicated that a wide variety of substances could increase the specific immune response to antigens, it was only a few that were to be the accepted adjuvants for decades: aluminum hydroxide in humans and other animals, oil in animals, such as poultry, and Freund's complete adjuvant (FCA) in laboratory animals. One of the main reasons for the retention of this limited repertoire was because of the general success of these adjuvants with inactivated virus cultures and bacterial products. With few exceptions research in adjuvants began with molecular biology. With the search for subunit vaccines, but in particular, after the introduction of recombinant DNA and chemical peptide antigen synthesis, it was realized that these new antigens in general were poor immunogens. In fact, many of the products could only be made immunogenic by FCA.

Even in laboratory animals, many researchers are today questioning the feasibility of using FCA because of the strong reactions inflicted, and a practical application in larger animals is totally out of the question. This situation has led to a great increase in adjuvant research during recent years. Most of the research has been concerned with purification of known adjuvants, such as oil, (myco)bacteria, and saponin, or based on known chemically well-defined adjuvants, such as aliphatic nitrogenous bases and polysaccharides. Out of this research new substances and antigen presentation systems are emerging.

II. Aluminum Salts

Aluminum salts, including $Al(OH)_3$ and $AlPO_4$, are the most widely used adjuvants in veterinary and human vaccines (Edelman, 1980). With oil emulsions they form a group of classical adjuvants as they have been applied for several decades. They are considered to be rather safe, although sterile abscesses (Butler et al., 1969) and persistent nodules are observed occasionally after subcutaneous administration (White et al., 1955). The capacity of aluminum salts to form complexes with biomaterials seemed to be crucial to adjuvanticity, but the precise modes of adjuvant action are still not completely understood. The formation of a depot of antigen from which the antigen releases slowly is considered to be an important mechanism, but there are several lines of evidence indicating that this is not the only prospect. Adsorption of antigen to $Al(OH)_3$ particles may alter the conformation of the antigen and thereby the accessibility of certain moieties to the immune system. Recognition and handling of antigen of the host immune system and processing and presentation by antigen-presenting cells is influenced by the adsorption to $Al(OH)_3$ gel in favor of the immune response. A similar mode of action was suggested for other adjuvants with the capability to bind antigens (Allison and Byars, 1986; Hunter and Bennett, 1986).

Histological studies of lymphoid organs revealed that complexes of antigen and small $Al(OH)_3$ particles are efficiently trapped in the lymph nodes (White et al., 1955) and trapping and retention of lymphocytes is also improved (Ramanathan et al., 1979). Al(OH)$_3$ can activate the complement system (Ramanthan et al., 1979) and since the complement system contributes to recruitment and stimulation of phagocytes, distribution and functions of these cells are modified. Macrophages play a pivotal role in the induction and regulation of the type and level of the immune response, and they can be affected by Al(OH)$_3$ as demonstrated by altered metabolic activity (Mundar et al., 1969) and synthesis of interleukin-1 (Bomford, 1986).

Absorptive properties of aluminum salts are important to binding of either antigen or (humoral) components of the host immune system. Binding of protein, i.e., antigen, depends on a number of factors (Hem and White, 1984; Lei, 1985): first, the nature of the protein (antigen), especially the ratio and distribution of hydrophobic and hydrophilic groups, the ratio of positively and negatively charged moieties, and the concentration in the medium; and second, the nature and concentration of either organic or inorganic substances that may interfere with the physical interaction of antigen and Al(OH)$_3$. Competition between antigen and other organic molecules for binding sites on the gel may result in blocking of the binding or even complete dislodgement of the antigen. Inorganic compounds such as phosphate, sulphate, and borate salts can modify the physicochemical properties of the surface and thereby the binding characteristics of the Al(OH)$_3$ particles. In addition, the binding of antigen depends on the pH of the medium, which determines directly the net charge of gel, antigen, and interfering substances. In practice, vaccines have physiological pH at which the Al(OH)$_3$ gel is positively charged. Substances with negative charge tend to bind strongly while positively or neutrally charged compounds form only weak and unstable complexes (Lei, 1985). Consequently, the adjuvanticity of Al(OH)$_3$ depends on the physicochemical properties of antigen and apparent differences between antigens can be expected (Bomford, 1984).

Al(OH)$_3$ is a strong adjuvant for humoral responses against various antigens including several viral and bacterial antigens but not against sheep red blood cells (Bomford, 1980a). Primary rather than secondary responses are enhanced (Jensen and Koch, 1988) and IgG1 rather than the other IgG subclasses are augmented (Mancino and Ovary, 1980). Al(OH)$_3$ and other aluminum salts are noneffective in the stimulation of cell-mediated immunity (Bomford, 1980b). A great number of effective veterinary vaccines contain Al(OH)$_3$ as an adjuvant, e.g., *Bordetella bronchiseptica* (McCandlish et al., 1978), *Bacterioides nodosus* (Thorley and Egerton, 1981), *Pasteurella multocida* (Nagy and Penn,

1974), *Leptospira interrogans* (Ris and Hamel, 1979), foot-and-mouth disease virus (Anderson *et al.*, 1971), bovine adenovirus (Bartha, 1974), canine parvo virus and canine herpes virus (Cornwell and Thompson, 1982), and bovine wart virus (Webster and Webster, 1985).

Combinations of aluminum salts with other adjuvants displayed distinct effects. Combinations with certain surfactants (Teerlink *et al.*, 1987) and oil-in-water emulsions (Wong and Barbaro, 1976; Muggleton and Hilton, 1967) resulted in enhanced adjuvanticity, while the addition of saponin to $Al(OH)_3$ resulted in either increased or decreased adjuvant effect depending on the antigen tested (Bomford, 1984).

Minor differences in the properties of commercially available aluminum hydroxide gels may be expected because of the complex nature of the gel structure. At the NATO ASI meeting on adjuvants in Cap Sunion, Greece, July 1988, a consensus among the participants was reached that Alhydrogel (Superfos, Denmark) should be used as a reference.

III. Oil Emulsions

That the immune response to an antigen may be modified by injecting it as an emulsion in oil has been known for a long time. Vallée (1924), Ramon (1925), Friedewald (1944), and Henle and Henle (1945) used oils in the preparation of bovine tuberculosis, diphtheria, and influenza vaccines. However, there is no doubt that Freund's works (1937 through 1960) actually demonstrated the value of oil adjuvants, and served as the basis for the whole series of fundamental studies on immunomodulators still under way (Freund and McDermott, 1942; Freund and Stone, 1959). Freund's incomplete adjuvant (FIA) is a mixture of mineral oil with mannitol monooleate, whereas Freund's complete adjuvant (FCA) contains additionally a mycobacterium. Both are still today's standard adjuvants in many laboratories.

The introduction over the last decade of noval purified mineral oils, and of new injectable emulsifying agents, has permitted the production of many oil-based veterinary vaccines. They are available as emulsions of antigenic media and oil mixtures stabilized by the addition of surface active principles.

The most commonly utilized oils are light mineral oils corresponding to the monograph of the *United States Pharmacopeia*. These contain no aromatic compounds but variable proportions of paraffinic and naphthenic principles generally approximating 70% and 30%, respectively. Vapor phase chromatographic analyses have shown a predominance of carbohydrates with 20 to 30 carbon atoms, although these occur with a wide range distribution pattern. Their viscosity must be low in order to ensure the fluidity of the vaccine. DRAKOEL 6 VR (Penreco, U.S.A.), MARCOL 52 and MARCOL 82 (ESSO, France), SONTEX 55 (Marathon Marco, U.S.A.), VESTAN A 50 B (Fina), and WHITREX 307 (Mobil) are some of the most popular in use in commercial vaccines.

The emulsifiers are required in order to promote the stability of the oil and aqueous phase mixture. Generally, the emulsifiers are nonionic surface active agents of reputed low toxicity. Mannitol monooleate was the first to be used. This is the emulsifying agent used in Freund's adjuvants. It is a viscous liquid (ca. 400 mPas), the composition of which is complex due to the possibilities of cyclization of mannitol into mannitan and mannide (O'Neill et al., 1972; Berlin, 1960; Vanselow, 1987). Although mannitol monooleates were initially produced for industrial purposes and contained many impurities, they are now available as products of injectable quality (Berlin, 1962; Gomes and Auge de Mello, 1978) (ARLACEL A Special, ICI, USA; MONTANIDE 80, Seppic, France).

Sorbitan oleates and ethoxy-derivatives are sometimes used. Trioleates in antigen-free vaccine emulsions have proved to be effective in stimulating nonspecific immunity in a study showing the protection of young pigs against diarrhea (Nabuurs et al., 1982). No reaction following intraperitoneal injections was reported. However, when antigens are added (Bokhout et al., 1981) granulomas have been observed to develop in rabbits and pigs. Sorbitan monooleates have been used in the preparation of vaccines, either alone (Woodard and Jasman, 1985; Box, 1985) or in combination with mannitol monooleates (Herbert, 1965; Solyom et al., 1977).

Ethylene and propylene oxide copolymers have prompted many basic studies. Some of these compounds seem to have intrinsic immunomodulating properties (Hunter et al., 1981; Hunter and Bennett, 1986). The properties of these products were reviewed by Zigterman et al. (1987). PLURONIC L 121 might be one of the most interesting (Snippe et al., 1981), although it is more of a wetting agent than an emulsifying one. It should therefore be combined with a surface active agent such as Polysorbate 80 to produce emulsions of acceptable stability (Allison, 1987).

Phospholipids are widely used for parenteral nutrition and, surprisingly, there have been few studies carried out on their role as emulsifying agents for the production of vaccines. They form the basis of one oil adjuvant containing glycerin and peanut oil, the efficacy of which has been demonstrated in both sheep and monkeys injected with equine encephalitis and Rift Valley Fever vaccines (Reynolds et al., 1980). Phospholipids are the elements of antigen-containing liposomes. Such preparations show promising characteristics as carriers in veterinary vaccines. The preparation of liposomes and their immunoadjuvant action has been recently reviewed by Gregoriadis (1988).

The type of oil emulsions used in verterinary vaccines are:

1. Water/oil (W/O) vaccines, which have a continuous oil phase. When these vaccines are made by either ARLACEL A or MONTANIDE 80, they are quite viscous (2000–5000 mPas) and difficult to inject. The development of new products, MONTANIDE 888 and MONTANIDE 103 has made it possible to obtain formulas of low viscosity (50–200 mPas) and high stability. The proportion of antigenic aqueous medium usually used ranges between 25 and 50% of the total volume. The viscosity of the vaccine increases rapidly as the quantity of medium used is augmented. W/O vaccines usually confer high-level, long-lasting immunity.
2. Oil/water (O/W) vaccines, which have a continuous aqueous phase. These vaccines contain hydrophilic emulsifiers. Their main advantage lies in their low viscosity and the ease with which they can be injected compared to early W/O-type vaccines. On the whole, O/W vaccines are less potent as far as the duration of immunity is concerned (Bomford, 1985). They are often well tolerated by pigs and cattle (Favre and Mougeot, 1981), but reactions have also been reported to this type of emulsions (Goto, 1978).
3. Double water/oil/water (W/O/W) emulsion formulas present a continuous aqueous phase wherein a W/O emulsion is dispersed. These were initially conceived to facilitate injecting W/O-type vaccine through secondary dispersion into an aqueous phase, so as to obtain double emulsions (Herbert, 1965). Such low-viscosity formulas have proved to be as effective as the FIA-containing vaccines in cases of bovine (Auge de Mello et al., 1980) or porcine (Anderson et al., 1971) foot-and-mouth disease. Technically, they are more difficult to produce and less stable than other types of emulsions.

A major drawback of vaccines prepared by the original constituents in FIA has been their local reaction and granuloma-inducing properties. However, by the application of the new oils and emulsifiers considerable advantages have been obtained. Comparative histological studies carried out on pigs vaccinated against Aujeszky's disease (Vannier, 1986) or foot-and-mouth disease (Favre and Mougoet, 1981) have shown that the local reactions associated with certain commercial vaccines could be substantially reduced. Archambault et al. (1988b) noted no clinical complications with rotavirus-containing vaccines following administration to calves. However, he emphasized the importance of stable formulas of low viscosity.

The list of veterinary vaccines based on oil emulsions is impressive and commercial products are available against practically all common bacterial and viral diseases in cattle, pigs, sheep, and poultry. Especially in poultry the use of oil emulsion vaccines is common because this species seems to be less sensitive to the potential adverse reactions of oil emulsions. Some countries have a more restrictive policy for the application of oil adjuvants, especially in cattle and pigs. One vaccine has been successful in the control of foot-and-mouth disease in South America (Olascoaga, 1978; Barei et al., 1979; Abracon et al., 1982; Bahnemann et al., 1988; Sadir et al., 1988). Recent work about the successful application of oil adjuvants has been reported for Aujeszky's disease in swine (Riviera et al., 1988; Vannier, 1986) and for dysentery in calves (Bellinzoni et al., 1989; Archambault et al., 1988a) or swine (Gerraty, 1988).

The mechanisms of action of the oil adjuvants are numerous and complex. They have been studied by many authors (Edelman, 1980; Stewart-Tull, 1983; Bomford, 1985; Dalsgaard, 1987; Vanselow, 1987; Warren and Chédid, 1988) discussing the following topics: (1) phenomena pertaining to the deposit and progressive release of the antigens; (2) the protection of the antigen within an "oily envelope" (W/O vaccines); (3) modulation of the activity of macrophages; (4) lymphocyte circulation; and (5) phenomena related to the presentation of antigens to macrophages.

Studies concerning the relationships between the physicochemical properties of the adjuvants or the vaccines, and their immunologic properties and safety are relatively rare. Former results, however, may become especially important in the light of recently published data concerning antigen adsorption and interface phenomena. Hunter and Bennett (1986) have shown the ethylene and propylene oxide copolymers exhibiting most pronounced adjuvant properties to be those which form highly developed structures at the water/oil interface. These results were confirmed by Allison (1988) who explained the activity of PLURONIC L 121 through its adsorption onto squalene-bound microdroplets of an H/E-type emulsion. Kreuter et al. (1986) showed that the activity of BSA adsorbed on polymetacrylate micropellets increases as the size of these micropellets decreases. The interface electric charge phenomenon (Zeta potential) responsible for modifying the quarternary structure of the adsorbed proteins exposing new antigenic sites may play a role (Jollès and Paraf, 1973). These surface phenomena are especially important in the case of oil emulsion vaccines, where the surface areas generated are considerable (1.5 m^2 approx. for a 1 ml dose of vaccine the dispersed phase of which would be constituted by 1-μm droplets).

IV. Surface Active Agents

A. LIPOPHILIC AMINES

Gall (1966) tested a variety of surface active agents on adjuvanticity. Among them, there were a number of lipophilic amines that demonstrated strong adjuvant activity for the humoral immune response against tetanus toxoid in guinea pigs. Since then, many investigators affirmed and extended these observations and research has concentrated on one of these lipophilic amines, namely dimethyldioctadecylammonium bromide (DDA) (Coon and Hunter, 1973; Snippe et al., 1977; Chiba and Egashira, 1978; Hilgers, 1987). Both cellular and humoral immune responses against various antigens could be augmented by DDA (Prager, 1985). Another lipophilic amine closely related to DDA, N, N-dioctadecyl-N', N'-bis(2-hydroxyethyl)propanediamine (also called CP 20,961 or avridine), demonstrated considerable adjuvanticity for humoral and cellular immune responses (Niblack et al., 1979; Anderson and Pearson, 1979).

DDA and avridine are low-molecular weight adjuvants (631 and 666 Dal, respectively) and both contain two long alkyl chains of 18 C atoms. They are poorly soluble in water and form suspensions. After heating or ultrasonic disruption DDA molecules form unstable micellar structures (Prager, 1985) and a precipitate is formed within a few days. As a consequence, difficulties appear with the formulation of stable vaccines containing the lipophilic amine and therefore they are often used in combination with a vehicle such as liposomes (Woodard et al., 1983; Pierce and Sacci, 1984; Jiskoot et al., 1986) or oil droplets. Depending on the route of administration, they exert preference for the stimulation of humoral or cellular immune responses. Humoral responses to antigens were enhanced by intraperitoneal injection of antigen and DDA or avridine (Hilgers et al., 1984a). Subcutaneous or intracutaneous injection of adjuvant and antigen failed to induce antibody responses but instead sensitized animals for cellular immunity manifested by delayed-type hypersensitivity reactions (Snippe et al., 1977; Chiba and Egashira, 1978; Kraaijeveld et al., 1982).

Although the adjuvant activity of DDA has been investigated extensively in laboratory animals, little information is available on the effects of large animals. In contrast, avridine has been tested with various bacterial, viral, and parasitic antigens in pigs or cattle (Jensen, 1986) and proved to be superior to various other adjuvants tested (Jensen, 1986). In chickens, avridine considerably augmented the immune response against Newcastle disease virus (Rweyemamu et al., 1986; Rijke et al., 1988). In addition to the stimulation of antibody titers in serum, avridine also enhanced the local immune response to various antigens, i.e., sheep red blood cells (SRBC) (Anderson et al., 1985), cholera toxin (Anderson et al., 1985; Pierce and Sacci, 1984), procholeragenoid (Pierce and Sacci, 1984), and reovirus (Anderson et al., 1985; Rubin et al., 1983). Increased uptake, localization, and retention of antigen in Peyer's patches and decreased rate of antigen degradation (Anderson et al., 1985) suggest important modes of adjuvanticity of avridine for local immune responses. Incorporation of avridine into liposomes improved the adjuvanticity for the IgA response (Pierce and Sacci, 1984).

The mechanism(s) underlying immunostimulation of the lipophilic amines are complex and include effects on both antigen and components of the host immune system (Hilgers, 1987; Klerx, 1985). DDA can bind to different types of antigens by either hydrophobic or electrostatic interactions (Baechtel and Prager, 1982). The importance of the physical interaction between antigen and lipophilic adjuvants was unambiguously demonstrated by the effects on cellular immunity against a small, lipophilic antigen (Hilgers et al., 1987b). Complexes of DDA or avridine and this monovalent antigen induced high levels of cell-mediated immunity, but if the formation of such complexes was blocked no responses could be detected. The lipophilic character of DDA and avridine is believed to be decisive to the stimulation of cell-mediated immunity. The importance of lipophilic moieties is affirmed by the observation that strong responses against proteins could be induced by protein–lipid conjugates (Coon and Hunter, 1973). Apparently, induction of cell-mediated immunity is favored by the presence of hydrophobic moieties in the antigen that can be introduced by either physical interaction with lipophilic compounds or covalent linkage of carbon chains.

In addition to interaction with antigen, DDA and avridine evoke a variety of immune reactions in the host. Intraperitoneal (I.P.) injection of DDA elicits an inflammatory response in mice, characterized by an increase in the number of peritoneal cells (Hilgers et al., 1984b; Gonggrijp et al., 1985), an influx of polymorphonuclear and mononuclear phagocytes (Hilgers *et al.,* 1984b), and the appearance of serum amyloid protein P in serum (Hilgers *et al.,* 1988). Furthermore, DDA modifies both antigen and lymphocyte trapping, activates the complement system (Klerx, 1985) and interfaces with antigen handling and processing by phagocytic cells (Bloksma *et al.,* 1983; Willers *et al.,* 1979). Low levels of nonspecific resistance against Semliki Forest virus and encephalomyelitis virus (Kraaijeveld *et al.,* 1982) could be observed shortly after I.P. administration of plain adjuvant. Avridine and, to a lesser extent, DDA gave rise to interferon levels in peritoneal exudate fluid and in serum (Kraaijeveld *et al.,* 1982). Furthermore, peritoneal cells harvested after I.P. injection of DDA exhibited increased levels of candidacidal activity (Hilgers *et al.,* 1984b), which correlated closely with an increased percentage of polymorphonuclear cells. Avridine enhanced the antibody-dependent bactericidal activity of neutrophils in calves (Woodard, *et al.,* 1983). Obvious nonspecific resistance to bacterial infections could be induced by combinations of DDA plus RNA (Gonggrijp *et al.,* 1985) or DDA plus poly (A : U) (Antonissen, 1986).

B. Nonionic Block Polymers

Another group of surface active agents with apparent adjuvanticity is the nonionic block polymers (NBPs) first described by Hunter and associates (Hunter *et al.,* 1981; Hunter and Bennett, 1984, 1986). NBPs are copolymers of hydrophilic polyoxyethylene and hydrophobic polyoxypropylene. The group includes a variety of molecules that differ in molecular weight, ratio of polyoxyethylene and polyoxypropylene, and orientation of the different polymers (Hunter *et al.,* 1981). They exert adjuvanticity as plain adjuvant but are more effective when used in combination with an oil phase. In general, the adjuvant-active NBPs have low hydrophilic/lipophilic-balance (HLB) values indicating predominantly lipophilic character. In an oil-in-water system, these NBPs have a tendency to reside at the interface separating the two immiscible liquids and form a hydrophilic surface around the oil droplets (Allison and Byars, 1986).

The adjuvanticity of the NBPs depends on the antigen used. The antibody response against dinitrophenyl (DNP)-haptenated liposomes or DNP-haptenated bovine serum albumin (DNP-BSA) was enhanced strongly by L81 and 31R1 and only moderately by L101, L121, and T1501 (Zigterman *et al.,* 1987). In contrast, antibody responses against BSA and hexasaccharide-BSA conjugate were not stimulated by L81 or 31R1 while L101, L121, and T1501 proved to be quite effective (Hunter and Bennett, 1986). In aqueous solutes, NBPs L81 and 31R1 form spherical drops while L101, L121, and T1501 form fibrous structures, and a correlation between structure in water and adjuvanticity for BSA was suggested (Hunter and Bennett, 1986). Such a relationship was clearly not valid for DNP-liposomes or DNP-BSA. In general, NBPs are not effective in the induction of cellular responses. L101 significantly augmented the cellular responses against two different antigens but only in combination with cyclophosphamide treatment of the animals (Snippe et al., 1981).

Mechanisms underlying the adjuvant activity of NBPs are not completely understood. Data suggest that physical interaction of NBPs with antigen is important (Allison and Byars, 1986) but other observations suggest direct effects on components of the host immune system (Atkinson et al., 1988; Hunter and Bennett, 1984, 1986; Zigterman, 1988). NBPs can bind different types of proteins, which can be either antigen or protein components of the host, such as the third component of the complement system or fibrinogen.

An adjuvant formulation that proved to be effective in various animal models is the so-called Syntex Adjuvant Formulation (SAF-1; Allison and Byars, 1986; Allison, 1987; Byars and Allison, 1987). It is composed of a squalene-in-water emulsion, NBP L121, and a MDP-derivative (muramyl-threonyl-isoglutamin). The emulsion is a strong adjuvant for both humoral and cellular immune responses (Byars and Allison, 1987) and proved to be of low toxicity (Byars, 1984). The potency to enhance cellular immunity was attributed to the presence of the MDP-derivative (Byars and Allison, 1987).

C. Sulpholipopolysaccharides

The synergistic adjuvant activity of combinations of lipophilic and polyanionic adjuvant (Hilgers et al., 1985, 1986b) was the main reason to synthesize a novel group of compounds with the chemical moieties of both types of adjuvants. Ficoll was derivatized with sulphate and lipid groups at various ratios yielding numerous different so-called sulpholipopolysaccharides (SLPs). The adjuvanticity of these compounds was tested with different antigens in mice (Hilgers et al., 1987a). The humoral immune response to a particulate antigen (red blood cells) was increased strongly by SLPs with high-sulphate and low-lipid contents and SLPs with high-lipid and low sulphate contents (Hilgers et al., 1987a). Effects of the SLPs on the humoral immune response to a soluble antigen (DNP-BSA) were apparently distinct as all SLPs with a certain minimal number of lipid groups enhanced the response, irrespective of their sulphate contents. Effects of the SLPs on the immune response to viral and various bacterial antigens have not been published but are under investigation. The mechanism(s) underlying the immunostimulatory effects of the SLPs has not been elucidated but similarities with that of other surface active adjuvants on one hand and polyanions the other hand may be expected.

D. Saponins

The adjuvant activity of certain saponins has been known since the early experiments with formalin-inactivated bacterial toxins (Ramon, 1926). Saponins are very common secondary constituents of plants. Chemically they are glycosides composed of several (hydrophilic) sugars in association with a (hydrophobic) molecule, which can be either of steroid or triterpenoid structure. Such compounds are usually surface active, and some of the saponins are strong detergents ("sapon" = soap). Among the steroid saponins the cardiac glycosides from *Digitalis lanata* have been studied extensively and their medical application is well known. Some of these compounds are also immunologically active as stimulators of B cell proliferation *in vitro* (Hammarström and Edward Smith, 1978), but they have not been applied *in vivo* as adjuvants because of their strong pharmacological effect on the heart. The triterpenoid saponins are widely used in industry as emulsifiers, e.g., of photographic films, foam-producing agents, e.g., in shampoos, beverages, and fire extinguishers. Because the bulk of the commercially available saponin is produced for these technical purposes, manufacturers do not discriminate between from which plant source their saponin is derived. Thus, "saponin" has become a general term in the catalogues of suppliers of chemicals, although the products may vary considerably and be extracted from different plant materials.

There are four major sources of technical saponin: *Smilax ornata* (sarsaparilla), *Gypsophilla paniculata* (bride's veil), *Saponaria officianalis* (soap root), and *Quillaja saponaria* (soap bark). Each of these plant materials are collected, extracted, and evaporated to dryness and sold as "saponin." It is among the triterpenoid saponins that compounds with adjuvant activity have been described. Considering the diversity of saponin sources it is understandable that the adjuvant activity was found unpredictable in early experiments (Ramon, 1926). Because of their surface activity many saponins are hemolytic to red blood cells, and induce severe local reactions when injected parenterally. These properties resulted in the almost complete negligence of saponins as adjuvants except in one field: foot-and-mouth disease (FMD) vaccines.

Espinet (1951) demonstrated strong adjuvant activity in FMD vaccines of the saponin purchased by him in South America. This actually resulted in the widespread application of saponin in commercial FMD vaccines. This was done on a trial and error basis, until a TLC-fingerprint method was developed (Dalsgaard, 1970). Using this method, it could be shown that all of the commercially available saponins being used as adjuvants with demonstrated activity were derived from the South American tree *Quillaja saponaria* Molina. From the bark of this tree Dalsgaard (1974) later isolated a homogeneous fraction, which was denoted "Quil A." Quil A had strong adjuvant activity in FMD vaccines (Dalsgaard and Jensen, 1977; Dalsgaard, 1978) and showed less local reactions at the site of injection than crude saponins. The optimum dose in cattle was estimated at about 1 mg per dose of vaccine, which is about 20% of the dose generally considered to be needed for crude saponins.

These observations led to the production of commercially available Quil A (Superfos, Denmark). This product has the advantage of being standardized, and the adjuvant activity is predictable. Its composition is still complex when analyzed by modern high-resolution techniques, high performance liquid chromatography (HPLC) and high performance thin-layer chromatography (HPTLC) (Dalsgaard, unpublished data). Further separation of quillaja saponins was achieved using these techniques. Kensil *et al.* (1988) detected 22 peaks with saponin activity in a HPLC separation of a methanol extract of crude quillaja bark. Adjuvant activity could be demonstrated in 14 peaks in mice using BSA as antigen. Four of these peaks were major and could be further purified in milligram amounts. Fast-atom bombardment mass spectroscopy was performed on three of the peaks and results indicated approximate pseudo-molecular ion masses of 1870, 1980, and 2310. Nuclear magnetic resonance spectra were too complex for a complete determination of molecular structure, but the sugar moieties could be analyzed in further detail. The sugars detected were rhamnose, fucose, arabinose, xylose, galactose, glucose, apiose, and glucuronic acid. There was substantial similarity in the carbohydrate composition of the different saponins, but subtle differences distinguish the individual substances.

Higuchi (1987) proposed a structural formula for a partially hydrolyzed component from quillaja saponin. This substance was not tested for adjuvant activity, but similar hydrolysis products were obtained by Kensil *et al.* (1988), none of which were adjuvants, indicating that even mild alkaline hydrolysis should be avoided. Although the saponin adjuvants are complicated molecules, it is to be expected that ongoing research soon will result in the description of the complete structural formula of a quillaja saponin with adjuvant activity.

In the literature, when saponin is used as an adjuvant it is rare to see indications of the origin of the plant material from which the saponin was extracted, except when Quil A was used. However, it is likely that most authors have used saponins extracted from *Quillaja saponaria* Molina since these saponins are the most commonly available, adjuvant-active saponins produced on a large scale. Saponins from other plants may be active as well, but considering the difficulties in growing, collecting, and extracting the plant material, adjuvant research on saponins has been almost exclusively limited to saponins from quillaja bark. Adjuvant effect has been obtained normally when the saponin is mixed with the antigen and applied parenterally, but Chavali and Campbell (1987) studied the influence of saponins from different defined sources when given by the oral route. The saponins were derived from quillaja, licorice, and ginseng. It was demonstrated that oral application in mice exhibited nonspecific immunostimulatory activities, i.e., the production of interferon and/or other cytokines. Also, mice vaccinated intraperitoneally against rabies showed increased resistance to challenge after oral administration of quillaja saponins (Chavali and Campbell, 1987). Application by the oral route represents an interesting approach because by this route saponins are widely nontoxic and permitted as food additives (Chavali and Campbell, 1987). This is in contrast to the normal way of application as adjuvants, subcutaneously or intramuscularly, where saponins exert a strong local reaction when applied in excessive doses. However, in most cases it is possible to find a balance between the antigen in question and the saponin dose where the saponin is well tolerated and still has strong adjuvant activity. Compared to technical crude saponins, Quil A is enriched in adjuvant-active saponins, and the dose of Quil A needed is usually about 20% of what is described for the crude preparations. The dose should always be adjusted to the antigen preparation and the animal species used. As a guideline for experiments, Quil A may be applied using a dose of 10 μg in mice, 50 μg in guinea pigs, 200 μg in rabbits, 500 μg in pigs, and 1000 μ in cattle (Dalsgaard, 1978, 1984). Horses, dogs, and cats seem to be somewhat more sensitive to Quil A, but commercial vaccines containing Quil A are available against equine influenza virus, canine parvovirus, and feline leukemia virus.

Several papers deal with the adjuvant activity of saponin/Quil A in foot-and-mouth disease vaccines (Dalsgaard and Jensen, 1977; Dalsgaard, 1978), and this vaccine is still by far the largest application for saponin adjuvants. Usually saponin is used in combination with aluminum hydroxide gel as adjuvant (Dalsgaard, 1978). It could probably replace aluminum hydroxide, but this is added not only because of its adjuvant activity but also because of its stabilizing effect on the viral antigen (Lei, 1985). Combination of saponin with oil adjuvants is rare but possible (Gerber, 1987). Quil A was successfully applied in a bovine ephemeral fever vaccine (Vanselow et al., 1985).

The second important area where saponin adjuvants have been applied successfully is in parasite immunology. Effective immunization using saponin as adjuvant has been achieved against *Schistosoma mansoni* (Smithers et al., 1989; James and Pearce, 1988), *Plasmodium knowlesi* (Deans et al., 1988), *Plasmodium yoelii* (Playfair and de Souza, 1986; Freeman and Holder, 1983; McColm et al., 1982), *Trypanosoma cruzi* (Scott et al., 1984; Neal and Johnson, 1977; McHardy, 1977), *Trypanosoma brucei* (Wells et al., 1982), *Babesia bovis* (Kuttler et al., 1981, 1983; Smith et al., 1981), and *Babesia canis* (Molinar et al., 1982). Scott and Neal (1984) reported that protection against *Trypanosoma cruzi* in mice was completely dependent on saponin adjuvant. Both specific antibody and cell-mediated immunity were potentiated strongly by saponin. In a comparative study (Scott et al., 1984) a wide range of adjuvants (Alhydrogel, saponin, *Corynebacterium parvum*, DDA, avridine, oil adjuvants, and several MDP analogs) were tested in mice with a *T. cruzi* 90-kDa cell surface glycoprotein for the ability to protect against a lethal challenge infection. Only saponin was effective. No particular Ig isotope was promoted preferentially, and saponin was unique in its ability to promote cell-mediated immunity against the 90-kDa glycoprotein.

Saponin was used in a mycoplasma strain F-38 sonicated vaccine in goats (Mulira et al., 1988) and compared to Alhydrogel and FIA. The goats were challenged after 4 months, and it was concluded that saponin and FIA were similar in their immune potentiation ability and were superior to Alhydrogel.

In bacteria, saponin/Quil A also has potent adjuvant activity. Quil A was used in sheep in a vaccine against *Bacterioides nodosus* (Egerton et al., 1978). Quil A was combined with Alhydrogel. The sheep had higher agglutinin antibody titers and higher recovery rates from infection, when Quil A was included. A 68-kDa protein antigen from *Bordetella bronchiseptica* was identified (Montaraz et al., 1985). When mice were immunized with this preparation in combination with saponin or FIA, significant protection against challenge was induced. A cattle vaccine based on *E. coli* K99 pilus antigen was tested in combination with different adjuvants for the induction of colostrum and milk secretory antibodies (Bachmann et al., 1984). It was concluded that the highest titers and the longest lasting secretion was obtained when the antigen was adsorbed to Alhydrogel and saponin was added. A sheep vaccine against *Corynebacterium pseudotuberculosis* was prepared (Cameron and Bester, 1984). Various adjuvants could not significantly improve the immunogenicity, but the combination of Alhydrogel and saponin did have a beneficial effect, and the vaccine was dependent on the adjuvant.

In a study on the enhancement of the immunogenic activity of ribosomal preparations from *Haemophilus influenzae* (Cabrera-Contreras *et al.*, 1985) various adjuvants were tested. Saponin, Alhydrogel, and diphtheria-pertussis-tetanus vaccine significantly enhanced the immunoprotective response in mice. The response was equal to or better than that of FIA. Muramyldipeptidepoly (A : U), and a mycobacterial extract failed to provide adjuvant activity in this system. Quil A enhanced the immune response to a pneumococcal type 14 capsular polysaccharide–bovine serum albumin conjugate (Verheul *et al.*, 1989) in mice. The immunogenicity of the conjugate was dependent on the coupling procedure. An interesting approach to modern vaccines is the use of anti-idiotypes. In an experiment (Oosterlaken *et al.*, 1988) where neutralizing monoclonal antibodies against Semliki Forest virus were coupled to keyhole limpet hemocyanin (KLH) and injected into BALB/c mice, potent antisera were obtained using Quil A as an adjuvant.

The mechanism of action of saponin/Quil A was studied by several authors. In a study on the comparative selectivity of adjuvants for humoral and cell mediated-immunity (Bomford, 1980a,b) significant differences among the various adjuvants tested were recorded. The humoral antibody response was studied using BSA and SRBC as antigens. In mice a relatively poor response was obtained using BSA and saponin as adjuvant, whereas saponin was outstandingly the best adjuvant for SRBC. Considering the success of saponin with parasite antigens it is concluded that saponin may be a particularly effective adjuvant for antigens in cell membranes. Cell-mediated immunity was tested by the delayed-type hypersensitivity test (DTH) in mice. DTH response against SRBC could not be obtained with saponin. Only *Propionibacterium acnes* was able to induce this response, and only when injections were made in the footpad rather than in the flank. However, saponin potentiated a DTH response to ovalbumin when injected as an aqueous solution. In a paper on the cellular site of action of the adjuvant activity of saponin for SRBC (Bomford, 1984), it was concluded that saponin attached to SRBC ghosts potentiated with humoral response in mice, but injection of saponin 1 or 2 days before or after SRBC at the same S.C. site was also effective. After the S.C. injection of saponin and SRBC the number of cells in the draining lymph node increased sixfold, and indirect plaque-forming cells appeared in it and in the spleen. Splenectomy increased the adjuvant activity of saponin, but T cell depletion abolished it. It was concluded that saponin does not have to be attached to the antigen, the effect is exerted on host cells in the draining lymph node, and it is T cell-dependent in this system. In a later paper (Scott et al., 1985) using KLH as antigen, it was shown that saponin increased the retention of antigen at the site of injection, and also increased the amount of (radiolabeled) antigen reaching the spleen. Both phenomena could be ascribed to the inflammatory response induced by the surface active saponin. When the saponin was "saturated" with cholesterol-containing liposomes both phenomena were inhibited. The most interesting observation was that this treatment did not inhibit adjuvant activity. This was supported by a parallel experiment using digitonin, a steroidal saponin that shares the hemolytic and cholesterol-binding activity of quillaja saponin. Digitonin caused similar antigen retention and splenic localization of antigen, but it was not adjuvant active.

The adjuvant activity of Quil A with T-dependent (DNP-KLH) and with T-independent TNP-brucella (TI-1 antigens) and TNP-Ficoll (TI-2 antigens) was studied in mice (Flebbe and Braley-Mullen, 1986a,b). As expected, Quil A potentiated the response to DNP-KLH, but it also augmented both the IgM and the IgG responses to TNP-brucella and TNP-Ficoll unlike most commonly used adjuvants, which have no effect on T-independent antigens. Quil A could augment both optimal and suboptimal doses of antigen, and it was also active when given in separate injections from the antigen. Quil A was also effective in augmenting the primary response to TNP-Ficoll in athymic nude mice. This effect could be inhibited by the mitotic inhibitor Velban indicating that Quil A at least partially exerts its effect through B cells and that the plaque-forming cell response primarily was obtained by stimulating cell proliferation and not by recruitment of antigen-reactive cells. By adoptive transfer experiments it was demonstrated that carrier-specific T cells were increased by Quil A in mice primed with the T-dependent antigen DNP-KLH. Quil A was unable to augment memory cell induction to the T-independent antigen, TNP-Ficoll, although both the primary IgM and IgG responses to this antigen were markedly increased. It was concluded that Quil A can mediate its adjuvant activity by a direct or indirect effect on B cells, although T cells may be affected to some extent. In an attempt to induce experimental autoimmune thyroiditis (EAT) in mice (Williams et al., 1987), mouse thyroglobulin (Mtg) was injected with different adjuvants. EAT was obtained by some adjuvants, but Quil A was ineffective. Quil A did not induce Mtg antibodies nor did it prime mice for the development of an *in vitro* proliferation response to Mtg, or *in vitro* activation and transfer of EAT.

Different adjuvants were compared for their ability to induce mouse polyclonal and monoclonal antibodies to human serum albumin (HSA) and interleukin-1α (Kenney et al., 1989). A number of important parameters were monitored i.e., titer, affinity, concentration, isotope, epitope specificity, and neutralizing activity. Quil A, Alhydrogel and threonyl-muramyldipeptide elicited the highest affinity antibodies to HSA. All adjuvants, particularly Quil A and Ribi adjuvant system, were superior to Freund's in eliciting antibodies that bound native versus denatured HSA. The study concluded that adjuvants selectively and independently enhance different qualities of the antibody response. Choosing the appropriate adjuvant can optimize production of monoclonal antibodies with desired qualities.

V. ISCOMS

The saponin adjuvant Quil A (Dalsgaard, 1974) contains components that apart from being adjuvant active have a unique capability to form stable complexes of extreme regularity with antigen and lipids. Evidence was presented in the previous section that Quil A does not necessarily have to be injected at the same site as the antigen to be adjuvant active. But if Quil A is allowed to interact with the antigen and certain lipids, especially cholesterol, under defined conditions, immunostimulating complexes (ISCOMs) are formed. ISCOMs are highly immunogenic, and the amount of Quil A needed to enhance the immune response is much lower in ISCOMs than with free Quil A. Apparently, the organization of the antigen in a multimeric regular form in an appropriate size for recognition by immunocompetent cells in combination with the simultaneous presentation of a potent adjuvant results in pronounced adjuvant activity.

Information on ISCOMs was published for the first time in 1984 (Morein et al., 1984). Since then about 50 papers on ISCOMs have appeared. One of the reasons for their popularity is that because the amount of Quil A included in ISCOMs is low, practically no adverse reactions have been reported. But the main reason is their high immunogenicity, which in comparative studies often has shown their superiority to most other adjuvants. There are two recent reviews (Morein et al., 1987; Höglund et al., 1989) that cover most of the aspects of ISCOM technology and applications. This section will cover the latest publications not included in the other reviews.

The humoral immune response in rats by measles virus antigens was investigated using ISCOMs, liposomes, or virus (Mougin et al., 1988). The rats were immunized with syngeneic peritoneal exudate cells fed *in vitro* with the various antigen preparations. A strong and persistent hemagglutination inhibiting and neutralizing antibody response was observed using any of the three preparations. The responses were very similar, but the dose of protein needed was 20 times lower for ISCOMs than for liposomes. Feeding of peritoneal exudate cells with soluble H and F glycoproteins resulted in a poor and transient response. Although the ISCOMs had a preferential incorporation of F antigen, they induced an equal anti-H and anti-F antibody response.

Bovine herpesvirus type-1 ISCOMs were prepared and characterized physicochemically (Merza et al., 1988). Glycosylated viral proteins were shown to be present in the ISCOMs, and a high degree of immunogenicity was observed in mice using this preparation. Trudel et al. (1988a) used similarly prepared BHV1 ISCOMs and compared the immunogenicity of 3×50 μg or 3×25 μg of these to a commercial live attenuated vaccine in calves. The ISCOM vaccine consistently gave a serological response superior to that of the attenuated vaccine, and calves vaccinated with ISCOMs were protected against challenge, whereas control animals showed signs of respiratory distress. Although the clinical course was milder after challenge of the group vaccinated with the attenuated vaccine, virus shedding was only reduced by a factor of 100 compared to a 10,000-fold reduction in the group of calves vaccinated with ISCOMs.

The purified envelope glycoprotein (gp 340) from Epstein-Barr virus (EBV) was inserted into ISCOMs (Ulaeto et al., 1988). Specific T cell proliferation was observed in blood mononuclear cell cultures from EBV-immune individuals when challenged with the ISCOM preparation or inactivated virus. Stable $CD3,^+$ $CD4,^+$ and $CD8^-$ T cell clones were generated. Rubella virus subunit ISCOMs were shown to be as effective as a commercial live attenuated vaccine in the induction of neutralizing and hemagglutination-inhibiting antibodies in rabbits (Trudel et al., 1988b). In a search for an animal model for demyelinating peripheral neuropathy associated with myelin-associated glycoprotein (MAG), cats were injected with MAG in Freund's adjuvant and in ISCOMs (Kahn et al., 1989). Freund's adjuvant did not induce antibody whereas 4 injections of ISCOMs induced IgM antibodies, which bound to human MAG and cat peripheral nerve myelin. Subunits from respiratory syncytial virus (RSV) were incorporated into ISCOMs. Preparations were made from the surface proteins of both human and bovine RSV. Both preparations induced antibodies in guinea pigs that were able to neutralize the human and the bovine virus. ISCOMs prepared from bovine RSV were significantly more effective than preparations containing the human virus. The glycoprotein gp51 from bovine leukemia virus (BLV) inserted into ISCOMs was highly immunogenic (Merza et al., 1988). The expression of neutralization epitopes on the surface of ISCOMs was determined using monoclonal antibodies. It was found to be highly dependent on the detergent used to solubilize gp51 from the virus. Tween-20, Tween-80, or octyl glucoside exposed sites on the ISCOM reacting with neutralizing monoclonals, whereas Triton X-100 and Mega-10 did not.

ISCOMs have created some hope for the development of effective vaccines against retroviruses. The glycoprotein gp70 and the transmembrane protein p15e of feline leukemia virus (FeLV) were incorporated into an ISCOM vaccine (Osterhaus et al., 1989). This vaccine was compared to a commercially available inactivated FeLV vaccine, and to a preparation not containing gp70 or p15e. Cats were immunized 3 times. Serological responses were measured by ELISA, membrane immunofluorescence, and virus neutralization. In contrast to the cats in the other groups, almost all cats vaccinated with ISCOM vaccine showed seroconversion with increased titers in all three tests. Western blots confirmed the presence of antibodies against gp70 and p15e. Further biochemical characterization of the FeLV ISCOMs, including the confirmation of the incorporation of the different proteins, was reported by Akerblom et al. (1989).

The success of FeLV ISCOM vaccines has initiated extensive research on the possibility of making ISCOM vaccines against human immunodeficiency virus (HIV). Pyle et al. (1989) constructed ISCOMs with the HIV-1 B external envelope glycoprotein gp120. This preparation induced a tenfold higher antibody response in mice than gp120 emulsified in Freund's. Rhesus monkeys immunized with ISCOM vaccine produced precipitating and neutralizing antibodies of titers equivalent to those seen in humans and chimpanzees after infection with HIV. After several injections with the ISCOM vaccine one rhesus monkey produced antibodies cross-neutralizing the HIV-1 RF and MN isolates, but not the CC isolate. The monkey antisera recognized gp120 on the membranes of HIV-1 B-infected H9 cells indicating that the correct epitope structure was preserved in the ISCOM preparation.

An antigen preparation from herpes simplex virus type-1 (HSV-1)-infected cell cultures was incorporated into ISCOMs (Erturk et al., 1989). In mice this preparation gave a higher antibody response than the same antigen adsorbed to Alhydrogel. The ISCOMs induced complete protection against an otherwise lethal systemic challenge with HSV-1 and HSV-2. Significant protection against a local challenge by skin scarification was also obtained.

Aujeszky's disease virus ISCOM vaccine was prepared and the efficacy tested in sheep (Morein et al., 1989). The vaccine was applied intradermally or intramuscularly in doses varying from 1 to 81 μg per animal. Vaccination was repeated on day 21, and on day 35 the animals were challenged by subcutaneous inoculation of 1000 TCID$_{50}$ of virulent *Phylaxia* virus. In a second experiment, only one vaccination with doses from 1 to 27 µg and with challenge on day 14 was applied. It was concluded that only one injection of 3 µg of ISCOMs provided protection against Aujesky's disease. No advantage of intradermal vaccination was seen. Western blots were able to discriminate vaccinated from challenged animals.

Using influenza virus ISCOMs and antigen micelles the inflammatory response and antigen localization was studied in mice (Watson *et al.*, 1989). Two hours after intraperitoneal injection polymorphonuclear leukocytes increased from 1 to 82% (ISCOMs) and 41% (micelles), returning to about zero 24 hours postinjection. The total recovery of radioactive antigen was significantly higher in ISCOM-vaccinated animals than in the corresponding group receiving micelles at the times tested, i.e., 1, 2, and 8 days postinjection. Animals vaccinated with ISCOMs had significantly more radioactive antigen in the spleen cells at all times tested. ISCOM structures could be detected by electron microscopy and it was found that they were closely attached to plasma membranes (externally), or internally in phagosomes of macrophages close to the membranes.

The literature cited has clearly demonstrated that ISCOMs have a great potential for the development of efficient second-generation vaccines in animals as well as in humans. One ISCOM vaccine against equine influenza virus is already on the market in Sweden and others are likely to follow. ISCOM vaccines have the capacity to stimulate antibody- as well as cell-mediated immunity including cytotoxic T-memory cells, a feature that is unique for nonreplicating vaccines, and of crucial importance in protection against disease. ISCOMs stimulate local immunity after application on mucosal membranes.

Most ISCOM vaccines have been prepared from antigen released from membranes. Such antigens have a natural affinity for hydrophobic interaction with the Quil A/lipid matrix, but techniques are available to modify soluble antigens in such a way that they can be incorporated into ISCOMs. This can be achieved by chemical exposure of intrinsic hydrophobic domains or by the introduction of acyl- or other groups into the antigen. Also, short antigens may be coupled to preformed ISCOMs carrying important T cell epitopes. The versatility of the ISCOM and its powerful adjuvant effect makes it an important antigen-presenting system.

VI. Muramyldipeptides

Analysis of the active components of Freund's complete adjuvant revealed that muramyldipeptide (MDP, *N*-acetylmuramyl-L-alanyl-D-isoglutamine) is the smallest active unit of the mycobacterium (Ellouz et al., 1974). MDP is a small molecule and very soluble in water. It demonstrated moderate adjuvanticity when used as a plain substance and several strategies were followed to improve the adjuvanticity. Formulation in a water-in-oil emulsion, incorporated into liposomes (Kotani et al., 1977), covalent attachment of MDP to a carrier molecule (Chédid et al., 1979), or to the antigen (Audibert et al., 1982; Carelli et al., 1982) substantially increased the immunostimulatory effect. In addition to adjuvanticity, MDP evokes a variety of immunologic and pharmacologic reactions in the host, such as inflammation, pyrogenic reactions, necrosis, and granulomas. In order to identify molecules with strong adjuvant activity but devoid of adverse side effects, more than 300 MDP derivatives (MDPs) were synthesized. MDPs with substituted sugar moieties or amino acids and with lipophilic groups at different sites of the molecules were prepared. The MDPs obtained exhibited distinct effects and a relationship with the chemical structure was sought.

Lipophilic MDPs proved to be effective stimulators of antibody responses, cell-mediated immunity, and nonspecific resistance (Kotani et al., 1986). In addition to these activities, most of them exerted a wide range of other biologic effects and only a few (L-18-MDP, B30-MDP, MTP-cholesterol, and MDP-PE) exhibited strong immunomodulatory potentials with minor side effects (Kotani et al., 1986).

Substitution of the sugar moiety or amino acids yielded derivatives with distinct pharmacologic and immunologic profiles. Minor modifications in molecular structure substantially affected immunomodulatory or immunostimulatory potentials. For example, displacement of the terminal D-isoglutamin by L-isoglutamin, D- or L-glutamine dramatically reduced the adjuvant properties. Comparison of the distinct activity profiles of MDPs revealed two promising immunoadjuvants, namely threonyl-MDP and murabutide. Threonyl-MDP, in which L-alanyl is displaced by L-threonyl, proved to be a strong adjuvant without significant side effects and is a relevant component of SAF-1 for cellular immune responses (Byars and Allison, 1987).

VII. Polymeric Adjuvants

The adjuvants mentioned above form an interface separating two physical phases. Binding of protein antigens to this interface may be an important aspect of adjuvanticity. Distinct from these types of adjuvants is the group of water-soluble polymers, including polyanions, such as dextran sulphate (Diamantstein *et al.*, 1971a,b; Bradfield *et al.*, 1974; van der Meer *et al.*, 1977; McCarthy *et al.*, 1977), carrageenan (Mancino and Minucci, 1983), polynucleotides (Johnson *et al.*, 1986; Hovanessian *et al.*, 1988), polycarboxylates (Diamantstein *et al.*, 1970), and polycations, e.g., diethylaminoethyl (DEAE)-dextran (Joo and Emod, 1988; Wittmann *et al.*, 1970a,b; Wittmann, 1972; Wittmann and Jakubik, 1977; Skoda and Wittmann, 1973; Jakubik *et al.*, 1975). As a considerable quantity of information is available on adjuvanticity of dextran sulfate (DXS) and the possible mode(s) of action, we will focus on this polymer.

DXS is a semisynthetic polymer of glucose derivatized with sulphate groups. The molecular weight varies from less than 10,000 to 500,000 Da and adjuvant activity has been demonstrated for many different antigens in various animal models. DXS can modify specific immune responses, including cellular and humoral responses, and nonspecific resistance. In laboratory animals, DXS stimulated antibody response to various thymus-dependent antigens, such as sheep red blood cells (Diamantstein *et al.*, 1971b; Hilgers *et al.*, 1984a), and DNP-BSA (Hilgers *et al.*, 1987a), but not against the thymus-independent antigen DNP-Ficoll (Hilgers *et al.*, 1984a). Opposite effects on cellular immunity of DXS were noticed as cellular responses against SRBC (McCarthy *et al.*, 1977), ovalbumin (McCarthy *et al.*, 1977), and *Listeria monocytogenes* (van der Meer *et al.*, 1977) were enhanced, while those against A-PE plus DDA (Hilgers *et al.*, 1987b) and *Mycobacterium tuberculosis* (Babcock and McCarthy, 1977) were suppressed. Carrageenan, another high-molecular weight, sulphated polysaccharide based on galactose, demonstrated depressive (Neveu and Thierry, 1982; Murthy and Ragland, 1984; Elfaki *et al.*, 1987) rather than stimulatory (Mancino and Minucci, 1983) effects on either humoral or cellular immunity to various thymus-dependent antigens.

Little is known about the effects of polyanions in larger animals. In pigs, the humoral immune response to nonviable *Mycoplasma hyopneumoniae* was enhanced by DXS (Kishima *et al.*, 1985) and protection to an experimental infection was improved. DXS substantially stimulated the antibody response against ovalbumin (Beh and Lascelles, 1985) and *Staphylococcus aureus* in sheep (Watson, 1987), but only marginally stimulated the antibody response to bovine ephemeral fever vaccine in calves (Vanselow *et al.*, 1985).

The cationic polymer DEAE–dextran displayed significant adjuvant activity in large animals. It stimulated the humoral response against ovalbumin in sheep (Beh and Lascelles, 1985), foot-and-mouth disease virus, and pseudorabies virus in cattle (Wittmann *et al.*, 1970b; Jakubik *et al.*, 1975) and pigs (Wittmann *et al.*, 1971a; Wittmann, 1972; Wittmann and Jakubik, 1977; Skoda and Wittmann, 1973). Immune responses to bovine diarrhea virus plus $Al(OH)_3$ were further enhanced on addition of DEAE–dextran (Chen *et al.*, 1985). In contrast to DXS and DEAE–dextran, the polynucleotide poly(A : U) was not effective in the stimulation of antibody titers against ovalbumin in sheep (Beh and Lascelles, 1985).

The mechanisms underlying adjuvanticity of DXS have been studied extensively. DXS can bind to serum lipoproteins (Basu *et al.*, 1979), but binding to antigens has not been demonstrated. Physical interaction of antigen and DXS is therefore considered to be relatively unimportant. This assumption is supported by the finding that DXS can stimulate the immune response even if antigen and adjuvant are given via distinct routes (Hilgers *et al.*, 1986a). Many investigations indicate that DXS can influence the host immune system via different pathways and strong adjuvanticity of DXS is considered to be the result of the effects of lymphocytes, the complement system, and phagocytic cells.

In vivo, DXS induced lymphocytosis (Bradfield and Born, 1974) with an optimum at 3 hours after intraperitoneal injection (Sasaki *et al.*, 1987). It promotes the retention of antigen at the site of injection and in the draining lymph nodes (Nakashima *et al.*, 1981). *In vitro,* DXS proved to be an activator of immature and mature B cells (Nariuchi and Kakiuchi, 1981; Nakashima *et al.*, 1980, 1981). It also increased the responsiveness of B cells to other polyclonal activators (Bouwer and Hinrichs, 1986), and synergistic mitogenic stimulation of B cells by combinations of DXS and lipopolysaccharides could be observed (Wetzel and Kettman, 1981a,b; Bergstedt-Lindquist *et al.*, 1982). DXS has been shown to be mitogenic also for human T cells and to stimulate interleukin-2 production (Palacois *et al.*, 1982). Specific receptors for sulphated polysaccharides on murine lymphocytes have been detected (Parish *et al.*, 1984, 1988; Parish and Snowden, 1985) and might be involved in the mitogenic stimulation of these cells. Binding of DXS to specific cell-surface receptors on these cells resulted in an influx of Ca^{2+} indicating transmembrane signaling (Tellam and Parish, 1987), and phosphatidylinositol kinase is probably involved in the mitogenic activation (Morelec *et al.*, 1988).

DXS influences also various components of the nonspecific branch of the host immune system (Klerx, 1985; Hilgers, 1987). It is a strong activator of the complement system via the alternate pathway (Loos and Bitter-Suermann, 1976; Klerx *et al.*, 1983), which may cause recruitment and stimulation of lymphocytes and phagocytic cells. Functions of macrophages are influenced, especially those involved in the handling, processing, and elimination of antigen. Phagocytic activity, adherence of macrophages to a substrate (Tam and Hindsdill, 1984), fusion of phagosomes with lysosomes (Bloksma et al., 1980; Kielian and Cohn, 1981, 1982a), and lysosomal enzyme activity (Just et al., 1974; Hilgers, 1987) are impaired by DXS. The capacity of DXS to bind to the plasma membrane of phagocytes, to accumulate in phagosomes and secondary lysosomes (Kielian and Cohn 1982b), and to decrease membrane fluidity (Kielian and Cohn, 1982b) is probably related to the inhibition of phagocyte functions. After a single injection, DXS accumulates in the liver and prohibits the elimination of foreign materials by Kupffer cells in the liver (Patel et al., 1983; Souhami et al., 1981) causing accumulation of antigen in lymphoid organs (Diamantstein et al., 1971b). DXS persists for several months in phagocytes (Ehlers and Diringer, 1984). Apparently, scavenger activity of phagocytic cells is impaired by DXS via multiple pathways. The rate of antigen elimination is reduced and contact of antigen and the host immune system is prolonged and intensified by DXS, which may lead to high levels of immunity. DXS did not increase Ia expression by macrophages (Behbehani et al., 1985), suggesting that it does not promote antigen-presentation functions by these cells. Besides specific immune responses, nonspecific resistance can also be modified by DXS and other polyanions resulting in either increased or reduced susceptibility to certain pathogens. DXS decreased the susceptibility to human immunodeficiency virus (Mitsuya et al., 1988), scrapie virus (Ehlers and Diringer, 1984), *Listeria monocytogenes* (Hahn, 1974), and certain strains of herpes simplex virus, but increased the susceptibility to other HSV strains (Frank et al., 1978) and to *Salmonella typhimurium* (Hof et al., 1982). Several other sulphated polysaccharides exhibited antiviral activity (Gonzalez et al., 1987). These findings suggest that sulphated polysaccharides can be applied therapeutically against certain infectious diseases. The mechanisms of antiviral activity are probably quite similar to those underlying adjuvanticity and include inhibition of virus adsorption (Baba et al., 1988), internalization into cells, and fusion of membranes.

VIII. General Conclusions

Effective vaccination includes the induction and persistence of certain levels of specific immunity assessed in most cases by specific antibody titers in serum. Cellular and local immunity and immunologic memory that can be boosted by a natural infection, however, play important roles in immunity against certain infectious diseases. Stimulation of humoral immune responses by adjuvants is investigated extensively and a great number of active compounds have been described (Borek, 1977; Edelman, 1980; Vanselow, 1987; World Health Organization, 1976). Less attention has been paid to the improvement of cellular and local immunity by adjuvants. A few substances, e.g., FCA, SAF-1, various lipophilic amines (DDA and CP-20,961), and to a lesser extent DXS, are able to enhance cellular responses, and only one or two, including avridine (Anderson et al., 1985; Rubin et al., 1983; Pierce and Sacci, 1984) and cholera toxin (Lycke and Holmgren, 1986; McKenzie and Hasley, 1984), stimulate local immunity.

A number of the adjuvants demonstrated opposite effects on the immune response. According to the definition, an adjuvant enhances the immune response against an antigen injected in conjunction with the adjuvant, but under certain circumstances immune responses may be unaffected or even suppressed.

Mechanisms underlying adjuvanticity and factors affecting the efficacy are still only partially understood. Detailed knowledge of the immune system contributes to our insight in processes determining type and level of immunity and disclose pathways for immunostimulation. Most adjuvants known evoke a series of pharmacologic and immunologic reactions, and discrimination of relevant and nonrelevant processes is complex. Possible modes of adjuvanticity can be deduced from similarities in biological effects of chemically distinct adjuvants and from differences in biologic effects of adjuvant-active and -nonactive analogs (e.g., MDPs, NBPs, and SLPs).

Targets for adjuvants are antigen, the complement system, macrophages, and lymphocytes. Effects of adjuvants on other components of the host immune system have been documented incidentally, e.g., polymorphonuclear cells, NK cells, dendritic cells, Langerhans cells, interleukins, and the endocrine system. As macrophages play a central role in the induction and regulation of immune response, they are considered to be important targets for immunoadjuvants. Several different functions of macrophages can be modified by adjuvants, including phagocytosis and pinocytosis, antigen processing, presentation and elimination, and production of soluble factors.

Many types of adjuvants form an interface between an aqueous phase and another physical phase, e.g., liposomes (Gregoriadis et al., 1987), micelles (Morein and Simons, 1985), insoluble salts, oil droplets, and lipoidal amines. Physicochemical properties of the interface determine binding characteristics and thereby the adjuvant effect. Antigens, but also components of the host immune system, can bind to this inter-

Barei, S., Panina, G. F., Orfei, Z., Nardelli, L., and Castelli, S. (1979). Comparison of the potency for cattle of trivalent FMD vaccines adjuvanted by aluminum hydroxide or oil emulsions. *Zentralbl. Veterinaermed., Reihe B* **26,** 454–460.

Bartha, A. (1974). Immunization of cattle with a polyvalent bovine adenovirus vaccine. *Dev. Biol. Stand.* **26,** 15–18.

Basu, S. K., Brown, M. S., Ho, Y. K., and Goldstein, J. L. (1979). Degradation of low density lipoprotein-dextran sulphate complexes associated with deposition of cholesteryl esters in mouse macrophages. *J. Biol. Chem.* **254,** 7141–7146.

Beh, K. J., and Lascelles, A. K. (1985). The effect of adjuvants and prior immunization on the rate and mode of uptake of antigen into afferent popliteal lymph from sheep. *Immunology* **54,** 487–495.

Behbehani, K., Beller, D. I., and Unanue, E. R. (1985). The effects of beryllium and other adjuvants on Ia suppression by macrophages. *J. Immunol.* **134,** 2047–2049.

Bellinzoni, R. C., Blackhall, J., Baro, and Auza, N. (1989). Efficacy of an inactivated oil adjuvanted rotavirus vaccine in the control of calf diarrhea. in press.

Bergstedt-Lindquist, S., Fernandez, C., and Severrinson, E. (1982). A synergistic polyclonal response to dextran sulphate and lipopolysaccharide. Immunoglobulin secretion and cell requirements. *Scand. J. Immunol.* **15,** 439–443.

Berlin, B. S. (1960). Gross physical properties of emulsified influenza virus vaccines and the adjuvant response. *J. Immunol.* **58,** 81–89.

Berlin, B. S. (1962). Tests for biological safety of arlacel A. *Ann. Allergy* **20,** 472–479.

Bloksma, N., de Reuver, M. J., and Willers, J. M. N. (1980). Influence on macrophage functions as a possible basis of immunomodification by polyanions. *Ann. Immunol. (Paris)* **131,** 255–265.

Bloksma, N., de Reuver, M. J., and Willers, J. M. N. (1983). Impaired macrophage functions as a possible basis of immunomodification by microbial agents, tilorone and dimethyldioctadeylammonium bromide. *Antonie van Leeuwenhoek* **49,** 13–22.

Bokhout, B. A., Van Gaalen, C., and Van der Heijden, P. J. (1981). A selected W/O emulsion: Composition and usefulness as an immunological adjuvant. *Vet. Immunol. Immunopathol.* **2,** 491–500.

Bomford, R. (1980a). The comparative selectivity of adjuvants for humoral and cell-mediated immunity. I. Effect on the antibody response to bovine serum albumin and sheep red blood cells of Freund's incomplete and complete adjuvants, alhydrogel, *Corynebacterium parvum, Bordetella pertussis,* muramyl dipeptide and saponin. *Clin. Exp. Immunol.* **39,** 426–434.

Bomford, R. (1980b). The comparative selectivity of adjuvants for humoral and cell-mediated immunity. II. Effect on delayed-type hypersensitivity in the mouse and guinea pigs, and cell-mediated immunity to tumour antigens in the mouse of Freund's incomplete and complete adjuvants, alhydrogel, *Corynebacterium parvum, Bordetella pertussis,* muramyl dipeptide and saponin. *Clin. Exp. Immunol.* **39,** 435–441.

Bomford, R. (1984). Relative adjuvant efficacy of Al(OH)$_3$ and saponin is related to the immunogenicity of the antigen. *Int. Arch. Allergy Appl. Immunol.* **75,** 280–281.

Bomford, R. (1985). Adjuvants. *In* "Animal Cell Biotechnology" (R. E. Spier and J. B. Griffiths, eds.), Vol. 2, pp. 235–249. Academic Press, London.

Bomford, R. (1986). *In* "Progress towards Better Vaccines" (R. Bell and G. Torrigiani, eds.), pp. 177–194. Oxford Univ. Press, London.

Borek, F. (1977). Adjuvants. *In* "The Antigens" (M. Sela, ed.), Vol. 4, pp. 374–428. Academic Press, New York.

Bouwer, A. H. G., and Hinrichs, D. J. (1986). Dextran sulphate-mediated enhancement of mitogen-induced B cell proliferation. *Cell. Immunol.* **97,** 316–321.

Box, P. G. (1985). Biological preparations. European Patent 0.186.368.

Bradfield, J. W. B., and Born, G. V. R. (1974). Lymphocytosis is produced by heparin and other sulphated polysaccharides in mice and rats. *Cell. Immunol.* **14**, 22–26.

Bradfield, J. W. B., Souhami, R. L., and Addison, I. E. (1974). The mechanism of the adjuvant effect of dextran sulphate. *Immunology* **26**, 383–392.

Butler, N. R., Voyce, M. A., Burland, W. L., and Hilton, M. L. (1969). Advantages of aluminum hydroxide adsorbed combined diphtheria tetanus and pertussis vaccines for immunization of infants. *Br. Med. J.* **1**, 663–669.

Byars, N. E. (1984). Two adjuvant-active muramyl dipeptide analogs induce differential production of lymphocyte-activating factor and a factor causing distress in guinea pigs. *Infect. Immun.* **44**, 344–350.

Byars, N. E., and Allison, A. C. (1987). Adjuvant formulation for use in vaccines to elicit both cell-mediated and humoral immunity. *Vaccine* **5**, 223–231.

Cabrera-Contreras, R., Plescia, O., Solotorovsky, M., and Lynn, M. (1985). Enhancement of immunogenic activity of ribosomal preparations from *Haemophilus influenzae* by various adjuvants. *Vaccine* **3**, 103–108.

Cameron, C. M., and Bester, F. J. (1984). An improved *Corynebacterium pseudotuberculosis* vaccine for sheep. *Oonderstepoort J. Vet. Res.* **51**, 263–268.

Carelli, C., Audibert, F., Gaillard, J., and Chédid, L. (1982). Immunological castration of male mice by a totally synthetic vaccine administered in saline. *Proc. Natl. Acad. Sci. U.S.A.* **79**, 5392–5395.

Chavali, S. R., and Campbell, J. B. (1987). Adjuvant effects of orally administered saponins on humoral and cellular immune responses in mice. *Immunobiology* **174**, 347–359.

Chédid, L., Parant, M., Parant, F., Audibert, F., Lefrancier, F., Choay, J., and Sela, M. (1979). Enhancement of certain biological activities of muramyl dipeptide derivatives after conjugation to a multi-poly(DL-alanine)-poly(L-lysine) carrier. *Proc. Natl. Acad. Sci. U.S.A.* **12**, 6557–6561.

Chen, K. S., Johnson, D. W., and Muscoplat, C. C. (1985). Adjuvant enhancement of humoral immune response to chemically inactivated bovine viral diarrhea virus. *Can. J. Comp. Med.* **49**, 91–94.

Chiba, J., and Egashira, Y. (1978). Adjuvant effect of cationic surface-active lipid, dimethyl dioctadecyl ammonium bromide, on the induction of delayed-type hypersensitivity to sheep red blood cells in mice. *Jpn. J. Med. Sci. Biol.* **31**, 361–364.

Coon, J., and Hunter, R. (1973). Selective induction of delayed hypersensitivity by a lipid conjugated protein antigen which is localized in thymus dependent lymphoid tissue. *J. Immunol.* **110**, 183–190.

Cornwell, H. J. C., and Thompson, H. (1982). Vaccination in dogs. *In Practice* **4**, 151–158.

Dalsgaard, K. (1970). Thin-layer chromatographic fingerprinting of commercially available saponins. *Dan. Tidsskr. Farm.* **44**, 327–331.

Dalsgaard, K. (1974). Saponin adjuvants. III. Isolation of a substance from *Quillaja saponaria* Molina with adjuvant activity in foot-and-mouth disease vaccines. *Arch. Gesamte Virusforsch.* **44**, 243–254.

Dalsgaard, K. (1978). A study of the isolation and characterization of the saponin Quil A. *Acta Vet., Scand., Suppl.* **69**, 1–40.

Dalsgaard, K. (1984). Assessment of the dose of the immunological adjuvant Quil A in mice and guinea pigs using sheep red blood cells as model antigen. *Zentralbl. Veterinärmed., Reihe B* **31**, 718–720.

Dalsgaard, K. (1987). Adjuvants. *Vet. Immunol. Immunopathol.* **17**, 145–152.

Dalsgaard, K., and Jensen, M. H. (1977). Saponin adjuvants, Part 6: The adjuvant activity of Quil-A in trivalent vaccination of cattle and guinea-pigs against foot-and-mouth disease. *Acta Vet. Scand.* **18**, 367–373.

Deans, J. A., Knight, A. M., Jean, W. C., Waters, A. P., Cohen, S., and Mitchell, G. H. (1988). Vaccination trials in rhesus monkeys with a minor invariant *Plasmodium knowlesi* 66-kD merozoite antigen. *Parasite Immunol.* **10**, 535–552.

Diamantstein, T., Wagner, B., Beyse, I., and Odenwald, M. V. (1970). Zum Mechanismus der Stimulierung der humoralen Antikörperbildung durch Polyanionen. *Z. Klin. Chem. Klin. Biochem.* **8**, 632–636.

Diamantstein T., Wagner, B., Beyse, I., Odenwald, M. V., and Schultz, G. (1971a). Stimulation of humoral antibody formation by polyanions. II. The influence of sulphate esters of polymers on the immune response in mice. *Eur. J. Immunol.* **1**, 340–346.

Diamantstein, T., Meinhold, H., and Wagner, B. (1971b). Stimulation of humoral antibody formation by polyanions. V. Relationship between enhancement of sheep red blood cell uptake by the spleen and adjuvant action of dextran sulfate. *Eur. J. Immunol.* **1**, 429–433.

Edelman, R. (1980). Vaccine adjuvants. *Rev. Infect. Dis.* **2**, 370–383.

Egerton, J. R., Laing, E. A., and Thorley, C. M. (1978). Effect of Quil A, a saponin derivative, on the response of sheep to alum precipitated *Bacteroides nodosus* vaccine. *Vet. Sci. Commun.* **2**, 247–252.

Ehlers, B., and Deringer, H. (1984). Dextran sulphate 500 delays and prevents mouse scrapie by impairment of agent replication in spleen. *J. Gen. Virol.* **65**, 1325–1330.

Elfaki, M. G., Daw, D. L., Murthy, K. K., Fletcher, O. J., and Ragland, W. L. (1987). Suppression of humoral immunity in chickens with carrageenan. *Vet. Immunol. Immunopathol.* **16**, 139–150.

Ellouz, F., Adam, A., Ciorbaru, R., and Lederer, E. (1974). Minimal structural requirements for adjuvant activity of bacterial peptidoglycan derivates. *Biochem. Biophys. Res. Commun.* **59**, 1317–1325.

Erturk, M., Jennings, R., Hockley, D., and Potter, C. W. (1989). Antibody responses and protection in mice immunized with herpes simplex virus type 1. Antigen immunestimulating complexes preparations. *J. Gen. Virol.* **70**, 2149–2156.

Espinet, R. G. (1951). Nuevo tipo de vacuna antiaftosa a complejo glucovirico. *Gac. Vet.* **74**, 1–13.

Favre, H., and Mougeot, H. (1981). Appréciation de l'innocuité et de l'efficacité des vaccins anti-aphteux en adjuvants huileux. *Proc. Int. Meet. O.I.E.*, Paris, pp. 145–166.

Flebbe, L. M., and Braley-Mullen, H. (1986a). Immunopotentiating effects of the adjuvants SGP and Quil A. 1. Antibody response to T-dependent and T-independent antigens. *Cell. Immunol.* **99**, 119–127.

Flebbe, L. M., and Braley-Mullen, H. (1986b). Immunopotentiation by SGP and Quil A. 2. Identification of responding cell populations. *Cell. Immunol.* **99**, 128–139.

Frank, U., Caspary, L., Nahn, H., and Falke, D. (1978). The effect of dextransulfate 500 on the pathogenesis of Herpes Simplex virus infections in weaning mice. *Arch. Virol.* **58**, 259–268.

Freeman, R., and Holder, A. A. (1983). Characteristics of the protective response of Balb-C mice immunized with a purified *Plasmodium yoelii* schizont antigen. *Clin. Exp. Immunol.* **54**, 609–616.

Freund, J., and McDermott, K. (1942). Sensitization to horse serum by means of adjuvants. *Proc. Soc. Exp. Biol. Med.* **49**, 548–553.

Freund, J., and Stone, S. H. (1959). The effectiveness of Tuberculo-plycolipid as an adjuvant in eliciting allergic encephalomyelitis and aspermatogeneis. *J. Immunol.* **82**, 560–567.

Friedewald, W. R. (1944). Adjuvants in immunization with influenza virus vaccines. *Science* **99**, 453–454.

Gall, D. (1966). The adjuvant activity of aliphatic nitrogenous bases. *Immnunology* 11, 369–386.

Gerber, J. D. (1987). Vaccine for stimulating immune response—containing an immunostimulating antigen and a saponin in an oil and water emulsion. Patent Appl. EP 242,205.

Gerraty, N. L. (1988). *Proc. I.P.V.D.S. Symp.*, Rio de Janeiro, Brasil.

Gomes, I., and Auge de Mello, P. (1978). Comparison of oil adjuvanted vaccines prepared with arlacel A Montanide 80. *Bull. C.P.F.A.* 31, 43–44.

Gonggrijp, R., Mullers, W. J. H. A., Dullens, H. F. J., and van Boven, C. P. A. (1985). Antibacterial resistance, macrophage influx and activation induced by bacterial rRNA with dimethyldioctadecylammonium bromide. *Infect. Immun.* 50, 728–733.

Gonzalez, M. E., Alarcon, B., and Carrasco, L. (1987). Polysaccharides as antiviral agents: Antiviral activity of carrageenan. *Antimicrob. Agents Chemother.* 31, 1388–1393.

Goto, N. (1978). Comparative studies on effects of incomplete oil adjuvants with different physical properties. *Jpn. J. Med. Sci. Biol.* 31, 53–79.

Gregoriadis, G. (1988). The immuno adjuvant action of liposomes. *E.A.G. Newsl.* 4, 3–21.

Gregoriadis, G., Davis, D., and Davies, A. (1987). Liposomes as immunological adjuvants: Antigen incorporation studies. *Vaccine* 5, 145–151.

Hahn, H. (1974). Effects of dextran sulphate 500 on cell-mediated resistance to infection with *Listeria monocytogenes* in mice. *Infect. Immun.* 10, 1105–1109.

Hammarström, L., and Edward Smith, C. I. (1978). A new polyclonal B-cell activator. *Cell. Immunol.* 36, 377–382.

Hem, S. L., and White, J. L. (1984). Characterization of aluminum hydroxide for use as an adjuvant in parenteral vaccines. *J. Parenter. Sci. Technol.* 38, 2–10.

Henle, W., and Henle, G. (1945). Effect of adjuvants on vaccination of human beings against influenza. *Proc. Soc. Exp. Biol. Med.* 59, 179–181.

Herbert, W. J. (1965). Multiple emulsions. *Lancet* 16, 771.

Higuchi, R. (1987). Structure of desacylsaponins obtained from the bark of *Quillaja saponaria*. *Phytochemistry* 26, 229–235.

Hilgers, L. A. T. (1987). Immunomodulating properties of synthetic adjuvants. Thesis, State University of Utrecht, Utrecht, The Netherlands.

Hilgers, L. A. T., Snippe, H., Jansze, M., and Willers, J. M. N. (1984a). Immunomodulating properties of two synthetic adjuvants; dependence upon type of antigen, dose and time of administration. *Cell. Immunol.* 86, 393–401.

Hilgers, L. A. T., Snippe, H., Jansze, M., and Willers, J. M. N. (1984b). Effect of *in vivo* administration of different adjuvants on the *in vitro* candidacidal activity of mouse peritoneal cells. *Cell. Immunol.* 90, 14–21.

Hilgers, L. A. T., Snippe, H., Jansze, M., and Willers, J. M. N. (1985). Combination of two synthetic adjuvants: Synergistic effects of a surfactant and a polyanion on the humoral immune response. *Cell. Immunol.* 92, 203–209.

Hilgers, L. A. T., Snippe, H., Jansze, M., and Willers, J. M. N. (1986a). Route-dependent immunomodulation: Local stimulation by a surfactant and systemic stimulation by a polyanion. *Int. Arch. Allergy Appl. Immunol.* 79, 388–391.

Hilgers, L. A. T., Snippe, H., Jansze, M., and Willers, J. M. N. (1986b). Synergistic effects of synthetic adjuvants on the humoral response. *Int. Arch. Allergy Appl. Immunol.* 79, 392–396.

Hilgers, L. A. T., Snippe, H., Jansze, M., and Willers, J. M. N. (1987a). Synthesis (sulfo-) (lipo-) polysaccharides: Novel adjuvants for humoral immune responses. *Immunology* 60, 141–146.

Hilgers, L. A. T., Snippe, H., van Vliet, K. E., Jansze, M., and Willers, J. M. N. (1987b). Suppression of the cellular adjuvanticity of quarternary amines by a polyanion. *Int. Arch. Allergy Appl. Immunol.* **80**, 320–325.

Hilgers, L. A. T., de Reuver, M. J., Vaandrager, A. R., Ong, T., Snippe, H., and Willers, J. M. N. (1988). Serum amyloid P component induction by immunomodulators. *Natl. Immunol. Cell. Growth Regul.* **7**, 328–333.

Hof, H., Emmerling, P., Hacker, J., and Hughes, C. (1982). The role of macrophages in primary and secondary infection of mice with *Salmonella typhimurium*. *Ann. Immunol. (Paris)* **133**, 21–32.

Höglund, S., Dalsgaard, K., Lövgren, B., Sundquist, B., Osterhaus, A., and Morein, B. (1989). Iscoms and immunostimulation with viral antigens. *Subcell. Biochem.* **15**, 39–68.

Hovanessian, A. G., Galabru, J., Riviere, Y., and Montagnier, L. (1988). Efficiency of poly(A)·poly(U) as an adjuvant. *Immunol. Today* **9**, 161–162.

Hunter, R. L., and Bennett, B. (1984). The adjuvant activity of nonionic block polymer surfactants. II. Antibody formation and inflammation related to the structure of triblock and octablock copolymers. *J. Immunol.* **133**, 3167–3175.

Hunter, R. L., and Bennett, B. (1986). The adjuvant activity of nonionic block polymer surfactants. III. Characterization of selected biologically active surfaces. *Scand. J. Immunol.* **23**, 287–300.

Hunter, R. L., Strickland, F., and Kezdy, F. (1981). The adjuvant activity of nonionic block polymer surfactants. I. The role of the hydrophile-lipophile balance. *J. Immunol.* **127**, 1244–1250.

Jakubik, J., Wittmann, G., and Skoda, R. (1975). Immunisierung von kalbern mit der EEI-DEAE-dextran-vakzine gegen die Aujeskysche krankheit. *Zentralbl. Veterinaermed., Reihe B* **22**, 827–832.

James, S. L., and Pearce, E. J. (1988). The influence of adjuvant on induction of protective immunity by a non-living vaccine against schistosomiasis. *J. Immunol.* **140**, 2753–2759.

Jensen, O. M., and Koch, C. (1988). On the effect of Al(OH)$_3$ as an immunological adjuvant. *Acta Pathol. Microbiol. Immunol. Scand.* **96**, 257–264.

Jensen, K. E. (1986). Synthetic adjuvants: Avridine and other interferon inducers. In "Advances in Carriers and Adjuvants for Veterinary Biologics" (R. M. Nervig, P. M. Gouch, M. L. Kaeberle, and C. A. Whetstone, eds.), pp. 79–89. Iowa State Univ. Press, Ames.

Jiskoot, W., Teerlink, T., van Hoof, M. M. M., Bartels, K., Kanhai, V., Crommelin, D. J. A., and Beuvery, E. C. (1986). Immunogenic activity of gonococcal protein I in mice with three different lipoidal adjuvants delivered in liposomes and in complexes. *Infect. Immun.* **54**, 333–338.

Johnson, A. G., Mohrman, M., Odean, M., and Petrequin, P. (1986). Adjuvant action of synthetic polynucleotides. In "Advances in Carriers and Adjuvants for Veterinary Biologics" (R. M. Nervig, P. M. Gouch, M. L. Kaeberle, and C. A. Whetstone, eds.), pp. 71–78. Iowa State Univ. Press, Ames.

Jollès, R., and Paraf, A. (1973). Chemicals and biological basis of adjuvants. *Mol. Biol. Biochem. Biophys.* **13**, 85–90.

Joo, I., and Emod, J. (1988). Adjuvant effect of DEAE–dextran on cholera vaccines. *Vaccine* **6**, 233–237.

Just, W. W., Leon-V., J. O., and Werner, G. (1974). Effect of polyanions on lysosomes and lysosomal enzymes of rat liver *in vitro*. *Hoppe-Seyler's Z. Physiol. Chem.* **355**, 1565–1568.

Khan, S. N., Stanton, N. L., Sumner, A. J., Brown, M. J., Spitalnik, S. L., and Morein, B. (1989). Analysis of the feline immune response to human myelin-associated glycoprotein. *J. Neurol. Sci.* **89,** 141–148.

Kenney, J. S., Hughes, B. W., Masada, M. P., and Allison, A. C. (1989). Influence of adjuvants on the quantity, affinity, isotype, and epitope specificity of murine antibodies. *J. Immunol. Methods* **121,** 157–166.

Kensil, C., Marciani, D. J., Belz, G. A., and Hung, C. H. (1988). Saponin adjuvant. Patent Appl. WO 88/09336.

Kielian, M. C., and Cohn, Z. A. (1981). Modulation of phagosome–lysosome fusion in mouse macrophages. *J. Exp. Med.* **153,** 1015–1027.

Kielian, M. C., and Cohn, Z. A. (1982a). Intralysosomal accumulation of polyanions. I. Fusion of pinocytic and phagocytic vacuole with secondary lysosomes. *J. Cell Biol.* **93,** 866–874.

Kielian, M. C., and Cohn, Z. A. (1982b). Intralysosomal accumulation of polyanions. II. Polyanion internalization and its influence on lysosomal pH and membrane fluidity. *J. Cell Biol.* **3,** 875–882.

Kishima, M., Ross, R. F., and Kuniyasu, C. (1985). Cell-mediated and humoral immune response to *Mycoplasma hyopneumoniae* in pigs enhanced by dextran sulfate. *Am. J. Vet. Res.* **46,** 456–462.

Klerx, J. P. A. M. (1985). Immunological adjuvant activity: Complement-dependent and independent processes. Thesis, State University of Utrecht, Utrecht, The Netherlands.

Klerx, J. P. A. M., Van Dijk, H., Damen, H., Rademaker, P. M., and Willers, J. M. N. (1983). Effects of immunological adjuvants on the mouse complement system. I. The inability of the polyanion heparin to act as an adjuvant is paralleled by inefficient alternative complement pathway inhibition. *Int. J. Immunopharmacol.* **5,** 549–553.

Kotani, S., Kinoshita, F., Morisaki, I., Shimono, T., Okunaga, T., Takada, H., Tsujimoto, M., Watanabe, Y., Kato, K., Shiba, T., Kusumoto, S., and Okada, S. (1977). Immunoadjuvant activities of synthetic 6-O-acyl-N-acetyl-muramyl-L-alanyl-D-isoglutamine with special reference to the effect of its administration with liposomes. *Biken J.* **20,** 95–103.

Kotani, S., Tsujimoto, M., Koga, T., Nagao, S., Tanaka, A., and Kawata, S. (1986). Chemical structure and biological activity relationship of bacterial cell walls and muramyl peptides. *Fed. Proc., Fed. Am. Soc. Exp. Biol.* **45,** 2534–2540.

Kraaijeveld, C. A., Snippe, H., Harmsen, T., and Benaissa-Trouw, B. (1982). Enhancement of delayed-type hypersensitivity and induction of interferon by the lipophilic agents DDA and CP-20,961. *Cell. Immunol.* **74,** 277–283.

Kreuter, J., Berg, U., Liehl, E., Soliva, M., and Speiser, P. P. (1986). Influence of the particle size on the adjuvant effect of particulate polymeric adjuvant. *Vaccine* **4,** 125–129.

Kuttler, K. L., Levy, M. G., James, M. A., and Ristic, M. (1981). Efficacy of a nonviable culture derived *Babesia bovis* vaccine. *Am. J. Vet. Res.* **43,** 281–284.

Kuttler, K. L., Levy, M., G., and Ristic, M. (1983). Cell culture derived *Babesia bovis* vaccine. Sequential challenge exposure of protective immunity during a 6 month post vaccination period. *Am. J. Vet. Res.* **44,** 1456–1459.

Lei, J. C. (1985). Aluminum hydroxide gel—guidelines for adsorption. *Vaccine* **3,** 154–155.

Loos, M., and Bitter-Suermann, D. (1976). Mode of interaction of different polyanions with the first (C1, C1) the second (C2) and the fourth (C4) component of complement. III. Inhibition of C4 and C2 binding site(s) on C1s by polyanions. *Immunochemistry* **13,** 789–791.

Lycke, N., and Holmgren, J. (1986). Strong adjuvant properties of cholera toxin on gut mucosal immune responses to orally presented antigens. *Immunology* **59**, 301–308.

Mancino, D., and Minucci, M. (1983). Adjuvant effects of 1, k and h carrageenans on antibody production in BALB/c mice. *Int. Arch. Allergy Appl. Immunol.* **72**, 359–361.

Mancino, D., and Ovary, Z. (1980). Adjuvant effects of amorphous silica and of aluminum hydroxide on IgE and IgG_1 antibody production in different inbred mouse strains. *Int. Arch. Allergy Appl. Immunol.* **61**, 253–258.

McCandlish, I. A. P., Thompson, H., and Wright, N. G. (1978). Vaccination against canine bordetellosis using an aluminum hydroxide adjuvant vaccine. *Res. Vet. Sci.* **25**, 51–57.

McCarthy, R. E., Arnold, L. W., and Babcock, G. F. (1977). Dextran sulphate: An adjuvant for cell-mediated immune responses. *Immunology* **32**, 963–974.

McColm, A. A., Bomford, R., and Dalton, L. (1982). A comparison of saponin with other adjuvants for the potentiation of protective immunity by a killed *Plasmodium yoelii* vaccine in the mouse. *Parasite Immunol.* **4**, 337–348.

McHardy, N. (1977). Immunization of mice against *Trypanosoma cruzi*. The effect of size of dose and route of injection of immunizing and challenge inocula. *Tropenmed. Parasitol.* **28**, 11–16.

McKenzie, S. J., and Hasley, J. F. (1984). Cholera toxin b subunit as a carrier protein to stimulate a mucosal immune response. *J. Immunol.* **133**, 1818–1824.

Merza, M., Belak, S., and Morein, B. (1988). Characterization of an iscom prepared with envelope glycoproteins of bovine herpesvirus type 1. *J. Vet. Med., Ser. B* **35**, 695–703.

Mitsuya, H., Looney, D. J., Kuno, S., Ueno, R., Wong-Staal, F., and Broder, S. (1988). Dextran sulfate suppression of viruses in the HIV family: Inhibition of virion binding to CD4+ cells. *Science* **240**, 646–649.

Molinar, E., James, M. A., Kakoma, I., Holland, C., and Ristic, M. (1982). Antigenic and immunogenic studies on cell culture derived *Babesia canis*. *Vet. Parasitol.* **10**, 29–40.

Montaraz, J. A., Novotny, P., and Ivanyi, J. (1985). Identification of a 68 kD protective protein antigen from *Bordetella bronchiseptica*. *Infect. Immun.* **47**, 744–751.

Morein, B., Löugren, K., Höglund, S., and Sundquist, B. (1987). The ISCOM: An immunopotentiating complex. *Immunol. Today* **8**, 333–338.

Morein, B., and Simons, K. (1985). Subunit vaccines against enveloped viruses: Virosomes, micelles and other protein complexes. *Vaccine* **3**, 83–93.

Morein, B., Sundquist, B., Höglund, S., Dalsgaard, K., and Osterhaus, A. (1984). Iscom, a novel structure for antigenic presentation of membrane proteins from enveloped viruses. *Nature (London)* **308**, 457–460.

Morein, B., Belak, S., Soos, T., Rusvai, M., McCwire, B. S., and Bognar, K. (1989). Iscom of viral envelope proteins protect against Aujeszky's disease. *Vet. Microbiol.* **20**, 143–154.

Morelec, M.-J., Enserguiex, D., Pedron, T., Girard, R., and Chaby, R. (1988). Opposite effects of lipopolysaccharide and dextran sulfate on membrane phospholipid metabolism of murine B lymphocytes. *Eur. J. Immunol.* **18**, 301–307.

Mougin, B., Bakouche, O., and Gerlier, D. (1988). Humoral immune response elicited in rats by measles viral membrane antigens presented in liposomes and iscoms. *Vaccine* **6**, 445–449.

Muggleton, P. W., and Hilton, M. L. (1967). Some studies on a range of adjuvant systems for bacterial vaccines. *Immunobiol. Stand.* **6**, 29–38.

Mulira, G. L., Masiga, W. N., and Nandokha, E. (1988). Efficacy of different adjuvants to potentiate the immune response to mycoplasma strain F-38. *Trop. Anim. Health Prod.* **20**, 30–34.

Munder, P. G., Ferber, E., Modolell, M., and Fisher, H. (1969). The influence of various adjuvants on the metabolism of phospholipids in macrophages. *Int. Arch. Allergy Appl. Immunol.* **36**, 117–128.

Murthy, K. K., and Ragland, W. L. (1984). Modification of humoral immune response in chicken following treatment with carrageenan. *Vet. Immunol. Immunopathol.* **7,** 347–357.

Nabuurs, M. J. A., Bokout, B. A., and van der Heijden, P. J. (1982). Intraperitoneal injection of an adjuvant for the prevention of post-weaning-diarrhea: A field study. *Prev. Vet. Med.* **1,** 65–76.

Nagy, L. K., and Penn, C. W. (1974). Protective antigens in bovine pasteurellosis. *Dev. Biol. Stand.* **26,** 65–76.

Nakashima, I., Nagase, F., Matsuura, A., and Kato, N. (1980). Adjuvant actions of polyclonal lymphocyte activators. II. Comparison and characterization of their actions in initiation and potentiation of immune responses to T-dependent and T-independent soluble antigens. *Cell. Immunol.* **49,** 360–371.

Nakashima, I., Matsuura, A., Nagase, F., Yokochi, T., and Kato, N. (1981). Adjuvant actions of polyclonal lymphocyte activators. IV. Augmentation of antigen retention occurring early and transiently at the site of injection and in the draining lymph node. *Cell. Immunol.* **57,** 477–485.

Nariuchi, H., and Kakiuchi, T. (1981). Response of spleen cells from mice with X-linked B-cell defect to polyclonal B-cell activators, purified protein derivate of tuberculin and dextran sulphate. *Cell. Immunol.* **61,** 375–380.

Neal, R. A., and Johnson, P. (1977). Immunization against *Trypanosoma cruzi* using killed antigens and with saponin as adjuvant. *Acta Trop.* **34,** 87–96.

Nevue, P. J., and Thierry, D. (1982). Effects of carrageenan—a macrophage toxic agent—on antibody synthesis and on delayed hypersensitivity in the guinea pig. *Int. J. Immunopharmacol.* **4,** 175–179.

Niblack, J. F., Otterness, I. G., Hemsworth, G. R., Wolff, J. S., Hoffmann, W. W., and Kraska, A. R. (1979). A structurally novel, synthetic adjuvant. *J. Reticuloendothel. Soc.* **26,** 655–666.

Olascoaga, R. C. (1978). Résumé des Travaux du C.P.F.A. sur les vaccins avec adjuvants huileux. *Proc. Conf. O.I.E. Foot Mouth Dis., 15th,* Paris.

O'Neill, H. J., Yamauchi, T. N., Cohen, P., and Hardegree, M. C. (1972). Characterisation of mannide monooleate. *J. Pharm. Sci.* **61,** 863–867.

Oosterlaken, T. A. M., Harmsen, M., Tangerman, C., Schielen, P., Kraaijeveld, C. A., and Snippe, H. (1988). A neutralization inhibition enzyme immunoassay for anti-idiotypic antibodies that block monoclonal antibodies neutralizing Semliki Forest virus. *J. Immunol. Methods* **115,** 255–262.

Osterhaus, A., Weijer, K., Uytdehaag, F., Knell, P., Jarrett, O., Akerblom, L., and Morein, B. (1989). Serological responses in cats vaccinated with FELV iscom and an inactivated FELV vaccine. *Vaccine* **7,** 137–141.

Palacois, R., Suguwara, I., and Fernandez, C. (1982). Dextran-sulfate: A mitogen for human T lymphocytes. *J. Immunol.* **128,** 621–624.

Parish, C. R., and Snowden, J. M. (1985). Lymphocytes express a diverse array of specific receptors for sulfated polysaccharides. *Cell. Immunol.* **91,** 201–214.

Parish, C. R., Rylatt, D. B., and Snowden, J. M. (1984). Demonstration of lymphocyte surface lectins that recognize sulphated polysaccharides. *J. Cell Sci.* **67,** 145–158.

Parish, C. R., McPhun, V., and Warren, H. S. (1988). Is a natural ligand of the T lymphocyte CD2 molecule a sulfated carbohydrate? *J. Immunol.* **141,** 3498–3504.

Patel, K. R., Li, M. P., and Baldeschwieler, J. D. (1983). Suppression of liver uptake of liposomes by dextran sulfate 500. *Proc. Natl. Acad. Sci. U.S.A.* **80,** 6518–6522.

Pierce, N. F., and Sacci, J. B. (1984). Enhanced mucosal priming by cholera toxin and procholeragenoid with a lipoidal amine adjuvant (avridine) delivered in liposomes. *Infect. Immun.* **44,** 496–473.

Playfair, J. H. L., and de Souza, J. B. (1986). Vaccination of mice against malaria with soluble antigens. 1. The effect of detergent, route of injection, and adjuvant. *Parasite Immunol.* **8,** 409–414.

Prager, M. D. (1985). DDA as an immunologic adjuvant. *Kodak Lab. Chem. Bull.* **56,** 1–4.

Pyle, S. W., Morein, B., Bess, J. W., Jr., Akerblom, L., Nara, P. L., Nigida, S. M., Jr., Lerche, N. W., Robey, W. G., Fischinger, P. J., and Arthur, L. O. (1989). Immune response to immunostimulatory complexes, iscoms prepared from human immunodeficiency virus type 1, HIV-1 or the HIV-1 external envelope glycoprotein gp120. *Vaccine* **7,** 465–473.

Ramanathan, V. D., Badenoch-Jones, P., and Turk, J. L. (1979). Complement activation by aluminum and zirconium compounds. *Immunology* **37,** 881–888.

Ramon, G. (1925). Sur l'augmentation anormale de l'antitoxine chez les chevaux producteurs de sérum anti-diphtérique. *Bull. Mem. Soc. Cent. Méd. Vét.* **78,** 227–234.

Ramon, G. (1926). Procédés pour accroitre la production des antitoxines. *Ann. Inst. Pasteur, Paris* **40,** 1–10.

Reynolds, J. A., Harrington, D. G., Crabbs, C. L., Peters, C. J., and Diluzio, N. R. (1980). Adjuvant activity of a novel metabolizable lipid emulsion. *Infect. Immun.* **28,** 937–943.

Rijke, E. O., Loeffen, A. H. C., and Lutticken, D. (1988). In "Advances in Immunomodulation" (B. Bizzini and E. Bonmassar, eds.), pp. 433–444. Pythagora Press, Roma-Milan.

Ris, D. R., and Hamel, K. L. (1979). *Leptospira interrogans* serovar pomona vaccines with different adjuvants in cattle. *N. Z. Vet. J.* **27,** 169–171.

Riviera, E., Karlsson, K. S., and Olofson, A. S. (1988). Comparison of the potentiating effect of different adjuvants in pseudorabies vaccines. *Proc. I.P.V.S. Cong.,* Rio de Janeiro, Brazil.

Rubin, D. H., Anderson, A. O., Lucis, D., and Michalek, S. M. (1983). Potentiation of the secretory IgA response by oral and enteric administration of CP-20,961. *Ann. N.Y. Acad. Sci.* **409,** 866–870.

Rweyemamu, M. M., Umehara, O., de Lucca Neto, D., Baltazar, M. de C., Vincente, F. E., and Medeiros Meto, R. da R. (1986). Efficacy of avridine as an adjuvant for Newcastle Disease virus antigen in chickens. *Am. J. Vet. Res.* **47,** 1243–1248.

Sadir, A. M., Schudel, A. A., and Laporte, O. (1988). Response to FMD. vaccines in newborn calf. *Epidem. Inf.* **100,** 135–144.

Sasaki, T., Maede, Y., and Namioka, S. (1987). Immunopotentiation of the mucosa of the small intestine of weaning piglets by peptidoglycan. *Jpn. J. Vet. Sci.* **49,** 235–243.

Scott, M. T., and Neal, R. A. (1984). The vaccine potential of cell surface glycoproteins from *Trypanosoma cruzi*. *Philos. Trans. R. Soc. London, B Ser.* **307,** 63–72.

Scott, M. T., Bahr, G., Moddaber, F., Afchain, D., and Chédid, L. (1984). Adjuvant requirements for protective immunization of mice using a *Trypanosoma cruzi* 90 kilodalton cell surface glycoprotein. *Int. Arch. Allergy Appl. Immunol.* **74,** 373–377.

Scott, M. T., Gross-Sampson, M., and Bomford, R. (1985). Adjuvant activity of saponin. Antigen localization studies. *Int. Arch. Allergy Appl. Immunol.* **77,** 409–412.

Skoda, R., and Wittmann, G. (1973). Die immunisierung von schweinen mit vakzinen aus inaktiviertem Aujesky-virus. *Zentralbl. Veterinaer-med., Reihe B* **20,** 127–138.

Smith, R. D., James, M. A., Ristic, M., Aikawa, M., Vega, Y., and Murguia, C. A. (1981). Bovine babesiasis. Protection of cattle *Bos taurus* with culture derived soluble *Babesia bovis* antigen. *Science* **212,** 335–338.

Smithers, S. R., Hacket, F., Ali, P. O., and Simpson, A. J. (1989). Protective immunization of mice against *Schistosoma mansoni* with purified adult worm surface membranes. *Parasite Immunol.* **11**, 301–318.

Snippe, H., Belder, M., and Willers, J. M. N. (1977). Dimethyldioctadecylammonium bromide as adjuvant for delayed type hypersensitivity in mice. *Immunology* **33**, 931–936.

Snippe, H., de Reuver, M. J., Strickland, F., Willers, J. M. N., and Hunter, R. L. (1981). Adjuvant effect of nonionic block polymer surfactants in humoral and cellular immunity. *Int. Arch. Allergy Appl. Immunol.* **65**, 390–398.

Solyom, F., Fazekas, A., Czelleng, F., Makar, A., and Roith, J. (1977). Efficiency testing of FMD vaccines prepared from strain C with different adjuvants. *Dev. Biol. Stand.* **35**, 113–115.

Souhami, R. L., Patel, H. M., and Ryman, B. E. (1981). The effect of reticuloendothelial blockade on the blood clearance and tissue distribution of liposomes. *Biochim. Biophys. Acta* **674**, 354–371.

Stewart-Tull, D. E. S. (1983). Immunologically important constituents of mycobacteria: Adjuvants. *In* "The Biology of the Myobacteria" (C. Ratledge and J. L. Stanford, eds.), vol. 2, pp. 3–84. Academic Press, London.

Tam, P. E., and Hinsdill, R. D. (1984). Evaluation of immunomodulatory chemicals: Alteration of macrophage function *in vitro*. *Toxicol. Appl. Pharmacol.* **76**, 183–194.

Teerlink, T., Beuvery, E. C., Evenberg, D., and van Wezel, T. L. (1987). Synergistic effect of detergents and aluminum phosphate on the humoral immune response to bacterial and viral membrane proteins. *Vaccine* **5**, 307–314.

Tellam, R. L., and Parish, C. R. (1987). The effect of sulfated polysaccharides on the free intracellular calcium ion concentration of lymphocytes. *Biochim. Biophys. Acta* **930**, 55–64.

Thorley, C. M., and Egerton, J. R. (1981). Comparison of alum-absorbed or non-alum-absorbed oil emulsion vaccines containing either pilate or non-pilate *Bacteroides nodosus* cells in inducing and maintaining resistance of sheep to experimental foot rot. *Res. Vet. Sci.* **30**, 32–37.

Trudel, M., Boulay, G., Sequin, C., Nadon, F., and Lussier, G. (1988a). Control of infectious bovine rhinotraceitis in calves with a BHV-1 subunit-iscom vaccine. *Vaccine* **6**, 525–529.

Trudel, M., Nadon, F., Seguin, C., and Payment, P. (1988b). Neutralizing response of rabbits to an experimental rubella subunit vaccine made from immunostimulating complexes. *Can. J. Microbiol.* **34**, 1351–1354.

Ulaeto, D., Wallace, L., Morgan, A., Morein, B., and Rickinson, A. B. (1988). *In vitro* T cell responses to a candidate Epstein-Barr virus vaccine. Human CD4-positive T cell clones specific for the major envelope glycoprotein GP 340. *Eur. J. Immunol.* **18**, 1689–1698.

Vallée, M. H. (1924). *Bacille tuberculeux* et excipient irresorbable. *C. R. Hebd. Seances Acad. Sci.* **178**, 152–154.

van der Meer, C., Hofhuis, F. M. A., and Willers, J. M. N. (1977). Killed *Listeria monocytogenes* vaccine becomes protective on addition of polyanions. *Nature (London)* **269**, 594–595.

Vannier, P. (1986). Immunisation des porcs charcutiers contre la maladie d'Aujeszky avec 2 vaccins huileux. *Journ. Rech. Porcine Fr.* **18**, 371–380.

Vanselow, B. A. (1987). The application of adjuvants to veterinary medicine. *Vet. Bull.* **57**, 881–896.

Vanselow, B. A., Abetz, I., and Trenfield, K. (1985). A bovine ephemeral fever vaccine incorporating adjuvant quil A: A comparative study using adjuvants quil A, aluminum hydroxide gel and dextran sulphate. *Vet. Rec.* **117**, 37–43.

Verheul, A. F. M., Versteeg, A. A., de Reuver, M. J., Jansze, M., and Snippe, H. (1989). Modulation of the immune response to pneumococcal type 14 capsular polysaccharide protein conjugates by the adjuvant Quil A depends on the properties of the conjugates. *Infect. Immun.* **57,** 1078–1083.

Warren, H. S., and Chédid, L. A. (1988). Future prospect for vaccine adjuvants. *CRC Crit. Rev. Immunol.* **8**(2), 83–101.

Watson, D. L. (1987). Serological response of sheep to live and killed *Staphylococcus aureus* vaccines. *Vaccine* **5,** 275–278.

Watson, D. L., Lovgren, K., Watson, N. A., Fossum, C., Morein, B., and Hoglund, S. (1989). Inflammatory response and antigen localization following immunization with influenza virus iscoms. *Inflammation* **13,** 641–650.

Webster, C. J., and Webster, J. M. (1985). Treatment of equine sarcoids with BCG. *Vet. Rec.* **116,** 131–132.

Wels, P. W., Emery, D. L., Hinson, C. A., Morrison, W. I., and Murray, M. (1982). Immunization of cattle with a variant specific surface antigen of *Trypanozoma brucei*. Influence of different adjuvants. *Infect. Immun.* **36,** 1–10.

Wetzel, G. D., and Kettman, J. R. (1981a). Activation of murine B cells. II. Dextran sulphate removes the requirement for cellular interaction during lipopolysaccharide-induced mitogenesis. *Cell Immunol.* **61,** 176–181.

Wetzel, G. D., and Kettman, J. R. (1981b). Activation of murine B cells. III. Stimulation of B. lymphocyte clonal growth with lipopolysaccharide and dextran sulphate. *J. Immunol.* **126,** 723–731.

White, R. G., Coons, A. H., and Connolly, J. M. (1955). Studies on antibody production. III. The alum granuloma. *J. Exp. Med.* **102,** 73–82.

Willers, J. M. N., Bloksma, N., van der Meer, C., Snippe, H., van Dijk, H., de Reuver, M. J., and Hofhuis, F. M. A. (1979). Regulation of the immune response by macrophages. *Antonie van Leeuwenhoek* **45,** 41–48.

Williams, W. V., Kyriakos, M., Sharp, G. C., and Braley-Mullen, H. (1987). Effects of the adjuvants SGP and Quil A on the induction of experimental autoimmune thyroiditis in mice. *Cell. Immunol.* **104,** 296–303.

Wittmann, G. (1972). Fruhstadien der immunitat nach impfung von schweinen mit einer maul- und klauenseuche DEAE-dextran vakzine. *Zentralbl. Veterinäermed., Reihe B* **19,** 406–411.

Wittmann, G., and Jakubik, J. (1977). Fruhstadien de immunitat nach impfung von ferkeln mit einer inaktiviertem Aujeskyvirus-vakzine. *Zentralbl. Veterinaermed., Reihe B* **24,** 569–575.

Wittmann, G., Bauer, K., and Mussgay, M. (1979a). Versuche zur schutzimpfung von schweinen mit vaksinen aus inaktiviertem maul-und klauenseuche (MKS)-virus. *Arch. Gesamte Virusforsch.* **29,** 139–158.

Wittmann, G., Bauer, K., and Mussgay, M. (1970b). Versuche zur schutsimpfung von rindern mit einem äthyläthylenimin(EEI) diäthylaminoäthyl-dextran (DEAE- D)-vakzine gegen maul- und klauenseuche vom virustyp 01. *Zentralbl. Veterinäermed., Reihe B* **17,** 106–111.

Wong, D. T. O., and Barbaro, J. F. (1976). Production of guinea pig IgG1 homotropic antibodies to hapten-conjugated homologous serum albumin with different adjuvant combinations. *Int. Arch. Allergy Appl. Immunol.* **50,** 155–163.

Woodard, L. F., and Jasman, R. L. (1985). Stable oil-in-water emulsions: Preparation and use as vaccine vehicles for lipophilic adjuvants. *Vaccine* **3,** 137–143.

Woodard, L. F., Jasman, R. L., Farrington, D. O., and Jensen, K. E. (1983). Enhanced antibody-dependent bactericidal activity of neutrophils from calves treated with a lipid amine immunopotentiator. *Am. J. Vet. Res.* **44,** 389–394.

World Health Organization (1976). Immunological adjuvants. *H. O. Tech. Rep. Ser.* **595.**

Zigterman, G. J. W. (1988). Nonionic block polymer surfactants enhance vaccine efficacy. Thesis, State University of Utrecht, Utrecht, The Nethelands.

Zigterman, G. J. W. J., Snippe, H., Jansze, M., and Willers, J. M. N. (1987). Adjuvant effects of nonionic block polymers surfactants on liposome-induced humoral immune response. *J. Immunol.* **138,** 220–225.

A Thymosin–Tuftsin Conjugate As a New Potential Immunomodulator in Cattle

DAVID NEMAT KHANSARI AND PARVIZ JAFARI

Immunobiological Laboratories, Inc., New York, New York 10018

I. Introduction
II. Tuftsin: A Macrophage Activator
   A. Biochemistry of Tuftsin
   B. Metabolism of Tuftsin
   C. Biological Activities of Tuftsin
   D. Summary
III. Thymosin-α: A T Cell Activator
   A. Biochemistry of Thymosin-α
   B. Effect of Thymosin-α on Lymphocytes
   C. Effect of Thymosin-α on Cyclic Nucleotides
   D. Clinical Applications of Thymosin-α
   E. Summary
IV. Thymosin–Tuftsin Conjugate (IMP-1)
   A. Synthesis
   B. Biological Activity *in vitro* on Bovine Immunocytes
   C. Biological Activity *in vivo*
V. Conclusion
   References

I. Introduction

Many infectious diseases in beef and dairy cattle have a multifactor etiology and involve the interaction of a stressed host with a viral and/or bacterial challenge. This interaction concept is particularly well accepted in the case of respiratory disease complex in calves which causes annual losses of more than $500 million in the United States alone (Roth, 1982; Filion *et al.*, 1984; von Tungeln, 1986).

Bovine respiratory disease (BRD), commonly known as "shipping fever", is especially prevalent among animals that have been weaned, transported, and placed in a feedlot. In spite of the development of numerous vaccines and antibiotic therapy for the prevention and treatment of BRD, a successful strategy for management of this disease has not been developed. The clinical symptoms, lesions, and mortality of shipping fever are commonly attributed to bacterial pneumonia caused by *Pasteurella haemolytica, Pasteurella multocida,* or *Hemophilus somnus* and to numerous viral agents (Roth, 1984). These agents are generally nonpathogenic if the host's defense system is not compromised (Lopez *et al.,* 1976), suggesting that immunosuppression is an important contributing factor in the pathogenicity of these organisms (Frank, 1986). The mechanism(s) of induced immunosuppression is not fully understood. There is, however, a great deal of evidence suggesting that environmental and/or physical stress can lead to induction of immunosuppression, which in turn can lead to greater susceptibility to infections (Kelley, 1980).

Infections can be controlled by either direct chemotherapy or agents capable of enhancing the specific or nonspecific immune responses of the host. Attempts by many investigators to intervene in the immunosuppression of stressed animals with synthetic or recombinant immunomodulators have produced encouraging results (Roth and Kaeberle, 1984; Larsson *et al.,* 1985; Blecha, 1986). These findings suggest that this approach, the administration of immunopotentiators, may be an effective strategy for prevention or treatment of BRD. Using this strategy requires the identification of the major compartments of the immune system that are necessary for defense against pathogenic organisms, that is, the potential areas of modulation. The large amount of communication between elements of the immune network can then be put to an advantage with respect to modulation. Not all of the compartments of the immune system act directly on the pathogenic organisms and this must be considered when a direct effect on the organism is sought. In cases such as shipping fever, where any number of stressors may act as triggers that set a variety of infectious agents on their pathogenic course, appropriate stimulation of the regulatory network and the effector circuits of a nonspecific immune response should be considered. Among the nonspecific effectors that hold the first line of defense, especially in the respiratory tract, are granulocytes and macrophages. Once activated, they phagocytose any foreign particles and/or destroy infected cells. T cells and their secretory products play a crucial role in the activation of these effector cells by virtue of specific (memory) or nonspecific (polyclonal) activation. This type of communication and network system has allowed us to be able to modulate both phagocytic and T cells. For instance, interleukin-2 (IL-2) activates phagocytic cells by triggering T helper cells to produce macrophage-activating factor and/or leukocyte migration inhibition factor (MIF) (indirect activation). In contrast, interferon-gamma (IFN-γ) activates phagocytic cells directly. Most of the biological response modifiers currently used for intervening in immunosuppression fall in these two categories. IL-2 and IFN-γ have received most of the attention as biological response modifiers (BRM) in both human and veterinary medicine over the past few years. The major disadvantages of using these modifiers are toxicity and a cost-effectiveness ratio. Even though recombinant technology of these compounds has improved the latter, the toxicity and severe side effects caused by high doses or long periods of administration have not been resolved.

Host mediators such as interleukins and other molecules are covered in other chapters. In this chapter we introduce a newly developed broad spectrum immunopotentiator produced by cross-linking two well-known immunomodulators: tuftsin, a macrophage activator, and thymosin-α, a T cell activator. This new conjugate retained the biological properties of its constituent molecules, thus it is a nonspecific polyvalent immunopotentiator.

II. Tuftsin: A Macrophage Activator

A. Biochemistry of Tuftsin

Tuftsin is a naturally occurring tetrapeptide (Thr-Lys-Pro-Arg) first described by Najjar and Nishioka (1970). This molecule forms an integral part of the heavy chain of human IgG, residues 289–292. The presence of this tetrapeptide facilitates binding of the IgG to various cells, inducing phagocytosis by monocytes, macrophages, and polymorphonuclear leukocytes (PMNs). Tuftsin is fully active only when it is free from its carrier leukokinin (Najjar, 1983), although it can still bind to its specific receptors on the cell membrane. There are two enzymes that are required to release tuftsin from leukokinin: tuftsin-endocarboxypeptidase cleaves the peptide bond linking arginine to glutamic acid residues 292 to 293, and leukokininase, found on the outer surface of the cell membrane, cleaves tuftsin at the amino terminal residue between lysine and threonine residues 288 and 289 (Najjar, 1985).

B. Metabolism of Tuftsin

Tuftsin is a self-regulated bioactive compound. It is not clear, however, how this regulation takes place. One mechanism reported is that whenever an excess of tuftsin is formed or added above the level sufficient to occupy the specific receptor, tuftsin will be cleaved to a tripeptide, Lys-Pro-Arg. This tripeptide has a high affinity for the tuftsin receptor and competes with intact tuftsin molecules for binding to its receptor (Spirer *et al.*, 1975).

Two aminopeptidases are responsible for inactivation of tuftsin. One is present on the outer surface of the membrane (Nagoaka and Yamsashita, 1981) and cleaves off the threonine residue to yield the tripeptide inhibitor (Fridkin *et al.*, 1977). After tuftsin binds to its receptor, it is internalized and becomes susceptible to action by another aminopeptidase found in the cell cytoplasm. Finally, in the cytoplasm tuftsin is digested to its constituent amino acids (Rauner *et al.*, 1976).

Removal of arginine by a carboxypeptidase B enzyme in serum also inactivates tuftsin. This serum enzyme is not very active, however, so tuftsin has a chance to remain in circulation without losing much of its activity (Najjar and Constantopoulos, 1972).

C. Biological Activities of Tuftsin

The first biological activities of tuftsin that were studied were the stimulation kinetics of polymorphonuclear leukocytes (neutrophils). Nishioka *et al.* (1973) demonstrated that neutrophils exposed to tuftsin migrated significantly faster and farther in capillary tubes than did the controls. Horsmanheimo *et al.* (1978) reported a significant increase in monocyte migration in the presence of tuftsin.

Kavai *et al.* (1981) showed that tuftsin and some of its analogues have an enhancing effect on the chemotaxis of human monocytes. They also demonstrated that tuftsin could restore monocyte chemotactic activity in patients suffering from Hodgkin's disease and systemic lupus erythematosus. Later, Babcock *et al.* (1983) reported a similar phenomenon using human mononuclear leukocytes.

The effects of tuftsin on phagocytosis were studied using human and canine leukocytes, rabbit peritoneal granulocytes, and macrophages from mice and guinea pigs (Constantopoulos and Najjar, 1972). Tuftsin stimulated the phagocytic activity of both macrophages and neutrophils almost to the same extent (Hisatsune and Nozaki, 1983). Interestingly, Fisher *et al.* (1983) reported that another phagocytic cell, retinal pigment epithelium in rats, was also stimulated by tuftsin when injected intraocularly.

Chemiluminescence of neutrophils and macrophages is markedly enhanced by the addition of tuftsin to the culture (Florentin et al., 1983). Macrophages, however, were less luminescent than neutrophils. Additionally, reduction of nitroblue tetrazolium (NBT), which is an indicator of glucose monophosphate shunt activity, was also increased (Spirer et al., 1975).

D. Summary

The tetrapeptide tuftsin is naturally present in serum either free or bound to its carrier IgG_1. This molecule stimulates virtually all functions of phagocytic cells: phagocytosis, antigen processing, migration, and bactericidal and cytotoxic activity. It also augments the number of antibody-forming cells. Tuftsin is a self-regulating endogenous immunomodulator. Deficiency of tuftsin causes signs and symptoms of frequent, severe infection.

III. Thymosin-α: A T Cell Activator

A. Biochemistry of Thymosin-α

The thymosins were discovered by Goldstein and his colleagues in 1966. Hooper et al. (1975) reported a procedure for the isolation of thymosin fraction V, which consisted of a family of small heat-stable peptides with molecular weights ranging from 1000–15,000. Low and Goldstein (1979) purified and sequenced thymosin-α_1, a component of fraction V, which is produced in thymic epithelial cells, circulates in the blood, and controls a number of physiological processes. Thymosin-α is similar to other biologically active hormones in that it appears to have multiple sources. Although thymosin-α was originally isolated from fraction V of thymus tissue, subsequent studies revealed that it may be present in other tissues as well. Determination of thymosin-α levels using a radioimmunoassay has revealed cross-reactivity between thymus, spleen, and a number of other tissues (McClure et al., 1981). Similar cross-reactivity has also been detected in the pituitary gland, as well as in discrete brain regions in a variety of rodent species. The use of fluorescent antibody techniques has revealed that thymosin-α is present in lymphocytes (Haynes et al., 1983). Thymosin-α has been synthesized by solution (Wang et al., 1978) and solid-phase (Wang et al., 1980) procedures. Although thymosin-α can be readily prepared by recombinant DNA technologies (Wetzel et al., 1980), chemical synthesis has been the method of choice. Thymosin-α is a peptide consisting of 28 amino acids. It has a molecular weight of 3000 and an isoelectric point of 4.2. The amino terminus of thymosin-α is blocked by an acetyl group (Chen and Goldstein, 1985).

Haritos et al. (1984) have isolated a polypeptide from rat thymus that contains 113 amino acid residues. This peptide has a complete thymosin-α sequence at its amino terminus. The new peptide, known as prothymosin-α, appears to be the precursor polypeptide from which the smaller fragments, including thymosin-α, are generated.

B. Effect of Thymosin-α on Lymphocytes

There is now substantial evidence that thymosin-α affects all three major compartments of the lymphoid system (bone marrow, thymus, and peripheral blood lymphocytes) by influencing maturation and differentiation of T cells (Ahmed et al., 1978; Fasca et al., 1982; Goldstein et al., 1983). The major biological properties of thymosin-α are its role in induction of T helper cells (Frasca et al., 1982) and expression of phenotypic T cell markers (Twomey and Kouttab, 1982). Table I represents a summary of the biological properties of thymosin-α.

Collectively, the observations suggest that thymosin-α acts on precursor and/or mature T cells responsible for providing helper function for B cells. It also is responsible for differentiation of thymocytes to T cells that are acting as cytotoxic cells and producing lymphokines, which participate in regulation and maintenance of normal immunity.

C. Effect of Thymosin-α on Cyclic Nucleotides

The mechanism by which thymosin-α influences the functional status of T cells is not well understood. Early steps of activation involve changes in the calcium ion flux (Naylor et al., 1976), stimulation of the cyclic GMP pathway (Naylor et al., 1979), and induction of prostaglandin synthesis (Goldstein et al., 1983).

Goldstein et al. (1983) found that after *in vitro* incubation of thymosins with thymocytes, the level of cyclic GMP increased significantly, whereas the level of cyclic AMP did not. Stimulation of intracellular GMP was minimal after incubation of cells with thymosins and reached a maximum between 5 and 10 minutes. They concluded that this did not eliminate cyclic AMP as an important second messenger for specific T

TABLE I

SOME BIOLOGICAL PROPERTIES OF THYMOSIN-α

In vitro
    Enhances T helper cell activity
    Expresses Thy-1,2 and Lyt-1,2,3 antigens
    Increases E-rosette-forming cells
    Increases the number of TdT^a-positive cells in bone marrow and spleen
    Increases the production of IL-2, IFN-α and MIF following mitogen or antigen stimulation
    Increases production of antibody
    Increases lymphocyte response to mitogens

In vivo
    Increases the number of cytotoxic cells
    Enhances the lymphocyte response to antigens and mitogens
    Increases the production of IFN-α following viral challenge
    Increases the number of NK cells
    Increases the number of T helper cells in aged animals
    Enhances IL-2 production

^{a} TdT, terminal deoxynucleotidyl transferase

cell responses since cyclic AMP can mimic thymosins in some *in vitro* systems, such as induction of spontaneous rosette-forming cells in the splenocytes from thymectomized adults (Bach *et al.*, 1975) and the appearance of TL and Thy-1 molecules in pre-T cell-enriched bone marrow cells.

D. CLINICAL APPLICATIONS OF THYMOSIN-α

Preclinical and clinical experiments have shown that thymosin-α, a broad spectrum biological response modifier, is useful in the treatment of diseases associated with deficiencies or imbalances of the immune system.

Many cancers are associated with deficiencies in cell-mediated immunity, especially following chemotherapy and/or radiotherapy. Recent animal studies revealed that thymosin-α restores immunity and resistance to progressive tumor growth or compensates for the immunosuppressive effect of chemotherapy. Thymosin-α has also been found to enhance the disease-free interval and prolong survival in patients with lung cancer when administration complements conventional radiotherapy.

Thymosin-α may be useful in the treatment and/or control of autoimmune diseases. A common feature of many of these diseases is a lack of sufficient numbers of suppressor T cells. In preclinical studies, high dose thymosin-α has been found to increase levels of suppressor T cells. Recent studies suggest that animals with juvenile onset diabetes or other endocrine abnormalities caused by autoimmune processes may benefit from thymosin-α therapy.

Children born with immune deficiencies usually suffer from numerous infections, and those who survive develop unmanageable malignancies. Most of these congenital immune deficiencies are T cell related, meaning that the defect is in T cell functions or a lack of mature T cells. Clinical experiments have shown that thymosin therapy has fully or partially restored immune functions in these patients (Goldstein et al., 1983).

E. Summary

Thymosin-α is a small peptide hormone secreted primarily by thymus epithelium. The source, however, is not limited to the thymus but includes many other tissues, including lymphocytes. The major biological activity of this hormone is its effect on the maturation and activation of the T cell compartment of the immune system; therefore, it has clinical applications for augmenting T cell functions in immune deficiency conditions or aging. Studies have also shown that thymosin-α enhances T cell functions in response not only to tumor cells, but to pathogens, thus reducing the incidences of infections that frequently accompany cancer treatment.

Administration of thymosin-α locally or systemically, alone or in combination with other biological response modifiers as an adjuvant, is being explored. It has been shown to be an efficient adjuvant and immunopotentiator in many animal models with experimental immune deficiencies.

IV. Thymosin–Tuftsin Conjugate (IMP-1)

A. Synthesis

Synthetic hybrid proteins with the specificity of hormones, antibodies, or toxins of diphtheria have been introduced as a new class of pharmaceuticals (Moolten and Cooperband, 1970; Chang and Neville,

1977; Youle and Neville, 1980). We recently constructed a thymosin–tuftsin conjugate employing m-maleimidobenzoyl-N-hydroxysuccinimide ester (MBS) as the coupling reagent. The conjugate prepared in this way retained a majority of the biological activities of both constituent peptides. Conjugation of the thymosin–tuftsin complex was accomplished using the procedure described by O'Sullivan et al. (1979) with modification. The procedure is briefly described below.

Thymosin-α and dimethylformamide were purchased from the Sigma Chemical Company (St. Louis, Missouri). Tuftsin was synthesized and purified in our laboratory according to the method described by Gottlieb et al. (1983). Cross-linker MBS was purchased from the Pierce Chemical Company Rockford, Illinois). Sephadex G-25 was purchased from Pharmacia Fine Chemical (Uppsala, Sweden) and acrylamide electrophoresis reagents were purchased from Bio-Rad Laboratories (Richmond, California).

Four mg of purified thymosin-α_1 (purified by HPLC) in 3 ml of 10 mM Na_2HPO_4 (pH 7.5) were mixed, while a vortex, with 400 μl of dimethylformamide containing MBS (2.5 μg/ml). The mixture was incubated at 21°C for 30 minutes, then passed over a Sephadex G-25 column to remove excess MBS. The quality of malemide groups incorporated was determined according to the method of Liu et al. (1979).

Six-hundred μg of tuftsin in 400 μl of phosphate buffer was mixed, while a vortex, with 13 μl of MBS solution, then incubated at 20°C for 2 hours. At the end of the incubation period, this mixture was added to modified thymosin-α and incubated at 20°C for 3 hours. Finally, the conjugate mixture was dialyzed against phosphate-buffered saline overnight at 4°C using a 3000-Dal cut-off dialysis bag. The conjugate was characterized and quality assurance was performed using HPLC and GC-MS chromatography procedures.

B. Biological Activity in Vitro on Bovine Immunocytes

Tetrapeptide tuftsin has been shown by numerous laboratories to be immunoligially active on phagocytic cells. Thymosin-α has been shown to activate both thymocytes and mature T cells. Our laboratory was able to cross-link these two peptides to make a broad spectrum immunopotentiator capable of activating both cell types. We have undertaken a series of investigations to evaluate the effect of thymosin–tuftsin conjugate (IMP-1) on monocytes by evaluating chemotaxis, cytotoxicity, and cytokine production. T cell activation was assessed by measuring mitogen stimulation, mixed lymphocyte reaction, and lymphokine production.

1. Effect of IMP-1 on Monocytes

Peripheral blood lymphocytes from an apparently healthy normal calf were prepared from heparinized blood by Ficoll-Hypaque centrifugation (Khansari et al., 1989). Monocytes were separated from lymphocytes by two sequential 1-hour plastic adherence steps to a purity of greater than 97%, as determined by nonspecific esterase staining.

a. Chemotaxis. Chemotaxis was performed using a blind well chamber by the method described by Synderman and Pike (1976). Monocytes were placed in the top compartment while the immunopotentiator, or chemotactic activating medium, or medium alone, was placed in the bottom well. After a 90 minute incubation at 37°C the

TABLE II

Effect of Tuftsin, Thymosin-α, and IMP-1 on Monocyte and Lymphocyte Function *in Vitro*

Assay	Treatment			
	None	Tuftsin	Thymosin-α	IMP-1
Monocyte chemotaxis[a] (cell no.)	10 ± 2	28 ± 3	11 ± 2	31 ± 5
Phagocytosis[b] (% surviving bacteria)	89 ± 4	51 ± 18	87 ± 7	55 ± 11
Superoxide anion[b] (cytochrome c reduction) × 10^{-6} M	8.8	12.3	9.5	10.5
IL-1 production[c] (cpm)	4332 ± 675	6191 ± 581	4845 ± 901	5801 ± 691
Lymphocyte proliferation[d] (SI)				
Phytohemagglutinin (PHA)	18.3	16.5	38.8	37.7
Mixed lymphocyte culture	12.2	15.2	23.0	20.7
Lymphokine production[e]				
IL-2 (U)	2.3	3.8	6.3	5.8
IFN-γ (U)	3.5	4.2	8.1	7.0

[a] 1 µg/ml of immunopotentiators were added to cultures.

[b] 100 µg/ml of immunopotentiators were added to cultures.

[c] Monocytes were stimulated with 15 µg/ml of lipopolysaccharide (LPS) for 48 hours. In this assay, CTLL cell proliferation in response to IL-1-stimulated culture supernatant of LBRM-33 cell line procedure was used.

[d] 2 µg/ml of immunopotentiators were added to cultures.

[e] Lymphocytes were stimulated with 2 µg/ml PHA for 48 hours. 2 µg/ml of immunopotentiators were used. Data was expressed as arbitrary unit.

filters were fixed and stained, and the average number of cells per microscopic field was determined. Results are shown in Table II.

These data suggest that IMP-1 is as active as tuftsin in that the conjugation process had little or no effect on the biological activity of the product.

b. Phagocytic Activity. Phagocytic activity of monocytes in the presence of immunopotentiators was evaluated by treating monocytes with either medium or medium containing the immunopotentiators for 2 hours at 37°C. After incubation, a suspension of live *Staphylococcus aureus* organisms was added to the mixture and incubated at 37°C for 30 minutes with shaking. The surviving bacteria were counted by plating. Percent of bacterial survival was calcuated by the formula:

$$\% \text{ bacterial survival} = \frac{\text{survivors of incubation with monocytes}}{\text{survivors of incubation without monocytes}}$$

Table II shows the effect of immunopotentiator treatment on phagocytosis of the *S. aureus*. Both tuftsin and IMP-1 enhanced the bacteriocidal activity of the monocytes.

The bactericidal activity following phagocytosis is via generation of superoxide anions as well as NBT reduction. Monocyte O_2^- production increases following treatment with either tuftsin or IMP-1. The results of these studies are summarized in Table II.

c. Cytokine Production. Interleukin-1 production by monocytes in response to bacterial lipopolysaccharide (LPS) in the presence or ab-

TABLE III

Effect of *In Vivo* Injections of IMP-1 on Immunocyte Function from Dexamethasone[a]-Treated Calves

Treatment	Immunocyte function[b]			
	IgG (ng/ml)	IL-2 (cpm)	PHA (cpm)	MLC (cpm)
Saline	18 ± 3	8116 ± 765	172,271 ± 8321	44,861 ± 5014
Dexamethasone	16 ± 4	5238 ± 450	90,441 ± 16,078	28,511 ± 7118
Dexamethasone + IMP-1[c]	24 ± 3	7662 ± 981	123,865 ± 18,433	36,099 ± 8317

[a] Three injections of 40 μg/kg/day, I.M.
[b] Six calves for each experiment.
[c] 10 μg/kg/day, I.M.

sence of immunopotentiator was assessed as described earlier (Khanasari et al., 1985). The IL-1 activities of the monocyte culture supernatants were determined using the method described by Conlon (1983). As shown in Table II, IMP-1 was as effective as tuftsin for enhancing monocyte IL-1 production. Once again these data suggest that the product of thymosin–tuftsin conjugation is in fact a monocyte activator similar to its constituent, tuftsin.

2. Effect of IMP-1 on T Cells

Because one of the subunit molecules of the IMP-1 is thymosin-α, a T cell activator, we also studied the effect of the new hybrid compound on T cell functions.

a. Blast Transformation Assay. Monocyte-depleted lymphocytes were cultured in the presence of phytohemagglutinin (PHA), a T cell activator and immunopotentiator, followed by [^{3}H]-thymidine uptake determination as described elsewhere (Khansari et al., 1984). As shown in Table II, In the presence of 2 μg/ml thymosin-α or IMP-1, the [^{3}H]-thymidine uptake was increased significantly. The magnitude of this enhancement, however, was less with IMP-1 than with thymosin-α. Tuftsin did not have any effect on lymphocyte response to T cell mitogen. These data suggest that the new compound has a potentiating effect on T cells.

b. Mixed Lymphocyte Reaction. Allogenic mixed lymphocyte reactions have been used widely to assess the cell-mediated immune status in humans and animals (Ling and MacLennan, 1981). Major histocompatibility-restricted cytotoxic T cells, which kill tumor or virus-infected cells, are stimulated in this assay. The proliferation of these cells can be determined by [^{3}H]-thymidine uptake in response to allogenic B cells. Mixed lymphocyte culture (MLC) was performed using the procedure described by Khansari et al. (1983). The data generated from these experiments are summarized in Table II. It is apparent that both thymosin-α and IMP-1 increased MLC while tuftsin had little effect on proliferative response of cytotoxic cells to allogenic non-T cell stimuli.

c. Lymphokine Production by T Cells. Peripheral blood lymphocytes were cultured in the presence of 2 μg/ml PHA with and without immunopotentiators. The cell-free culture supernatants were recovered by centrifugation and assayed for IL-2 and IFN-γ content. The IL-2 activities were assayed by the method of Gillis et al. (1978). Interferon-γ activities of the culture supernatant were determined by radioimmunoassay. Table II shows a summary of the results of these experiments. Production of IL-2 and IFN-γ was enhanced if either thymosin-α or

IMP-1 was present in the system. Tuftsin also increased IL-2 and INF-γ production but not to as high a level as did thymosin-α or IMP-1.

Taken all together, the results of our *in vitro* experiments suggest that thymosin–tuftsin conjugate has a potentiation effect on both T cells and monocytes.

C. Biological Activity *In Vivo*

We have just begun to study the effect of IMP-1 on immunosuppressed calves. In our preliminary experiments 18 calves were separated into 3 groups of 6 calves each. Groups 1 and 2 were injected with dexamethasone (40 μg/kg/day, I.M.) for 3 days. The third group was injected with saline solution. On day 4, all calves were bled, then injected with IMP-1 (10 μg/kg/day, I.M.) for 2 days. Peripheral blood lymphocytes from the day 4 bleeding were separated and their immunologic functions were assessed. On day 7, all calves were bled again and peripheral blood lymphocytes were separated and immunologic functions were assessed. The results of these experiments are tabulated in Table III. These results indicate that dexamethasone-treated calves were immunosuppressed and that administration of IMP-1 partially restored this suppression. However, dose response experiments and kinetic studies need to be done before the beneficial effect of IMP-1 can be truly assessed.

V. Conclusion

Physical and/or environmental stress leads to a systemic immunosuppression. The immunocompromised subject becomes highly susceptible to various infections by microorganisms that otherwise are not pathogenic. Studies have shown that restoration of the immune response in the stressed subject is possible by administration of immunopotentiator(s); however, the search for an effective, nontoxic, low-cost immunopotentiator is continuing. We took advantage of two naturally occurring immunomodulators and developed a compound that potentiated two key elements of the immune system: phagocytic cells and T cells. *In vitro* experiments demonstrated that this new compound was very effective in stimulating target cells. *In vivo* experiments were not conclusive but preliminary studies lead us to believe that IMP-1 may have a beneficial effect on the restoration of immunologic functions in immunocompromised animals. If this is true it may be possible to prevent economically devastating stress-induced infections, such as shipping fever, by administration of IMP-1 before or during the stressful event.

ACKNOWLEDGMENTS

This study was funded by Immunobiological Laboratories, Inc. The authors thank Sylvia Kistner for typing this article.

REFERENCES

Ahmed, A., Smith, A. H., Wong, D. M., Thurman, G. B., Goldstein, A. L., and Sell, K. W. (1978). In vitro induction of Lyt surface markers on precursor cells incubated with thymosin polypeptides. *Cancer Treat. Rep.* **62,** 1739–1747.

Babcock, G. F., Amoscato, A. A., and Nishioka, K. (1983). Effect of tuftsin on the migration, chemotaxis and differentiation of macrophages and granulocytes. *Ann. N.Y. Acad. Sci.* **419,** 64–74.

Bach, M. A., Fournier, C., and Bach, J. F. (1975). Regulation of theta-antigen expressions by agents altering cyclic amp. *Ann. N.Y. Acad. Sci.* **249,** 316–327.

Blecha, F. (1986). The role of IL-2 in the immune response of incoming feeder cattle. *Bovine Proc.* **18,** 113–118.

Chang, T. M., and Neville, D. M., Jr. (1977). Artificial hybrid protein containing a toxic protein fragment and a cell membrane receptor-binding moiety in a disulfide conjugate. I. Synthesis of diphtheria toxin fragment A-S-S-human placental lactogen with methyl-5-bromovaler-imidate. *J. Biol. Chem.* **252,** 1505–1514.

Chen, J., and Goldstein, A. L. (1985). Thymosins and other thymic hormones. *In* "Biological Response Modifiers" (P. F. Torrence, ed.), pp. 121–140. Academic Press, Orlando, Florida.

Conlon, P. J. (1983). A rapid biologic assay for detection of interleukin-1. *J. Immunol.* **131,** 1280–1282.

Constantopoulos, A., and Najjar, V. A. (1972). Tuftsin a natural and general phagocytosis stimulating peptide affecting macrophages and polymorphonuclear granulocytes. *Cytobios* **6,** 97–100.

Filion, L. G., Willson, P. S., Bielefedt-Ohmann, H., Babink, L. A., and Thomson, R. G. (1984). The possible role of stress in the induction of pneumonic pasteurelosis. *Can. J. Comp. Med.* **48,** 268–274.

Fisher, L. J., Stevens, G., Jr., and McCann, P. M. (1983). Tuftsin stimulation of phagocytosis by the retinal pigment epithelium. *Ann. N.Y. Acad. Sci.* **419,** 227–233.

Florentin, I., Martinez, J., Maral, J., Pelletier, M., Chung, V., Roch-Arveiller, M., Bruley-Rosset, M., Giroud, J. P., Winternitz, F., and Matthé, G. (1983). Immunopharmacological properties of tuftsin and some analogues. *Ann. N.Y. Acad. Sci.* **419,** 177–191.

Frank, G. H. (1986). The role of pasteurella haemolytica in the bovine respiratory disease complex. *VM/SAC, Vet. Med. Small Anim. Clin.* **81,** 838–846.

Frasca, D., Garavini, M., and Doria, G. (1982). Recovery of T-cell functions in aged mice injected with synthetic thymosin-alpha-1. *Cell. Immunol.* **7,** 384–391.

Fridkin, M., Stabinsky, Y., Zakuth, V., and Spirer, Z. (1977). Tuftsin and some analogs: Synthesis and interaction with human polymorphonuclear leukocytes. *Biochim. Biophys. Acta* **496,** 203–211.

Gillis, S., Ferm, M. M., Ou, W., and Smith, K. A. (1978). T cell growth factor: Parameters of production and quantitative microassay for activity. *J. Immunol.* **120**, 2027–2032.

Goldstein, A. L., Slater, F. D., and White, A. (1966). Preparation, assay, and partial purification of a thymic lymphocytopoietic factor (thymosin). *Proc. Natl. Acad. Sci. U.S.A.* **56**, 1010–1017.

Goldstein, A. L., Low, T. L. K., Zatz, M. M., Hall, N. R., and Naylor, P. H. (1983). Thymosins. *Clin. Immunol. Allergy* **3**, 119–133.

Gottlieb, P., Stabinsky, Y., Zakuth, V., Spirer, Z., and Fredkin, M. (1983). Synthetic pathways to tuftsin and radioimmunoassay. *Ann. N.Y. Acad. Sci.* **419**, 12–22.

Haritos, A. A., Goodall, G. J., and Horecker, B. L. (1984). Prothymosin alpha: Isolation and properties of the major immunoreactive form of thymosin alpha 1 in rat thymus. *Proc. Natl. Acad. Sci. U.S.A.* **81**, 1088–1011.

Haynes, B. F., Robert-Guroff, M., Metzgar, R. S., Franchini, G., Kalyanararman, V. S., Palker, T., and Gallo, R. C. (1983). Monoclonal antibody against human T-cell leukemia virus P19 defines a human thymic epithelial antigen acquired during ontogeny. *J. Exp. Med.* **157**, 907–920.

Hisatsune, K., and Nozaki, S. (1983). A biochemical study of the phagocytic activities of tuftsin and its analogues. *Ann. N.Y. Acad. Sci.* **419**, 205–213.

Hooper, J. A., McDaniel, M. C., Thurman, G. B., Cohen, G. H., Shulof, R. S., and Goldstein, A. L. (1975). Purification and properties of bovine thymosin. *Ann. N.Y. Acad. Sci.* **249**, 125–144.

Horsmanheimo, A., Horsmanheimo, M., and Fudenberg, H. H. (1978). Effect of tuftsin on migration of polymorphonuclear and mononuclear human leukocytes in leukocyte migration agarose test. *Clin. Immunol. Immunopathol.* **11**, 251–255.

Kavai, M., Lukacs, K., Szegedi, G., Szegedi, M., and Erchegyi, J. (1981). Chemotactic and stimulating effect of tuftsin and its analogs on human monocytes. *Immunol. Lett.* **2**, 219–224.

Kelley, K. W. (1980). Stress and immune function: A bibliographic review. *Ann. Rech. Vet.* **11**, 445–478.

Khansari, D. N., Petrini, M., Ambrogi, F., Gold-Schmidt-Clermont, P., and Fudenberg, H. H. (1983). Role of autorosette forming cells in antibody synthesis *in vitro:* Suppressive activity of ARFC in humoral immune response. *Immunobiology* **166**, 1–11.

Khansari, D. N., Whitten, H. D., and Fudenberg, H. H. (1984). Phencyclidine-induced immunosuppression. *Science* **225**, 76–78.

Khansari, D. N., Chou, Y. K., and Fudenberg, H. H. (1985). Human monocytes heterogeneity: Interleukin 1 and prostaglandin E_2 production by separate subsets. *Eur. J. Immunol.* **15**, 48–51.

Khansari, D. N., Beauclair, K., and Gustad, T. (1989). Separation of bovine lymphocytes and granulocytes from blood by use of elutriation. *Am. J. Vet. Res.* **50**, 1263–1265.

Larsson, B., Fossum, C., Tornquist, M., Matsson, P., and Alenius, S. (1985). Evaluation of the prophylactic potential of an immunomodulator against respiratory disease in calves. *Acta Vet. Scand.* **26**, 262–272.

Ling, N. R., and MacLennan, I. C. M. (1981). Analysis of lymphocytes in blood and tissues. *In* "Techniques in Clinical Immunology" (R. A. Thompson, ed.), pp. 222–250. Blackwell, Oxford.

Liu, F. T., Zinnecker, M., Hamaoka, T., and Katz, D. (1979). New procedures for preparation and isolation of conjugates of proteins and a synthetic copolymer of D-amino acids and immunochemical characterization of such a conjugates. *Biochemistry* **18**, 690–693.

Lopez, A., Thomson, R. G., and Savan, M. (1976). The pulmonary clearance of Pasteurella hemolytica in calves infected with bovine parainfluenza-3 virus. *Can. J. Comp. Med.* **40**, 385–391.

Low, T. L. K., and Goldstein, A. L. (1979). The chemistry and biology of thymosin. II. Amino acid sequence analysis of thymosin alpha and polypeptide beta 1. *J. Biol. Chem.* **254,** 987–995.

McClure, J. E., Lameris, N., Wara, D. W., and Goldstein, A. L. (1981). Immunochemical studies on thymosin: Radioimmunoassay of thymosin alpha-1. *J. Immunol.* **128,** 368–375.

Moolten, F. L., and Cooperband, S. R. (1970). Selective destruction of target cells by diphtheria toxin conjugated to antibody directed against antigens on the cells. *Science* **169,** 68–70.

Nagoaka, I., and Yamashita, T. (1981). Inactivation of phagocytosis-stimulating activity of tuftsin by polymorphonuclear neutrophils. A possible role of leucine on ectoenzyme. *Biochim. Biophys. Acta* **675,** 85–93.

Najjar, V. A. (1983). Tuftsin, a natural activator of phagocyte cells: An overview. *Ann. N.Y. Acad. Sci.* **419,** 1–11.

Najjar, V. A. (1985). Tuftsin (Thr-Lys-Pro-Arg): A natural activator of phagocytic cells with antibacterial and antineoplastic activity. *In* "Biological Response Modifiers" (P. F. Torrence, ed.), pp. 141–167. Academic Press, Orlando, Florida.

Najjar, V. A., and Nishioka, K. (1970). Tuftsin a natural phagocytosis stimulating peptide. *Nature (London)* **228,** 672–673.

Najjar, V. A., and Constantopoulos, A. (1972). A new phagocytosis-stimulating tetrapeptide hormone, tuftsin, and its role in disease. *RES, J. Reticuloendothel. Soc.* **12,** 197–215.

Naylor, P. H., Sheppard, H., Thurman, G. B., and Goldstein, A. L. (1979). Increase of cyclic GMP induced in murine thymocytes by thymosin fraction-5. *Biochem. Biophys. Res. Commun.* **73,** 843–849.

Naylor, P. H., Thurman, G. B., and Goldstein, A. L. (1976). Effect of calcium on the cyclic GMP elevation induced by thymosin fraction-5. *Biochem. Biophys. Res. Commun.* **90,** 810–818.

Nishioka, K., Satoh, P. S., Constantopoulos, A., and Najjar, V. A. (1973). The chemical synthesis of the phagocytosis-stimulating tetrapeptide tuftsin (Thr-Lys-Pro-Arg) and its biological properties. *Biochim. Biophys. Acta* **310,** 230–237.

Rauner, R. A., Schmidt, J. J., and Najjar, V. A. (1976). Proline endopeptidase and ex-o-peptidase activity in polymorphonuclear granulocytes. *Mol. Cell. Biochem.* **10,** 77–80.

Roth, J. A. (1984). Immunosuppression and immunomodulation in bovine respiratory disease. *In* "Bovine Respiratory Disease" (R. W. Loan, eds.), pp. 143–192. Texas A&M Univ. Press, College Station.

Roth, J. A., and Kaeberle, M. L. (1984). Enhancement of lymphocyte blasto-genesis and neutrophil function by Avridine in dexamethasone-treated and non-treated cattle. *Am. J. Vet. Res.* **46,** 53–58.

O'Sullivan, M. J., Gnemmi, E., Morris, D., Chiregatti, G., Simmonds, A. D., Simmons, M., Bridges, J. W., and Marks, V. (1979). Comparison of two methods of preparing enzyme antibody conjugates: Application of these conjugates for enzyme immunoassay. *Anal. Chem.* **100,** 100–108.

Spirer, Z., Zakuth, V., Golander, A., Bogair, N., and Fridkin, M. (1975). The effect of tuftsin on the nitrous blue tetrazolium reduction of normal human polymorphonuclear leukocytes. *J. Clin. Invest.* **55,** 198–200.

Synderman, R., and Pike, M. (1976). Macrophage chemotaxis. *In* "*In Vitro* Methods in Cell-Mediated and Tumor Immunity" (B. R. Bloom and J. R. David, eds.), pp. 185–196. Academic Press, New York.

Twomey, J. J., and Kauttab, N. M. (1982). Selected phenotypic induction of null lymphocytes from mice with thymic agents. *Cell. Immunol.* **72,** 186–194.

von Tungeln, D. L. (1986). The effects of stress on the immunology of the stocker calf. *Bovine Pract.* **18,** 109–115.

Wang, S. S., Kulesha, I. D., and Winter, D. P. (1978). Synthesis of thymosin alpha-1. *J. Am. Chem. Soc.* **101,** 253–254.

Wang, S. S., Makopski, R., Bach, A. E., and Merrifield, R. B. (1980). Automated solid phase synthesis of thymosin alpha 1. *Int. J. Pept. Protein Res.* **15,** 1–4.

Wetzel, R., Heyneker, H. L., Goeddel, D. V., Jhurani, P., Shapiro, J., Crea, R., Low, T. L. K., McClure, J. E., and Goldstein, A. L. (1980). Production of biologically active or alpha-desacetylthymosin alpha 1 in *Escherichia coli* through expression of a chemically synthesized gene. *Biochemistry* **19,** 6096–6104.

Youle, R. J., and Neville, D. M., Jr. (1980). Anti-thy 1.2 monoclonal antibody linked to ricin is a potent cell-type-specific toxin. *Proc. Natl. Acad. Sci. U.S.A.* **77,** 5483–5486.

Part III
Cytokine Immunomodulation

The Molecular Biology of Large Animal Cytokines

CHARLES MALISZEWSKI, BYRON GALLIS AND PAUL E. BAKER

Immunex Research and Development, Seattle, Washington 98101

I. Cytokine Biology
   A. Introduction
   B. General Considerations
   C. Biological Characteristics of Selected Cytokines
   D. Cytokine Regulation of Hematopoiesis and the Immune Response
II. Recombinant Bovine and Porcine Cytokines
   A. Recombinant Bovine Interleukin-1
   B. Recombinant Bovine Interleukin-2
   C. Recombinant Bovine GM-CSF
   D. Recombinant Bovine Interferon-γ
   E. Recombinant Porcine Interleukin-1
   F. Common Structural Features of Cytokines and Their Genes
III. Conclusions
   References

I. Cytokine Biology

A. INTRODUCTION

The cytokines of large animals, humans, and rodents share numerous features at the levels of structure and biological function. Although considerably more data have been gathered in murine and human systems, we and other researchers have begun to develop a clearer understanding of the molecular biology, *in vitro* activities, and practical applications of several cytokines of domestic animals in general, and cattle in particular. Thus, as an introduction to this subject, comments presented in this section will deal with cytokine immunology of all mammals. In the second half of this chapter, we will consider a few of the specific cytokines of domestic animals of agricultural importance.

In introducing the subject of cytokines, a clarification of terminology is in order. The term "cytokine" will be used to include both lymphokines and monokines. Lymphokines include those hormones produced by lymphocytes (mostly produced by $T4^+$ helper or Th cells), and monokines are cytokines produced by monocytes. Of course, numerous other cell lineages that will not be dealt with in this chapter are also cytokine secretors. Strictly speaking, cytokines are true hormones in that they are products of one type of cell, which may have their influence on other cells. In addition, while hormones may include nonproteins, such as glucocorticoids, all cytokines thus far studied are, indeed, proteins or glycoproteins.

B. General Considerations

During the past ten years, a wealth of data has been generated in studies on soluble mediators of the immune response. To date, over twenty distinct cytokines have been identified, including the interleukins (IL-1 through IL-10), colony-stimulating factor-1 (CSF-1, also called macrophage-CSF or M-CSF), granulocyte-CSF (G-CSF), granulocyte/macrophage-CSF (GM-CSF), tumor necrosis factor-α and -β, TGF-α and -β (transforming growth factor), and interferon-γ. While the list of immunomodulatory peptides continues to grow, so does documentation of their wide array of biological activities. In fact, cytokines have been implicated in virtually every aspect of the immune response, including hematopoiesis, antibody secretion, inflammation, tumor cytotoxicity, allergy, and autoimmunity. Because of the enormous volume of information and the availability of numerous excellent reviews on the individual cytokines, emphasis in this chapter will be confined to those cytokines for which bovine and/or porcine genes have been cloned, i.e., IL-1, IL-2, interferon-γ, and GM-CSF.

With regard to cytokine receptors, it is clear that there is not a unique biochemical pathway for each growth factor that stimulates cell proliferation. Studies with the receptors for insulin, epidermal growth factor (EGF), CSF-1, and platelet-derived growth factor (PDGF) indicate that each receptor is a protein tyrosine kinase. Site-directed mutagenesis of a single key residue conserved in these receptors and required for binding of the ATP substrate of the kinase inactivates the ability of each receptor to transduce a signal and its intrinsic protein kinase activity. A number of the cytokines that stimulate growth of hematopoietic cells also stimulate protein tyrosine kinase activity, even though in some cases the receptors are not protein tyrosine kinases. This strongly suggests that a similar, if not identical, pathway exists by which most growth factors stimulate cell proliferation. Thus, knowledge about some of the biochemical pathways by which insulin, EGF, and PDGF stimulate cell proliferation may be taken as a paradigm for the study of hormones that stimulate the replication of cells of the immune system.

The vast amount of information available on the signaling mechanisms of these hormones has been recently reviewed (Kahn and White, 1988; Rosen, 1987; Czech et al., 1988; Williams, 1989). The signaling mechanisms of each hormone are of enormous complexity and subtlety, as indicated by the production of at least several "second messengers," which are rapidly generated after hormone binding (Kahn and White, 1988; Rosen, 1987; Czech et al., 1988; Williams, 1989; Wahl et al., 1988, 1989; Stralfors, 1988; Chan et al., 1988; Alemany et al., 1987; Sturgill et al., 1988). For example, in the cases of both insulin and EGF, at least two enzymatic activities that may act on many substrates are activated by protein tyrosine phosphorylation. Phospholipases C and protein serine kinases are activated to initiate secondary responses, which proceed along different pathways (Kahn and White, 1988; Rosen, 1987; Czech et al., 1988; Wahl et al., 1988, 1989; Sturgill et al., 1988). Protein tyrosine phosphorylation activates protein serine kinases, which in turn regulate the key enzymes in metabolic pathways (Kahn and White, 1988; Rosen, 1987; Czech et al., 1988; Sturgill et al., 1988). Protein tyrosine phosphorylation of phospholipases (Wahl et al., 1988, 1989) activates these enzymes to produce other messengers by hydrolysis of phosphatidylinositol, which releases inositol triphosphates (IP_3) that increase intracellular calcium, and diacyglycerol, which activates protein kinase C. In addition, activated phospholipase produces glycosylphosphatidylinositol, an effector of many phenotypes whose receptor is yet unknown (Stralfors, 1988; Chan et al., 1988; Alemany et al., 1987). These multiple signaling mechanisms are the means by which hormones exert their pleiotropic phenotypic effects in particular cell types of a distinctive differentiated state.

C. Biological Characteristics of Selected Cytokines

As indicated above, this review will deal specifically with IL-1, IL-2, GM-CSF, and interferon-γ (i.e., those cytokines for which domestic animal cloned homologs are now available). The following section describes structural and functional characteristics of human and mouse versions of these cytokines and their receptors.

1. Interleukin-1

Interleukin-1, a product of macrophages (i.e., a monokine) and numerous other cell types, acts as a mediator of a remarkable array of biological activities, including the acute-phase response, catabolism, sleep, hemodynamic regulation, and the chronic inflammatory response (Dinarello, 1989). Numerous immunoregulatory activities have been described as well. For instance, IL-1 induces maturation of T (Gery and Waksman, 1972; Gillis and Mizel, 1981) and B (Hoffman and Watson, 1979; Falkoff et al., 1983), and NK (Dempsey et al., 1982) cells, stimulates production of bone marrow hematopoietic cells (Mochizuki et al., 1987), and stimulates the production of a variety of other immunomodulatory factors (Dinarello, 1989). In vivo studies have identified two additional biological activities of IL-1 that may have useful immunopharmacological applications in economically important species such as swine and cattle: adjuvanticity (Staruch and Wood, 1983; Reed et al., 1989) and wound healing (Raines et al., 1989).

At least two distinct IL-1 genes have been demonstrated in mice and humans (Auron et al., 1984; March et al., 1985; Lomedico et al., 1984; Gray et al., 1986; Furutani et al., 1985). These two genes, IL-1α and IL-1β, encode intracellular precursor peptides having molecular weights of approximately 31,000 which are posttranslationally processed to products of 17,500 Da, representing the C-terminal portion of the precursor. These are the predominant secreted forms of IL-1, although numerous additional naturally produced IL-1 subfragments have also been identified (Dinarello 1989). Both human IL-1α and IL-1β bind to the same receptor with similar affinities (Dower et al., 1986). Despite their similarities in size, function, and binding specificity, IL-1α and IL-1β exhibit only limited amino acid homology (less than 30%). However, significant homologies exist across species for each form of IL-1 (Lomedico et al., 1987; Hopp et al., 1986), which suggests that the retention of analogous molecules may have been evolutionarily advantageous.

While much is known about the biology of IL-1 there is little that is understood about how it mediates such diverse biochemical and biological effects. [The 80,000-Da receptor for IL-1 from a murine thymoma cell line (Sims et al., 1988) has recently been cloned and sequenced]. It is clear that when IL-1 binds to its specific cellular receptor, it stimulates transcription of a number of genes, including those for IL-1 itself, CSFs, IL-2, and cyclooxygenase, the key enzyme involved in the synthesis of prostaglandin E_2 (Martin and Resch, 1988; Dinarello, 1988; Rosoff et al., 1988). The details of how IL-1 acts through its receptor on the cell surface to trigger transcription of genes remain unknown. However, it is known that IL-1 triggers a number of responses soon after binding to its receptor. In a human T cell leukemia line, IL-1 was shown to cause a rapid increase in levels of diacylglycerol and phosphorylcholine, but did not increase inositol triphosphate (Raz et al., 1988). In glomerular mesangial cells, IL-1 rapidly increased diacyglycerol and phosphorylethanolamine levels, but had no effect on levels of intracellular calcium, phosphorylcholine, or inositoltriphosphate (Kester et al., 1989). In a murine T lymphoma line, IL-1 neither increased intracellular calcium nor caused activation or translocation of protein kinase C (Abraham et al., 1987). Interleukin-1 also stimulates serine phosphorylation of a cytosolic 65,000-Da protein (Matsushima et al., 1987, 1988) and serine/threonine phosphorylation of a triad of 27,000-Da cytosolic proteins (Kaur and Saklatvala, 1988), as well as phosphorylation of the EGF receptor, the latter being phosphorylated by a protein kinase C-independent mechanism (Bird and Saklatvala, 1989).

Saklatvala and colleagues found that phosphorylation of the 27,000-Da proteins occurred 3 minutes after addition of IL-1, but not earlier. However, using a monoclonal antibody to the IL-1 receptor and cells which express 100,000 functional, recombinant IL-1 receptors/cell, it was demonstrated (Gallis et al., 1990) that IL-1 induced serine/threonine phosphorylation of its receptor within 1 minute after addition to cells. The rapid response to IL-1 suggests that one "second messenger" in this system involves activation of a serine/threonine kinase. From earlier studies, the kinase is clearly not protein kinase C nor the multi-functional Ca^{2+}-activated protein kinase (Schulman and Lou, 1989), since neither IP_3 nor calcium levels are raised by IL-1, nor is protein kinase C activated (Abraham et al., 1987; Bird and Saklatvala, 1989). The identification of this protein kinase and its substrates are a logical focus for further studies on the mechanisms by which IL-1 generates its pleiotropic effects.

2. Interleukin-2

Interleukin-2 is the most extensively characterized of the cytokines (Smith, 1988). First discovered by Morgan and her colleagues, IL-2 was called T cell growth factor due to its potent proliferative effect on T lymphocytes (Farrar et al., 1986). Subsequent studies have indicated that IL-2 also functions as an inducer of B cell growth and differentiation (Zubler et al., 1984; Maraguchi et al., 1985). Its purported role as an adjuvant in vivo makes IL-2 an attractive candidate for enhancing the effects of vaccines in large animals (Ramchaw et al., 1987; Flexner et al., 1987).

The cDNA clones for human and murine IL-2 include open reading frames encoding proteins of 15,000–17,000 Da (Taniguchi et al., 1983; Kashima et al., 1985), and the predicted amino acid sequences for both species share approximately 60% homology. The recombinant proteins have been expressed in prokaryotic expression systems (Taniguchi et al., 1983; Kashima et al., 1985), allowing extensive characterization of the molecule. The receptor for IL-2 consists of at least two noncovalently associated polypeptides, a 55,000-Da protein called Tac or α chain, and a 75,000-Da protein, the β chain. The α chain binds IL-2 with low affinity ($K_d \sim 10^{-8}$ M) and the β chain binds IL-2 with intermediate affinity ($K_d \sim {}^{-9}$ M), but both proteins are required for high-affinity binding ($K_d \sim 10^{-12}$ M) by IL-2. While either the α chain (Hatakeyama et al., 1985) or β chain (Mills and May, 1987) is sufficient to transduce a biological response, both are required to induce cell proliferation at low concentrations of IL-2 (Greene and Leonard, 1986).

IL-2 has been shown to activate Na^+/H^+ exchange (Mills and May, 1987) and cause increases in cytosolic calcium from extracellular as well as intracellular stores (Utsunomiya et al., 1986). The hormone also causes protein phosphorylation in cellular membranes (Gaulton and Eardley, 1986), in proteins associated with the IL-2 receptor (Benedict et al., 1987), and only in T cell lines that express high-affinity IL-2 receptors (Ishil et al., 1989). IL-2 also causes a rapid and concentration-dependent protein tyrosine phosphorylation of a number of proteins in T cells (Saltzman et al., 1988) and other cells (Morla et al., 1988), as well as ribosomal protein S6 phosphorylation (Farrar et al., 1986). The fact that IL-2 causes protein tyrosine phosphorylation and ribosomal protein S6 phosphorylation suggests that this hormone acts via one pathway for stimulation of synthesis of macromolecules demonstrated to exist in insulin and EGF-stimulated cells (Kahn and White, 1988; Rosen, 1987; Czech et al., 1988; Sturgill et al., 1988).

3. Granulocyte/Macrophage Colony-Stimulating Factor

The colony-stimulating factors are glycoproteins that regulate both proliferation and differentiation of hematopoietic precursor cells, as well as the functional activities of mature cells of these lineages (Metcalf, 1986; Clark and Kamen, 1987). One of these factors, GM-CSF, induces granulocyte, macrophage, and eosinophil colony formation. In addition to its role as a hematopoietic growth factor, GM-CSF has also been shown to regulate numerous biological activities *in vitro* including: antibody-dependent cell-mediated cytotoxicity (ADCC) (Vadas et al., 1983), superoxide anion production (Weisbart et al., 1985), inhibition of migration of neutrophils (Gasson et al., 1984); ADCC (Vadas et *al.*, 1983) and schistosomula killing (Dessein *et al.*, 1982) by eosinophils; tumor cell cytotoxicity (Grabstein *et al.*, 1986a), and the enhancement of B cell antibody production by macrophages (Grabstein *et al.*, 1986b). *In vivo* studies in monkeys and mice have demonstrated a marked neutrophilia induced by GM-CSF administration (Metcalf *et al.*, 1987; Donahue *et al.*, 1986; Mayer *et al.*, 1987). Recent results from therapeutic trials in humans have been extremely promising with regard to the ability of GM-CSF to restore myelopoiesis in patients with aplastic anemia (Vadhan-Raj *et al.*, 1988). These findings, along with the observation that antibacterial activity was markedly enhanced in granulocytes derived from GM-CSF-treated monkeys, suggest that GM-CSF may have immunotherapeutic potential in treatment of bacterial infections in domestic animals.

The cDNA clones for murine (Gough *et al.*, 1985) and human (Wong *et al.*, 1985; Cantrell *et al.*, 1985; Lee *et al.*, 1985) GM-CSF have been isolated. Both encode peptides of approximately 14,000 Da and display 60% amino acid sequence similarity. The availability of purified recombinant material has allowed for the proliferation of *in vitro* and *in vivo* studies on GM-CSF activities, including those described above.

While there is much information available describing the growth-promoting the differentiation effects of GM-CSF, very little is known about how GM-CSF transduces a signal to its target cells. A 130,000-Da receptor for GM-CSF (Park *et al.*, 1986) has been identified on a variety of murine cells. GM-CSF binding to putative receptors does not alter the resting transmembrane electrical potential, intracellular pH, or the concentration of intracellular calcium, but it causes rapid release of arachidonic acid from human granulocytes (Sullivan *et al.*, 1987). This result suggests that one or more phospholipases may be activated by GM-CSF. Similarly, it was found that GM-CSF does not cause activation of protein kinase C, an increase in intracellular calcium, or phosphatidylinositol turnover in human neutrophils, but does activate guanylate cyclase and reduce adenylate cyclase activity (Coffey *et al.*, 1988). Alterations in cyclase activities could effect levels of cyclic GMP and cyclic AMP, important second messengers, which might activate biochemical pathways that could regulate some of GM-CSF's effects on responsive cells. Finally, GM-CSF induces protein tyrosine phosphorylation in cells, which proliferate in response to it (Morla *et al.*, 1988).

4. *Interferon-γ*

Originally identified as a member of a family of antiviral agents, a number of immunoregulatory functions have been ascribed to interferon-γ (IFN-γ) (Trinchieri and Perussia, 1985). For instance,

IFN-γ-mediated activities on myeloid cells include up-regulation of the expression of Ia antigens (Wong et al., 1983), IgG Fc receptors (Guyre et al., 1983), and differentiation markers (Trinchieri and Perussia, 1985), and induction of ADCC (Trinchieri and Perussia, 1985), oxygen radical elaboration (Nathan et al., 1983), and tumoricidal activity (Celada et al., 1984). IFN-γ has also been implicated in B cell differentiation (Leibson et al., 1984; Nakagawa et al., 1985; Snapper and Paul, 1987). The myeloid cell activation and antiviral functions of IFN-γ make it an attractive candidate for therapeutic use in cattle and other large animals.

Cloned murine and human IFN-γ genes encode mature proteins of approximately 16,000–17,000 Da and display approximately 40% amino acid sequence similarity (Gray and Goeddel, 1983; Gray et al., 1982). Relatively lltttle is known about the receptor for IFN-γ or how IFN-γ transduces a signal through its receptor. The receptor for IFN-γ binds the cytokine with a K_d of 1×10^{-10} M and has a MW of approximately 100,000 (Langer and Pestka, 1988; Rubenstein et al., 1987). Treatment of a human monocyte line, U937, with IFN-γ causes rapid changes in intracellular calcium and membrane potential (Klein et al., 1987) as well as a rapid redistribution of protein kinase C (Fan et al., 1988). Transcription of several IFN-γ inducible genes (such as HLA-DR) is inhibited by protein kinase C inhibitors (Fan et al., 1988). Binding of IFN-γ to its receptor also stimulates IFN-γ receptor phosphorylation (Mao et al., 1987). It is not clear how these initial, rapid effects of IFN-γ are related to two interferon-induced, double-stranded, RNA-dependent enzymes, (2′-5′)-oligoadenylate synthetase and eIF-2α protein kinase, which regulate the degradation and translation of viral RNA, respectively (Pestka et al., 1987). Although IFN-γ does not induce *de novo* synthesis of these enzymes in normal cells, this synthesis is greatly increased by IFN-γ in cells already infected by viruses such as influenza, reovirus, and vaccinia. Whether the mechanisms by which IFN-γ increases mRNA synthesis of these two enzymes in virally infected cells is related to how it increases expression of MHC Class II remains to be elucidated.

D. Cytokine Regulation of Hematopoiesis and the Immune Response

The ability of cytokines to influence maturation, differentiation, and proliferation of hematopoietic cells occurs in at least two fashions. First, cytokines are responsible for the constitutive development of mature hematopoietic elements in the bone marrow and peripheral lymphoid organs. In the fetus, early precursors migrate from the developing liver to the bone marrow and later to the thymus. At various points in time and in various tissues, cytokines influence their development. During this process, the CSFs in question are produced largely, if not solely, by stromal cells. Interleukin-3, one of the cytokines that act early in development, is thought to have a significant impact in driving uncommitted cells toward the level of primitive hematopoietic stem cells. Under the influence of other CSFs, a commitment toward more mature lineages is made. For example, it is likely that IL-7 causes a commitment toward the lymphocytic series, while IL-1 may predispose a commitment in the myelomonocytic direction. Under the influence of GM-CSF, IL-4, IL-5, CSF-1 (M-CSF), G-CSF, and probably yet undiscovered other stromal cytokines, functional monocytes, neutrophils, eosinophils, and mast cells mature.

Second, just as natural or constitutive hematopoiesis is under the regulatory control of stromal cytokines, under conditions of immunologic perturbation caused by outside influences such as microorganisms, antigen presenting cells and Th cells can produce the same cytokines as stromal cells and thereby induce maturation, differentiation, and proliferation of hematopoietic elements (Miyajima et al., 1988). Thus, inducible hematopoiesis may be envisioned as a means by which the immune system can be readily up-regulated in order to provide the host defense mechanisms against infection. Examples of all the known regulatory effects of inducible cytokines in various circumstances of immunologic perturbation are beyond the scope of this chapter.

No great leap of faith is required to envision involvement of cytokines in any of hundreds of specific circumstances. Likewise, it is reasonable to assume that administration of exogenous cytokine to an individual might have beneficial or even detrimental effects. With the availability of practically unlimited amounts of purified recombinant cytokines, researchers and clinicians are now challenged with the task of determining conditions that might beneficially influence the outcome of disease processes.

II. Recombinant Bovine and Porcine Cytokines

As explained earlier, cytokines of one animal species almost always have their most pronounced effects on animals of the same species. For example, in our hands purified recombinant human IL-1 will function in a comitogenesis assay using bovine thymocytes, as will purified recombinant bovine IL-1. However, in order to induce equivalent effects, 10,000 times more human cytokine than bovine is needed. This is one reason for administration of bovine cytokines, as opposed to murine or human, for example, to cattle. In addition, there is a second consideration. Under any of several circumstances, it might be advantageous to administer cytokine over an extended period of time. Administration of nonbovine cytokine to cattle would undoubtedly induce a neutralizing immune response, thus further dampening the effect of that cytokine. In light of these considerations, numerous investigators in our laboratory have been involved in production of recombinant cytokines of cattle, and more recently, swine.

There are several ways to clone and identify the cDNAs encoding cytokines. In the case of bovine and porcine cytokines, mRNAs from various bovine cells and cell lines were isolated and cDNA libraries prepared. Using the technique of cross-species hybridization, cDNAs encoding specific cytokines were isolated using probes made from human cytokine cDNAs (Table I). Recombinant cytokines were made by placing their cDNAs into appropriate plasmids for bacterial, yeast, or mammalian expression. Using this approach, we have cloned and expressed bovine IL-1α and IL-1β (Maliszewski, et al., 1988a), IL-2 (Cerretti et al., 1986a), GM-CSF (Maliszewski et al., 1988b), IFN-γ (Cerretti et al., 1986b), and porcine IL-1 (Maliszewski et al., 1990), many of which have also been purified to homogeneity. Table II contains a brief summary of pertinent facts regarding these peptides.

A. Recombinant Bovine Interleukin-1

Bovine alveolar macrophages were cultured for 16 hours with *Salmonella typhimurium* lipopolysaccharide in order to elicit maximal IL-1-specific mRNA (Maliszewski et al., 1988a). An alveolar macrophage

TABLE I

Conditions for Cloning cDNA for Large Animal Cytokines

Cytokine	mRNA Source	Cloning vector
BoIL-1	Alveolar macrophage	λgt10
BoIL-2	Lymph node cells	Plasmid
BoIFN-γ	Lymph node cells	Plasmid
BoGM-CSF	BT2 T cell line	λgt10
PorIL-1	Alveolar macrophage	λgt10

TABLE II

RECOMBINANT BOVINE CYTOKINES

Cytokine	Mature amino acid length	Predicted MW	Expression system
BoIL-1α	150	17,210	*Escherichia coli*
BoIL-1β	151	17,732	*E. coli*
BoIL-2	135	15,452	*Saccharomyces cerevisiae*
BoGM-CSF	126	14,250	COS-7
IFN-γ	143	16,858	*E. coli*
PorIL-1α	152	17,420	COS-7

cDNA library was constructed in γgt10 and used to infect *Escherichia coli*. Independent plaques (50,000–100,000) were blotted onto nitrocellulose filters and hybridized with ^{32}P-labeled human IL-1α and IL-1β probes (corresponding, respectively, to nucleotides 49-896 and 23-645 of the published human IL-1 sequences). After rescreening positive plaques, cDNA inserts were isolated and subcloned into the pGEMBL plasmid.

The partial restriction map and nucleotide sequence for bovine IL-1α cDNA are shown in Fig. 1. An open reading frame, spanning 804 nucleotides, encodes a 268-amino acid protein with a predicted MW of 30,820. Comparison of the amino acid sequence with that of human IL-1α indicates that the amino terminal amino acid of mature bovine IL-1α may be Gln 119. Thus, the mature protein is composed of 150 amino acids, with a predicted MW of 17,210. Bovine IL-1α is 73% homologous with the human and 62% with the mouse sequence.

The open reading frame for bovine IL-1β, beginning at nucleotide 1 and ending at nucleotide 798, codes for 266 amino acids with a predicted MW of 30,760 (Fig. 2). The mature protein contains a single *N*-linked glycosylation site. Comparison of the bovine and human sequences indicates that the amino terminus of active bovine IL-1β is Ala 114. Thus, mature bovine IL-1β consists of 151 amino acids and has a MW of 17,732. The amino acid sequence displays 62% and 59% similarity with human and mouse sequences, respectively.

To determine whether the bovine IL-1 cDNA inserts encoded peptides with IL-1 activity, DNA fragments encoding amino acids 120–268 for IL-1α and amino acids 114–266 for IL-1β were inserted into *E. coli* expression plasmids under transcriptional control of the λP$_L$ promoter. (Fig. 3). The proteins synthesized by the transformed/induced *E. coli*

A

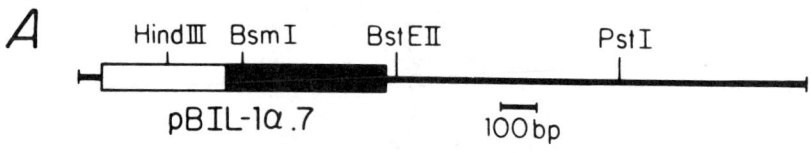

B

```
                                  GACGAGGGAGCCAGTCATCTCATTGTTGCTAGCTCGGTTCAGCAAAGAAGTGAAG          -1

     Met Ala Lys Val Pro Asp Leu Phe Glu Asp Leu Lys Asn Cys Tyr Ser Glu Asn Glu Asp          20
     ATG GCC AAA GTC CCT GAC CTC TTT GAA GAC CTG AAG AAC TGT TAC AGT GAA AAT GAA GAC          60

     Tyr Ser Ser Glu Ile Asp His Leu Ser Leu Asn Gln Lys Ser Phe Tyr Asp Ala Ser Tyr          40
     TAC AGT TCT GAA ATT GAC CAC CTC TCT CTC AAT CAG AAG TCC TTC TAT GAT GCA AGC TAT          120

     Glu Pro Leu Arg Glu Asp Gln Met Asn Lys Phe Met Ser Leu Asp Thr Ser Glu Thr Ser          60
     GAG CCA CTT CGT GAG GAC CAG ATG AAT AAG TTT ATG TCC CTG GAT ACC TCG GAA ACC TCT          180

     Lys Thr Ser Lys Leu Ser Phe Lys Glu Asn Val Val Met Val Ala Ala Ser Gly Lys Ile          80
     AAG ACA TCC AAG CTT AGC TTC AAG GAG AAT GTG GTG ATG GTG GCA GCC AGT GGG AAG ATT          240

     Leu Lys Lys Arg Arg Leu Ser Leu Asn Gln Phe Ile Thr Asp Asp Asp Leu Glu Ala Ile          100
     CTG AAG AAG AGA CGG TTG AGT TTA AAT CAG TTC ATC ACC GAT GAT GAC CTG GAA GCC ATT          300
                                                                                  *
     Ala Asn Asn Thr Glu Glu Glu Ile Ile Lys Pro Arg Ser Ala His Tyr Ser Phe Gln Ser          120
     GCC AAT AAT ACA GAA GAA GAA ATC ATC AAG CCC AGA TCA GCA CAT TAC AGC TTC CAG AGT          360

     Asn Val Lys Tyr Asn Phe Met Arg Val Ile His Gln Glu Cys Ile Leu Asn Asp Ala Leu          140
     AAC GTG AAA TAC AAC TTT ATG AGA GTC ATC CAC CAG GAA TGC ATC CTG AAC GAC GCC CTC          420
     ▲
     Asn Gln Ser Ile Ile Arg Asp Met Ser Gly Pro Tyr Leu Thr Ala Thr Thr Leu Asn Asn          160
     AAT CAA AGT ATA ATT CGA GAT ATG TCA GGT CCA TAC CTG ACG GCT ACT ACA TTA AAT AAT          480

     Leu Glu Glu Ala Val Lys Phe Asp Met Val Ala Tyr Val Ser Glu Glu Asp Ser Gln Leu          180
     CTG GAG GAG GCA GTG AAA TTT GAC ATG GTT GCT TAT GTA TCA GAA GAG GAT TCT CAG CTT          540

     Pro Val Thr Leu Arg Ile Ser Lys Thr Gln Leu Phe Val Ser Ala Gln Asn Glu Asp Glu          200
     CCT GTG ACT CTA AGA ATC TCA AAA ACT CAA CTG TTT GTG AGT GCT CAA AAT GAA GAC GAA          600

     Pro Val Leu Leu Lys Glu Met Pro Glu Thr Pro Lys Ile Ile Lys Asp Glu Thr Asn Leu          220
     CCC GTC TTG CTA AAG GAG ATG CCT GAG ACA CCC AAA ATC ATC AAA GAT GAG ACC AAC CTC          660

     Leu Phe Phe Trp Glu Lys His Gly Ser Met Asp Tyr Phe Lys Ser Val Ala His Pro Lys          240
     CTC TTC TTC TGG GAA AAG CAT GGC TCT ATG GAC TAC TTC AAA TCA GTT GCC CAT CCA AAG          720

     Leu Phe Ile Ala Thr Lys Gln Glu Lys Leu Val His Met Ala Ser Gly Pro Pro Ser Ile          260
     TTG TTT ATT GCC ACA AAG CAA GAA AAA TTG GTG CAC ATG GCA AGT GGG CCG CCC TCG ATC          780

     Thr Asp Phe Gln Ile Leu Glu Lys End                                                      268
     ACT GAC TTT CAG ATA TTG GAA AAA TAG CCTTGACTGTGCACTCTACTTACTTGTAAAGTGGTGACCATCC          850

     GTATGTACTATGTACATGAAGGAGTCGAGCCCTTCACTGTTAGTCACTCGCTGAGCATGTGCTGAGCTTTTGTAATTCT          929
     AAATGAATGTTTACTCTCTTTGTAAGAGAGAACACAAAGTCCAACACTAACATATAATGTTGCTTGTTATTTAAACAAC          1008
     ACCCTATACTTTGCAAACTACCAATCAATTTAATTATTATTCTGCACAATAATCTTGGGAGGACTGAGGCTACTATCTG          1087
     TGGCTACAAAAGGTTCTTTCCATATTATAGATGAGTAAACTAAGGCATAAGAATACTAATACCCATGACAGCAGTTGGA          1166
     ATAAGCCGTGGACACACAATTTCATTCCAACTGCTCAGCTTCTACTTTTAAGCCACTGATGGACCCTTTATCAAATACT          1245
     ATAAGTTTCTGGGGTCTCAGTTTTGCTGCTGCTGCTAAGTCACTTCAGTCATGTCCAACTCTGTGCGACCCCATAGACGG          1324
     CAGCCCACCAGGCTCCGCAGTCCCTGGGATTCTCCAGGCAAGAACACTGGAGTGGGTTGCCATTTCCTTCTCCAATGCA          1403
     TGAAAGTGAAAAGTGAAAGTGAAGTTGCTCAGTCATGTCCGACTCTTAGCGACCCCATGGACTGCAGCCTACCAGGCTCC          1482
     TCTGTCCATGGGATTTTCCAGGCAAGAGTACTGGAGTGGGGTGCCATTGCCTTCTCCCGGGGTCTCAGTTTGACCATCT          1561
     TCAAAATCAGGGTAATGATGACTATAGCCCTCCTACCTCAACAGTATTTTATGCCAATGAGTTCATTTAAGTAAAATTT          1640
     TTCTTGAAGCTGAGCCTCAAGAAGAATGCAAAGCATGAAATGTTATTTTAAGTTATTATTTATATGCATATATATTTAT          1719
     AAGCATTATTTCTAAGATATTATTATTTATTTATAACATATTATTATATTTATGGCAATTCCTTGCAATGTGTGAGTATG          1798
     ACCAGGTATCTTCAATAATAGTAGACAGTGTTTTCTAGGCTGAGTAAGTCCGAGGTACTAACGCACTTTGGTTCAAAGT          1877
     GCCTTTTCCATTGTCATGAACTTCTGTATTCCAGTACCTGGGAGCCCTGTGATTATGATAATAAATTTATATTAATTGC          1956
     CCTGTTAAAAAAAAAAAAAAAAAAAAAAAA                                                           1986
```

were analyzed by SDS-polyacrylamide gel electrophoresis (SDS-PAGE) (Fig. 4) and a new protein of the approximate expected MW was found. The cultures were assayed for bovine IL-1 activity as judged by a bovine thymocyte comitogenesis assay. This assay takes advantage of the fact that neither IL-1 nor submitogenic doses of lectin, such as phytohemagglutinin (PHA), alone induces significant blastogenesis of thymocytes. However, when thymocytes are cultured in the presence of IL-1 and PHA, both IL-2 and IL-2 receptors are induced, thereby providing a very potent proliferative signal that can be measured by incorporation of tritiated thymidine ($[^3H]$-Tdr). The assay can be quantified by comparison of the amount (i.e., cpm) of $[^3H]$-Tdr incorporated by thymocytes cultured in graded doses of recombinant protein-containing or control bacterial culture lysates. The results indicated that biologically active bovine IL-1α and IL-1β were synthesized by the appropriate bacterial cultures (Table 3). Recombinant bovine IL-1β has since been purified to homogeneity.

B. Recombinant Bovine Interleukin-2

A plasmid cDNA library was constructed from mRNA isolated from concanavalin A-stimulated bovine lymph node cells (Cerretti et al., 1986a). Small-scale plasmid DNA preparations from pools representing 2500 transformants were digested with Pst I to remove cDNA inserts and electrophoresed through agarose gels. The gels were blotted onto nitrocellulose filters and hybridized with a ^{32}P-labeled human IL-2 probe (corresponding to nucleotides 52–759 of the published human IL-2 sequence). Positive clones were divided into pools of 500, rescreened with radiolabeled probe, and secondary positive colonies were isolated. After selecting positive colonies, cDNA inserts were excised from purified plasmids, sequenced, and analyzed by computer. A partial restriction map for bovine IL-2 and the nucleotide sequence and predicted amino acid sequence are shown in Fig. 5. The open

---

FIG. 1. Restriction map and nucleotide sequence of bovine IL-1α cDNA. (A) Partial restriction map of the cDNA insert in pBIL-1α.7. The coding region for the precursor protein is boxed and the coding region for mature IL-1α is shaded. (B) Nucleotide sequence and predicted amino acid sequence of bovine IL-1α. DNA and protein sequences are numbered starting with the initator Met. The amino terminus (Ser 120) of recombinant mature IL-1α(*), potential N-glycosylation site (▲) the AT-rich regions (□), and the ATTTA sequence motif (overbar) are indicated. Reprinted with permission from Maliszewski et al. (1988a). Copyright 1988, Pergamon Press, Inc.

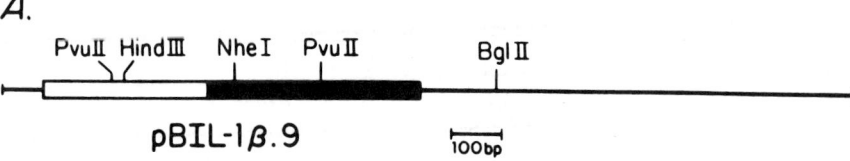

FIG. 2. Restriction map and nucleotide sequence of bovine IL-1β cDNA. (A) Partial restriction map of the cDNA insert in pBIL-1β.9. (B) Nucleotide sequence and predicted amino acid sequence of bovine IL-1β. Structural features are denoted as described in legend to Fig. 1. Reprinted with permission from Maliszewski *et al.* (1988a). Copyright 1988, Pergamon Press, Inc.

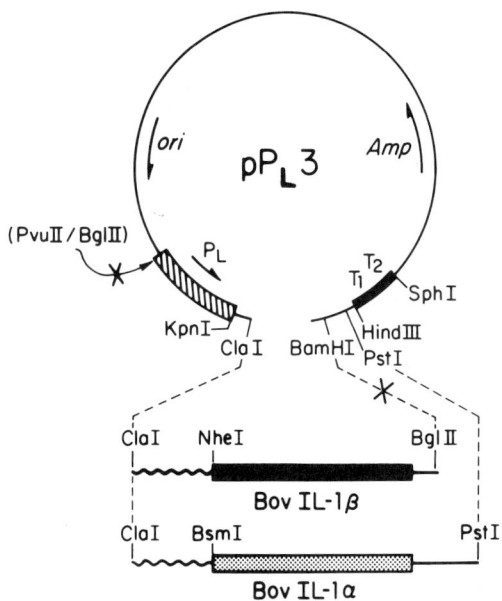

FIG. 3. Structure of *E. coli* expression plasmids pP$_L$3BIL-1α and pP$_L$3BIL-1β. The plasmids contain sequences derived form pBR322 including the origin of replication (ori) and the ampicillin resistance gene (Amp). Regions containing the λP$_L$ promoter used to direct transcription of IL-1 and the *rrnB* transcription terminators T$_1$ and T$_2$ are indicated. Waved lines represent synthetic oligonucleotides used to fuse the coding regions for IL-1α and IL-1β (boxed) to pP$_L$3. Reprinted with permission from Maliszewski *et al.* (1988a).

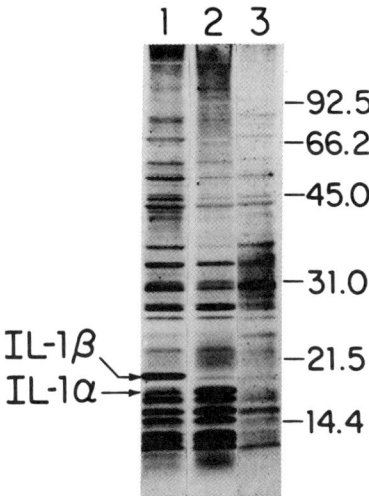

FIG. 4. Induction of bovine IL-1 synthesis in *E. coli*. Aliquots of *E. coli* cultures containing the following plasmids were centrifuged and prepared for SDS-PAGE: Lane 1, pP$_L$3BIL-1β; lane 2, pP$_L$3BIL-1α; lane 3, pP$_L$3 lacking IL-1 sequences. The position of protein MW markers are indicated as molecular weights × 10^{-3}. Arrows indicate position of recombinant bovine IL-1α and IL-1β. Reprinted with permission from Maliszewski *et al.* (1988a). Copyright 1988, Pergamon Press, Inc.

TABLE III
Bovine Thymocyte Costimulator Assay

Plasmid	Units/ml/OD of *E. coli*[a]	
	Experiment 1[b]	Experiment 2
pP$_L$3BIL-1α	812,693	223,903
pP$_L$3BIL-1β	98,581	69,632
pP$_L$3	0	0

[a] Activity is expressed in U/ml of induced *E. coli* cultures, normalized to OD 600.

[b] Numbers represent means of duplicate samples.

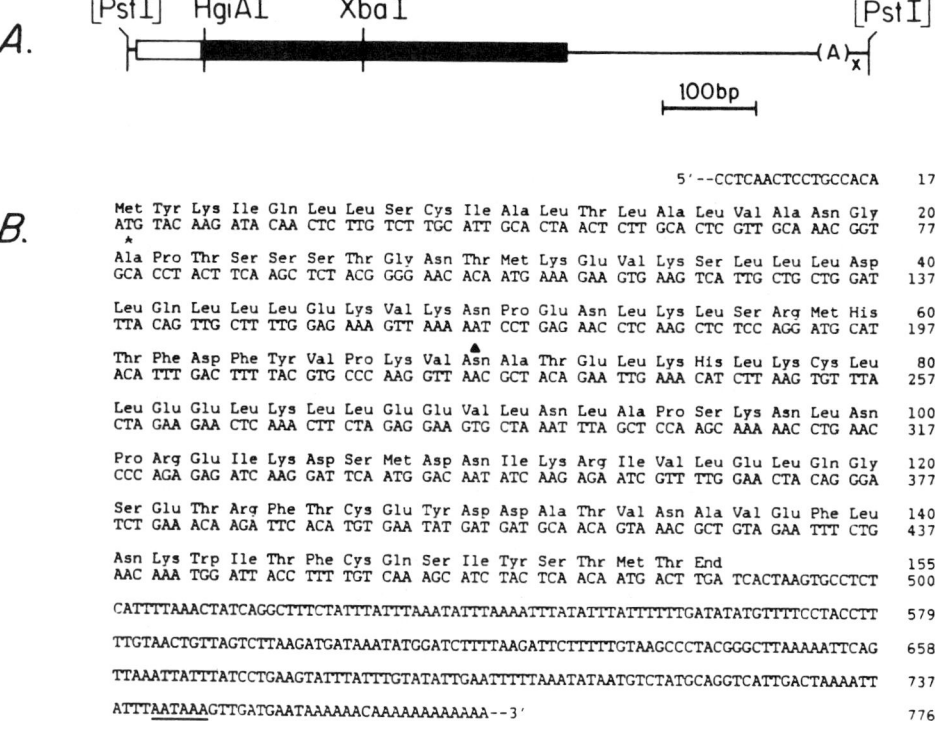

FIG. 5. Restriction map and nucleotide sequence of bovine IL-2 cDNA. (A) Partial restriction map of the cDNA insert in pBIL-2–4. The Pst I sites were generated by the cloning procedure. (B) Nucleotide sequence and predicted amino acid sequence of bovine IL-2. The predicted amino terminus (Ala-21, asterisk), possible *N*-linked glycosylation site (triangle), and polyadenylation/maturation signal (underline) are indicated.

reading frame, beginning at nucleotide 18 and ending at nucleotide 485, codes for 155 amino acids with a predicted MW of 17,555. Comparison of the bovine and human sequences indicates that the 20 amino acids at the 5' end of the open reading frame probably represent a signal sequence, making the Ala 21 the amino terminus of mature bovine IL-2. Therefore, mature bovine IL-2 would consist of 135 amino acids and would have a predicted MW of 15,452. Sequence comparisons reveal 65% and 50% similarity with human and mouse amino sequences, respectively.

To determine whether the cDNA insert from this clone encoded a peptide with IL-2 activity, a DNA fragment encoding amino acids 21–155 was inserted into an *E. coli* expression system under transcriptional control of the λP_L promoter (refer to Fig. 3). Cells transformed with this plasmid or a control plasmid were grown at 30°C, then shifted to 42°C for 3 hours for heat induction of the P_L promoter. The proteins synthesized by the transformed/induced *E. coli* were analyzed by SDS-PAGE and a new protein of the approximate expected MW was found (Fig. 6).

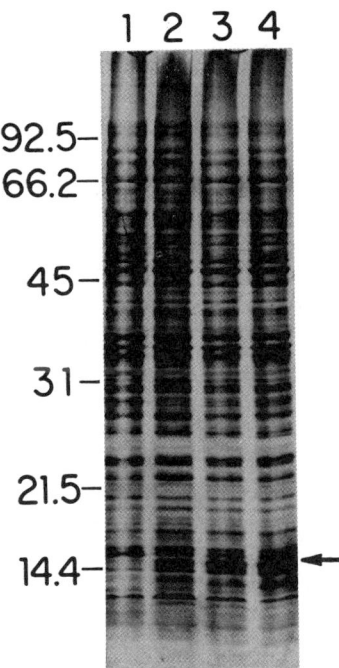

FIG. 6. Induction of bovine IL-2 synthesis in *E. coli*. Aliquots of *E. coli* cultures containing the indicated plasmids were centrifuged and prepared for SDS-PAGE at the times after induction listed below: Lanes 1, empty plasmid, 20 hours; lane 2, pLNBovIL-2, 1.5 hours; lane 3, pLBoviL-2, 4 hours; lane 4, pLNBovIL-2, 20 hours. The positions of protein MW markers are indicated at the far left. Arrow indicates position of recombinant bovine IL-2.

The above cultures were assayed for bovine IL-2 activity as judged by their ability to induce proliferation of a bovine IL-2-dependent cell line, BT2. The assay was quantified by comparison of the cpm of [^{3}H]-Tdr incorporated by BT2 cells cultured in graded doses of control cell lysate (from *E. coli* cultures transformed with the insertless plasmid) versus recombinant material (cell lysate from *E. coli* transformed with the IL-2-containing plasmid). The test material had approximately 2.8×10^6 units/ml of IL-2 activity, while no activity was measured in the control lysate.

Foreign proteins can be made to be secreted by the yeast *Saccharomyces cerevisiae*, thus simplifying large-scale purification procedures. The cDNA encoding mature bovine IL-2 was cloned into a yeast expression plasmid as a fusion gene, following the yeast α-factor leader (Urdal *et al.*, 1984) and under the control of the yeast ADH2 promoter. As the yeast grew in culture, depleting glucose in the medium, the ADH2 promoter was derepressed, allowing production and secretion of the fusion protein. The fusion protein was enzymatically cleaved to the α-factor leader and mature bovine IL-2. The secreted bovine IL-2 was purified to homogeneity, using a two-step HPLC technique, previously developed for purification of human IL-2 made in a similar fashion by yeast (Price *et al.*, 1987). The final yield of pure bovine IL-2 (as determined by silver stained gels) was on the order of 50 mg/liter of yeast broth.

C. Recombinant Bovine GM-CSF

Lectin-stimulated BT2 cells synthesize GM-CSF as determined by Northern blot analysis using a radiolabeled human GM-CSF cDNA probe (corresponding to nucleotides −15 to 540 of the published sequence). A λgt10 cDNA library was generated from BT2 mRNA and 100,000 plaques were screened with the human probe (Maliszewski *et al.*, 1988b). Of four positive clones identified by plaque filter hybridization, one was subcloned into the pGEMBL 18 plasmid for restriction mapping and sequence analysis. The nucleotide sequence identified an open reading frame encoding a protein of 143 amino acids, including a putative 17-residue signal sequence (Fig. 7). The mature secreted protein would thus be composed of 126 amino acids and have a predicted MW 14,250. The size of naturally synthesized bovine GM-CSF would likely exceed the predicted value, due to the presence of two *N*-linked glycosylation sites. The amino acid sequence displays 71% and 56% similarity with human and mouse sequences, respectively.

To determine if the bovine GM-CSF cDNA encodes a protein with the

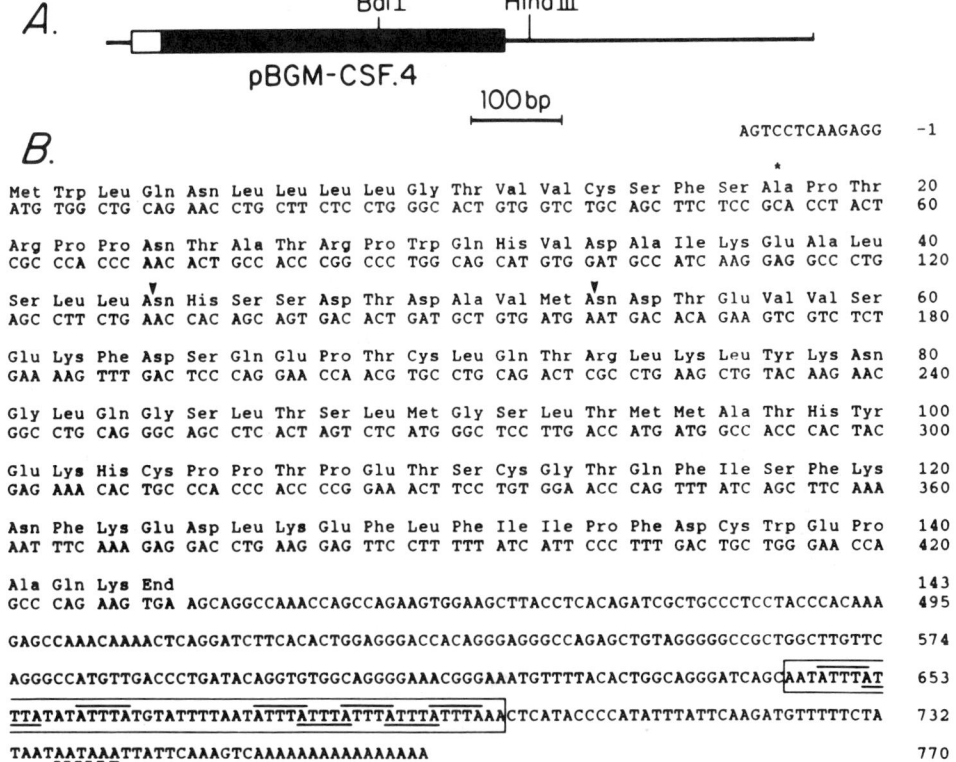

FIG. 7. Restriction map and nucleotide sequence of bovine GM-CSF. (A) Partial restriction map of the cDNA insert in pBGM-CSF.4. (B) Nucleotide sequence and predicted amino acid sequence of bovine GM-CSF. The predicted amino terminus (Ala 18), N-glycosylation sites, etc., are indicated as described in Fig. 1. Reprinted with permission from Maliszewski et al. (1988b). Copyright 1988, Pergamon Press, Inc.

biochemical and functional properties of GM-CSF, a fragment consisting of nucleotides −13 to 458 was inserted into a mammalian expression vector (pDC) (Fig. 8). COS-7 cells were transfected with the GM-CSF plasmid (pDC/BGM-CSF) or with an insertless control plasmid (pDC), and cultured for the final 6 hours of a 72-hour culture period in the presence of [^{35}S] methionine/cysteine. Radiolabeled culture supernatants were analyzed for the presence of newly synthesized soluble proteins by SDS-PAGE and autoradiography (Fig. 9). A major band with a MW of 22,500 was detected in supernatant fluid from cells

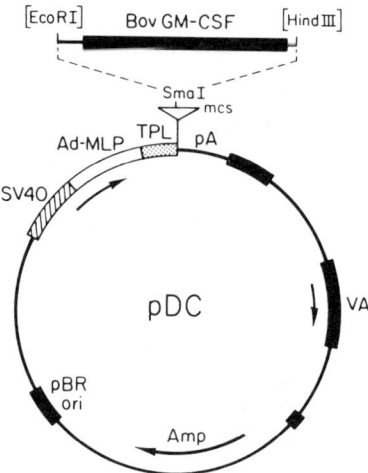

FIG. 8. Structure of bovine GM-CSF expression plasmid. The bovine GM-CSF cDNA was inserted into a site in the pDC mammalian expression plasmid flanked by sequences representing: (1) the SV40 origin of replication, enhancer, and early and late promoters; (2) the adenovirus-2 major late promoter and tripartite leader; (3) SV40 polyadenylation and transcription termination signals; and (4) adenovirus-2 virus-associated RNA genes (VAI and VAII).

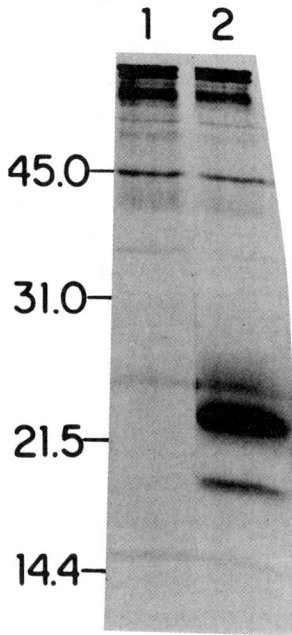

FIG. 9. SDS-PAGE of recombinant bovine GM-CSF. Supernatants from ^{35}S-labeled COS-7 cells, transfected with pDC (lane 1) or pDC/BGM-CSF (lane 2), were electrophoresed on an 18% gel and prepared for autoradiography. The positions of protein MW markers are indicated in kDa. Reprinted with permission from Maliszewski et al. (1988b). Copyright 1988, Pergamon Press, Inc.

transfected with pDC/GM-CSF, but not in control supernatant. In addition, the GM-CSF supernatant contained a minor band with a MW of approximately 18,000 and a protein smear above the major band, likely representing hypo- and hyperglycosylated proteins, respectively.

Recombinant bovine GM-CSF activity was monitored by a proliferation assay, which measures uptake of tritiated thymidine by 96-hour cultures of bovine bone marrow cells. Cells were cultured in the presence of threefold dilutions of control and GM-CSF containing supernatants from transfected COS cells. Bovine bone marrow cells proliferated in a dose-dependent manner in the presence of recombinant bovine GM-CSF supernatant (54,000 U/ml) (Fig. 10). There was no detectable activity in the control COS supernatant. In order to determine the species specificity of GM-CSF biological activity, similar assays were performed with human, murine, and bovine cells in the presence of recombinant GM-CSF from all three species. The results from these studies clearly indicate that GM-SCF from the three species displayed only very limited cross-reactivity (Table IV). Recombinant bovine GM-CSF has been expressed in the yeast system (described above) and purified to homogeneity.

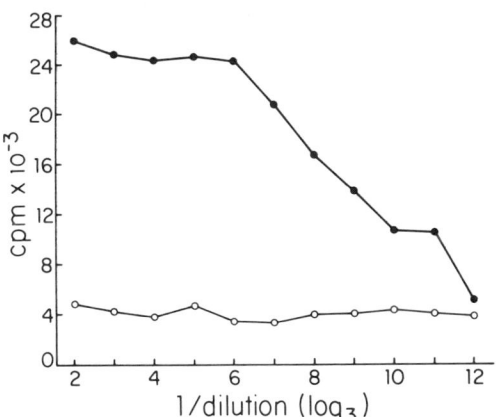

FIG. 10. Biological activity of recombinant bovine GM-CSF. Supernatants from COS-7 cells transfected with pDC (open circles) or pDC/BGM-CSF (solid circles) were assayed for GM-CSF in the bovine bone marrow proliferation assay. The y-axis represents incorporated cpm of [^{3}H]-thymidine and the x-axis represents the reciprocal $\log_3$ dilution of sample. Each point represents the mean of duplicate samples. Reprinted with permission from Maliszewski *et al.* (1988b). Copyright 1988, Pergamon Press, Inc.

TABLE IV

Cross-Species Reactivities of Bovine, Murine, and Human GM-CSF

Species of recombinant GM-CSF	Bone marrow proliferation assay (U/ml)[a]		
	Bovine	Human	Murine
Bovine	67,224	348	12
Human	334	99,351	0
Murine	0	0	13,830

[a] Proliferation assays using bovine, human, or murine bone marrow cells from 96-hour cultures. Numbers represent means of triplicate or quadruplicate samples. Reprinted with permission from Maliszewski et al. (1988b). Copyright 1988, Pergamon Press, Inc.

D. Recombinant Bovine Interferon-γ

The bovine lymph node cell library, from which the IL-2 cDNA was cloned, was screened in a similar manner with a radiolabeled human IFN-γ cDNA probe (corresponding to nucleotides 186 to 877 of the published sequence). The cDNA for bovine IFN-γ (Cerretti et al., 1986b) includes an open reading frame encoding a 166-amino acid protein of predicted MW 19,393 (Fig. 11). Included in the coding sequence is a putative signal sequence of 23 residues as well as two N-linked glycosylation sites. The bovine analogue displays 63% and 47% amino acid sequence similarity with human and murine sequences, respectively.

The identity of bovine IFN-γ was verified by inserting the cDNA into the pP_L3 expression plasmid and analyzing transformed E. coli lysates for biological activity. Functional activity was measured by the virus plaque reduction assay. Briefly, MDBK (bovine kidney-derived) cells were pretreated with twofold dilutions of control or recombinant IFN-γ-containing bacterial lysates (or with human IFN-α as a positive control), then incubated with known amounts of vesicular stomatitis virus, and overlayed with methylcellulose. After overnight incubation, the methylcellulose was removed and plaques were stained with crystal violet and counted. Cultures of E. coli containing the IFN-γ plasmid expressed the recombinant lymphokine at 115,300 U/ml, whereas control cultures (with insertless plasmid) displayed only background activity.

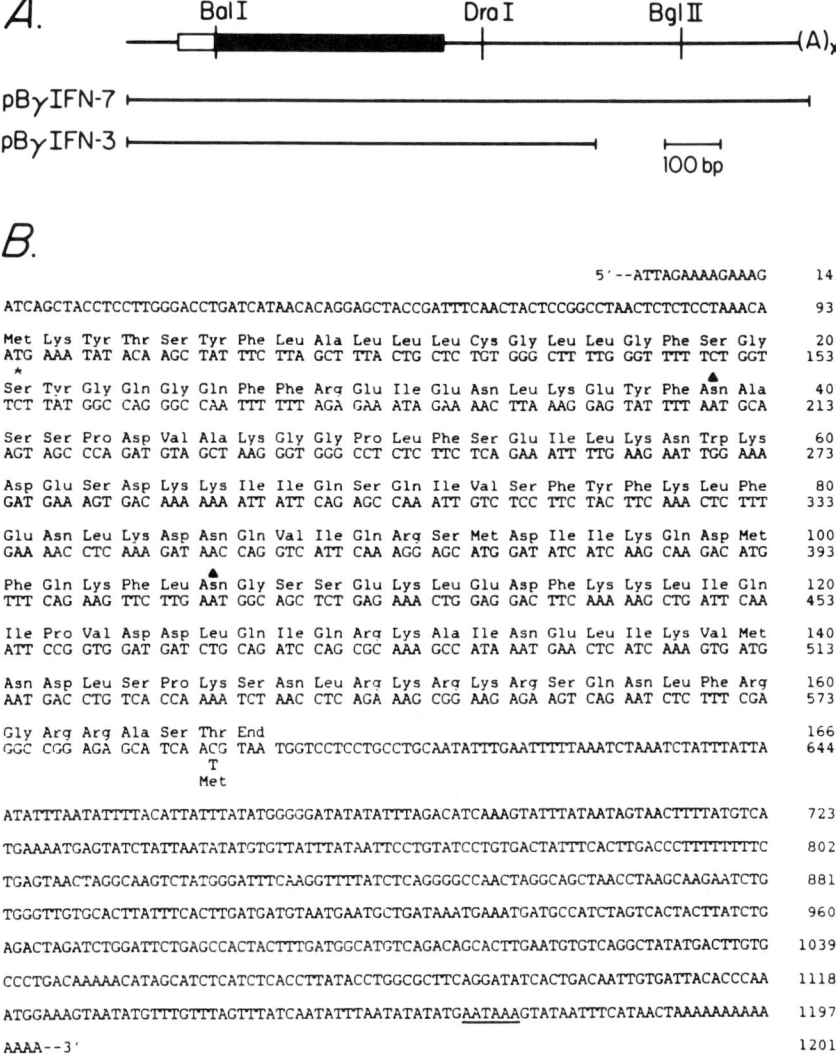

FIG. 11. Restriction map and nucleotide sequence of bovine IFN-γ cDNA. (A) Partial restriction map of the cDNA inserts encoding bovine IFN-γ. (B) Nucleotide sequence and predicted amino acid sequence of bovine IFN-γ. The predicted amino terminal end of mature bovine IFN-γ (Gln-24) and other structural features are appropriately indicated. Reprinted with permission from Cerretti *et al.* (1986b). Copyright 1986, American Association of Immunologists.

E. Recombinant Porcine IInterleukin-1

Porcine alveolar macrophage mRNA was used as the template for construction of a cDNA library in λgt10. Independent plaques (150,000) were hybridized with a ^{32}P-labeled bovine IL-1α probe (corresponding to nucleotides 245 to 894 of the published sequence). Five positive clones were isolated after three sequential rounds of screening, and one was selected for further analysis. The cDNA for porcine IL-1α includes an open reading frame of 270 amino acids with a predicted MW of 30,788 and containing three N-linked glycosylation sites (Maliszewski et al., 1990). Porcine IL-1α displays 71%, 84%, and 61% similarity with human, bovine, and murine analogues, respectively. COS-7 cells transfected with a procine IL-1α mammalian expression plasmid secreted detectable levels of active porcine IL-1α, as determined by a porcine thymocyte costimulator assay. Further characterization of recombinant porcine IL-1α is currently in progress.

F. Common Structural Features of Cytokines and Their Genes

Bovine cytokine genes appear to share a number of features with genes for other mammalian cytokines. For instance, Southern blot analysis of restriction endonuclease-digested bovine genomic DNA indicates that all five bovine genes (IL-1α, IL-1β, IL-2, IFN-γ, and GM-CSF) are present as single copies in the genome, as are their murine and human analogues. Sizes for bovine cytokine mRNAs also are consistent with those reported for analogous cytokines from other species. A common feature for all of these cytokine messages is the presence in the 3' noncoding region of AT-rich stretches, including multiple copies of the ATTTA motif (e.g., see Figs. 1 and 7). Such a motif has been implicated in the regulation of expression of cytokine genes (Shaw and Kamen, 1986; Cosman, 1987), a function that is obviously of critical importance for temporal control of levels of such powerful immunomodulatory proteins.

Bovine cytokines display 50–73% identity with murine and human analogues at the amino acid level (Table V). Such a high degree of sequence conservation is consistent with the critical roles that cytokines play in survival. Alignment of cytokine amino acid sequences from several species may be used to identify elements of primary and secondary protein structure that may be important for biological function and/or receptor binding. We have constructed such comparisons for all five of the cloned bovine cytokines. IL-1a is presented as an example,

TABLE V

Cross-Species Amino Acid Sequence
Similarities of Bovine and
Porcine Cytokines

Cytokine	Percent identity with	
	Human	Murine
BoIL-1α	73	62
BoIL-1β	62	59
BoIL-2	65	50
BoIFN-γ	63	47
BoGM-CSF	71	56
PorIL-1	71	61

because sequences from at least five mammalian species have been identified, thus presenting data for a fairly exhaustive cross-species alignment (Fig. 12). There is a total of 118 identities, representing approximately 43% of all residues. Of particular interest are identities present in the sequences for mature IL-1, which maintains receptor binding and biological activities. Establishing the importance of these conserved residues may be accomplished by mutational analysis of IL-1 at specific amino acid positions, followed by determination of binding and biological activities of the protein products. Such studies could elucidate the structural requirements for IL-1 function and lead to the development of IL-1 agonists and antagonists. Clearly, such analyses could also be applied to other cytokines for which amino acid sequences from two or more species are available.

III. Conclusions

At the heart of all cytokine actions is the interaction of ligand with its receptor. Without exception, these reactions have been found to be exquisitely specific. In fact, their affinities are generally several orders of magnitude greater than antigen–antibody interactions. After the receptor binds to its ligand, signals are sent across the cytoplasmic membrane, which result in a series of second messages. Although not presently known for certain, it is reasonable to assume that these second messages are not unlike those previously shown to be at play for

Interspecies Amino Acid Alignment of IL-1α

```
Bovine    MAKVPDLFED LKNCYSENED YSSEIDHLSL NQKSFYDASY EPLREDQMNK
Porcine   MAKVPDLFED LKNCYSENEE YSSDIDHLSL NQKSFYDASY EPLPGDGMDK
Rabbit    MAKVPDLFED LKNCFSENEE YSSAIDHLSL NQKSFYDASY EPLHEDCMNK
Human     MAKVPDMFED LKNCYSENEE DSSSIDHLSL NQKSFYHVSY GPLHEGCMDQ
Murine    MAKVPDLFED LKNCYSENED YSSAIDHLSL NQKSFYDASY GSLHETCTDQ

Bovine    FMSLDTSETS KTSKLSFKEN VWMVAA---S GKILKKRRLS LNQFITDDDL
Porcine   FMPLSTSKTS KTSRLNFKDS VWMAAA---N GKILKKRRLS LNQFITDDDL
Rabbit    VVSLSTSETS VSPNLTFQEN VWAVTA---S GKILKKRRLS LNQPITDVDL
Human     SVSLSISETS KTSKLTFKES MVVVAT---N GKMLKKRRLS LSQSITDDDL
Murine    FVSLRTSETS KMSNFIFKES RVTVSATSSN GKILKKRRLS FSETFIEDDL

Bovine    EAIANNIEEE IIKPRSAHYS FQSNVKYNFM RVIHQECIIN DALNQSIIRD
Porcine   EAIANDTEEE IIKPRSATYS FQSNMKYNFM RVINHQCIIN DARNQSIIRD
Rabbit    ETNVSDPEEG IIKPRSVPYT FQRNMRYKYL RIIKQEFTIN DALNQSLVRD
Human     EAIANDSEEE IIKPRSAPFS FLSNVKYNFM RIIKYEFILN DALNQSIIR-
Murine    QSITHDIEE- TIQPRSAPYT YQSDLRYKLM KLVRQKFVMN DSLNQTIYQD

Bovine    MSGPYLTATT INNLEEAVKF DMVAYVSE-E DSQLPVTLRI SKTQLFVSAQ
Porcine   PSGQYLMAAV INNLDEAVKF DMAAYTSN-D DSQLPVTLRI SETRLFVSAQ
Rabbit    TSDQYLRAAP LQNLGDAVKF DMGVYMTS-E DSILPVTLRI SQTPLFVSAQ
Human     ANDQYLTAAA IHNLDEAVKF DMGAYKSSKD DAKITMILRI SKTQLYVTAQ
Murine    VDKHYLSTTW INDLQQEVKF DMYAYSSGGD DSKYPVTLKI SDSQLFVSAQ

Bovine    NEDEPVLLKEM PEIPKIIKD -EINLLFFWE KHGSMDYFKS VAHPKLFIAT
Porcine   NEDEPVLLKEL PEIPKTIKD -ETSLLFFWE KHGNMDYFKS AAHPKLFIAT
Rabbit    NEDEPVLLKEM PEIPRIIITD SESDILFFWE TQGNKNYFKS AANPQLFIAT
Human     DEDQPVLLKEM PEIPKTIITG SETNLLFFWE THGTKNYFTS VAHPNLFIAT
Murine    GEDQPVLLKEL PEIPKLIITG SETDLIFFWK SINSKNYFTS AAMPELFIAT

Bovine    KQEKLVHMASG PPSITDFQI LEK--
Porcine   RQEKLVHMAPG LPSMTDFQI LENQS
Rabbit    KPEHLVHMARG LPSMTDFQI S----
Human     KQDYWVCIAGG PPSITDFQI LENQA
Murine    KEQSRVHILARG LPSMTDFQI S----
```

FIG. 12. Alignment of bovine, porcine, rabbit, human, and murine IL-1α amino acid sequences as deduced form their DNA sequences. Boxed residues indicate identity for all five species at a given sequence position.

other peptide hormones such as insulin and PDGF. Where target cells proliferate in response to a specific cytokine, we speculate that binding of cytokine to receptor results in activation of protein kinases, leading to phosphorylation and subsequent activation of various enzymes.

Using cross-species hybridization techniques, we have cloned the cDNAs encoding a number of cytokines of cattle and swine. Several of these cytokines have been expressed in yeast or bacteria. At a basic level, the availability of large quantities of these proteins will allow further experimentation into their mechanisms of action, perhaps elucidating various intracellular mechanisms involved in cell signaling. In a more practical sense, production of sufficient quantities of bovine and porcine cytokines may translate to novel methodologies to prevent or treat diseases of farm animals.

REFERENCES

Abraham, R. T., Ho, S. N., Barna, T. J., and McKean, D. J. (1987). Transmembrane signalling during interleukin 1-dependent T cell activation. *J. Biol. Chem.* **262,** 2719–1728.

Alemany, S., Mato, J. M., and Stralfors, P. (1987). Phospho-dephospho control by insulin is mimicked by a phospho-oligosaccharide in adipocytes. *Nature (London)* **330,** 77–79.

Auron, P. E., Webb, A. C., Rosenwasser, L. J., Mucci, S. F., Rich, A., Wolff, S. M., and Dinarello, C. A. (1984). Nucleotide sequence of human monocyte interleukin 1 precursor cDNA. *Proc. Natl. Acad. Sci. U.S.A.* **81,** 7909–7911.

Benedict, S. H., Mills, G. B., and Gelfand, E. W. (1987). Interleukin 2 activates a receptor-associated protein kinase. *J. Immunol.* **139,** 1694–1697.

Bird, T. A., and Saklatvala, J. (1989). IL-1 and TNF transmodulate epidermal growth factor receptors by a protein kinase C-independent mechanism. *J. Immunol.* **142,** 126–133.

Cantrell, M. A., Anderson, D., Cerretti, D. P., Price, V., McKereghan, K., Tushinski, R. J., Mochizuki, D. Y., Larsen, A., Grabstein, K., Gillis, S., and Cosman, D. (1985). Cloning, sequence, and expression of a human granulocyte-macrophage colony-stimulating factor. *Proc. Natl. Acad. Sci. U.S.A.* **83,** 6250–6254.

Celada, A., Gray, P. W., Rinderknecht, E., and Scheiber, R. D. (1984). Evidence for a gamma-interferon receptor that regulates macrophage tumoricidal activity. *J. Exp. Med.* **160,** 55–74.

Cerretti, D. P., McKereghan, K., Larsen, A., Cantrell, M. A., Anderson, D., Gillis, S., Cosman, D., and Baker, P. E. (1986a). Cloning, sequence, and expression of bovine interleukin 2. *Proc. Natl. Acad. Sci. U.S.A.* **83,** 3223–3227.

Cerretti, D. P., McKereghan, K., Larsen, A., Cosman, D., Gillis, S., and Baker, P. E. (1986b). Cloning, sequence, and expression of bovine interferon-γ. *J. Immunol.* **136,** 4561–4564.

Chan, B. L., Lisanti, M. P., Rodriquez-Boulan, E., and Saltiel, A. R. (1988). Insulin-stimulated release of lipoprotein lipase by metabolism of its phosphatidylinositol anchor. *Science* **241,** 1670–1672.

Clark, S. C., and Kamen, R. (1987). The human hematopoietic colony-stimulating factors. *Science* **236**, 1229–1237.

Coffey, R. G., Davis, J. S., and Djeu, J. Y. (1988). Stimulation of guanylate cyclase activity and reduction of adenylate cyclase activity by granulocyte-macrophage colony-stimulating factor in human blood neutrophils. *J. Immunol.* **140**, 2695–2701.

Cosman, D. (1987). Control of messenger RNA stability. *Immunol. Today* **8**, 16–17.

Czech, M. P., Klarland, J. K., Yagaloff, K. A., Bradford, A. P., and Lewis, R. E. (1988). Insulin receptor signaling. Activation of multiple serine kinases. *J. Biol. Chem.* **263**, 11017–11020.

Dempsey, R. A., Dinarello, C. A., Mier, J. W., Rosenwasser, L. J., Allegretta, M., Brown, T. E., and Parkinson, D. R. (1982). The differential effects of human leukocytic pyrogen/lymphocyte activating factor, T cell growth factor, and interferon on human natural killer activity. *J. Immunol.* **129**, 2504–2510.

Dessein, A. J., Vadas, M. A., Nicola, N. A., Metcalf, D., and David, J. R. (1982). Enhancement of human blood eosiniphil cytotoxicity by semipurified eosinophil colony-stimulating factor(s). *J. Exp. Med.* **156**, 90–103.

Dinarello, C. A. (1988). Biology of interleukin 1. *FASEB J.* **2**, 108–115.

Dinarello, C. A. (1989). Interleukin-1 and its biologically related cytokines. *Adv. Immunol.* **44**, 153–205.

Donahue, R. E., Wang, E. A., Stone, D. K., Kamen, R., Wong, G. G., Seghal, P. K., Nathan, D. G., and Clark, S. C. (1986). Stimulation of hematopoiesis in primates by continuous infusion of recombinant GM-CSF. *Nature (London)* **321**, 872–875.

Dower, S. K., Kronheim, S. R., Hopp, T. P., Cantrell, M., Deeley, M., Gillis, S., Henney, C. S., and Urdal, D. L. (1986). The cell surface receptors for interleukin-1α and interleukin-1β are identical. *Nature (London)* **324**, 266–268.

Falkoff, R. J. M., Muraguchi, A., Hong, J.-X., Butler, J. L., Dinarello, C. A., and Fauci, A. (1983). The effects of interleukin 1 on human B cell activation and proliferation. *J. Immunol.* **131**, 801–805.

Fan, X.-D., Goldberg, M., and Bloom, R. B. (1988). Interferon-γ induced transcriptional activation is mediated by protein kinase C. *Proc. Natl. Acad. Sci. U.S.A.* **85**, 5122–5125.

Farrar, W. L., Cleveland, J. L., Beckner, S. K., Bonvini, E., and Evans, S. W. (1986). Biochemical and molecular events associated with interleukin 2 regulation of lymphocyte proliferation. *Immunol. Rev.* **92**, 49–65.

Flexner, C., Hugin, A., and Moss, B. (1987). Prevention of vaccinia virus infection in immunodeficient mice by vector-directed IL-2 expression. *Nature (London)* **330**, 259–262.

Furutani, Y., Notake, M., Yamayoshi, M., Yamagishi, J., Momura, H., Ohue, M., Furuta, R., Fukui, T., Yamada, M., and Nakamura, S. (1985). Cloning and characterization of the cDNAs for human and rabbit interleukin-1 precursor. *Nucleic Acids Res.* **13**, 5869–5882.

Gallis, B., Prickett, K. S., Jackson, J., Slack, J., Schooley, K., Sims, J. E., and Dower, S. K. (1990). Interleukin 1 induces rapid phosphorylation of its own receptor. Submitted for publication.

Gasson, J. C., Weisbart, R. H., Kaufman, S. E., Clark, S. C., Hewick, R. M., Wong, G. G., and Golde, D. C. (1984). Purified granulocyte-macrophage colony-stimulating factor: Direct action on neutrophils. *Science* **226**, 1339–1342.

Gaulton, G., and Eardley, D. D. (1986). Interleukin-2 dependent phosphorylation of interleukin 2 receptors and other T cell membrane proteins. *J. Immunol.* **136**, 2470–2477.

Gery, I., and Waksman, B. H. (1972). Potentiation of the T-lymphocyte response to mitogens. II. The cellular source of potentiating mediator(s). *J. Exp. Med.* **136,** 143–155.

Gillis, S., and Mizel, S. B. (1981). T-cell lymphoma model for the analysis of interleukin-1 mediated T-cell activation. *Proc. Natl. Acad. Sci. U.S.A.* **78,** 1133–1137.

Gough, N. M., Metcalf, D., Gough, J., Grail, D., and Dunn, A. R. (1985). Structure and expression of the mRNA for murine granulocyte-macrophage colony stimulating factor. *EMBO J.* **4,** 645–653.

Grabstein, K. H., Urdal, D. L., Tushinski, R. J., Mochizuki, D. Y., Price, V. L., Cantrell, M. A., Gillis, S., and Conlon, P. J. (1986a). Induction of macrophage tumoricidal activity by granulocyte-macrophage colony-stimulating factor. *Science* **232,** 506–508.

Grabstein, K. H., Mochizuki, D., Kronheim, S., Price, V., Cosman, D., Urdal, D., Gillis, S., and Conlon, P. J. (1986b). Regulation of antibody production in vitro by granulocyte-macrophage colony-stimulating factor. *J. Mol. Cell. Immunol.* **2,** 199–207.

Gray, P. W., and Goeddel, D. V. (1983). Cloning and expression of murine immune interferon cDNA. *Proc. Natl. Acad. Sci. U.S.A.* **80,** 5842–5846.

Gray, P. W., Leung, D. W., Pennica, D., Yelverton, E., Najarian, R., Simonsen, C. C., Dernyck, R., Sherwood, P. J., Wallace, D. M., Berger, S. L., Levinson, A. D., and Goeddel, D. V. (1982). Expression of human immune interferon cDNA in *E coli* and monkey cells. *Nature (London)* **295,** 503–508.

Gray, P. W., Glaister, D., Chen, E., Goeddel, D. V., and Pennica, D. (1986). Two interleukin 1 genes in the mouse: Cloning and expression of the cDNA for murine interleukin 1β. *J. Immunol.* **137,** 3644–3648.

Greene, W. C., and Leonard, W. J. (1986). The human interleukin 2 receptor. *Annu. Rev. Immunol.* **4,** 69–95.

Guyre, P., Morganelli, P., and Miller, R. (1983). Recombinant immune interferon increases immunoglobulin G Fc receptors on cultured human mononuclear phagocytes. *J. Clin. Invest.* **72,** 393–400.

Hatakeyama, M., Minamoto, S., Uchiyama, T., Hardy, R. R., Yamada, G., and Taniguchi, T. (1985). Reconstitution of functional receptor for human interleukin-2 in mouse cells. *Nature (London)* **318,** 467–470.

Hoffman, M. K., and Watson, J. (1979). Helper T cell replacing factors secreted by thymus-derived cells and macrophages: Cellular requirements for B cell activation and synergistic properties. *J. Immunol.* **122,** 1371–1375.

Hopp, T. P., Dower, S. K., and March, C. J. (1986). The molecular forms of interleukin-1. *Immunol. Res.* **5,** 271–280.

Ishil, T., Takeshita, T., Nomata, N., and Sugamina, K. (1989). Protein phosphorylation mediated by byl-2/IL-2 receptor β-chain interaction. *J. Immunol.* **141,** 174–179.

Kahn, C. R., and White, M. F. (1988). The insulin receptor and the molecular mechanism of insulin action. *J. Clin. Invest.* **82,** 1151–1156.

Kashima, N., Nishi-Takaoka, C., Fujita, T., Taki, S., Yamada, G., Hamuro, J., and Taniguchi, T. (1985). Unique structure of murine interleukin 2 as deduced from cloned cDNA. *Nature (London)* **313,** 402–404.

Kaur, P., and Saklatvala, J. (1988). Interleukin 1 and tumor necrosis factor increase phosphorylation of fibroblast proteins. *FEBS Lett.* **241,** 6–18.

Kester, M., Simonson, M. S., Mene, P., and Sedor, J. R. (1989). Interleukin-1 generates transmembrane signals from phospholipids through novel pathways in cultured rat mesangial cells. *J. Clin. Invest.* **83,** 718–723.

Klein, J. B., McLeish, K. R., and Sonnenfeld, G. (1987). Alterations of membrane potential in U937 cells induced by interferon-γ. *J. Interferon Res.* **7,** 770 (abstr.).

Langer, J. A., and Pestka, S. (1988). Interferon receptors. *Immunol. Today* **9**, 393–400.

Lee, F., Yokota, T., Otsuka, T., Gemmell, L., Larson, N., Luh, J., Arai, K.-I, and Rennick, D. (1985). Isolation of cDNA for a human granulocyte-macrophage colony-stimulating factor by functional expression in mammalian cells. *Proc. Natl. Acad. Sci. U.S.A.* **82**, 4360–4364.

Leibson, H. J., Gefter, M., Zlotnik, A., Marrack, P., and Kappler, J. W. (1984). Role of γ-interferon in antibody-producing responses. *Nature (London)* **309**, 799–801.

Lomedico, P. T., Gubler, U., Hellman, C. P., Dukovich, M., Giri, J. G., Pan, Y.-C., Coller, K., Seminow, R., Chua, A. O., and Mizel, S. B. (1984). Cloning and expression of murine interleukin-1 cDNA in *Escherichia coli*. *Nature (London)* **312**, 458–462.

Lomedico, P. T., Gubler, U., and Mizel, S. B. (1987). Cloning and expression of murine, human and rabbit interleukin 1 genes. *Lymphokines (N.Y.)* **13**, 13.

Maliszewski, C. R., Baker, P. E., Schoenborn, M. A., Davis, B. S., Cosman, D., Gillis, S., and Cerretti, D. P. (1988a). Cloning, sequence and expression of bovine interleukin 1α and interleukin 1β complementary cDNAs. *Mol. Immunol.* **25**, 429–437.

Maleszewski, C. R., Schoenborn, M. A., Cerretti, D. P., Wignall, J. M., Picha, K. S., Cosman, D., Tushinski, R. J., Gillis, S., and Baker, P. E. (1988b). Bovine GM-CSF: molecular cloning and biological activity of the recombinant protein. *Mol. Immunol.* **25**, 843–850.

Maliszewski, C. R., Renshaw, B., and Baker, P. E. (1990). Nucleotide sequence of porcine interleukin 1α. In press.

Mao, C., Ballottii, R., Agnet, M., Falcoff, E., and Mulin, G. (1987). Studies on the phosphorylation of the human interferon gamma receptor. *J. Interferon Res.* **7**, 765 (abstr.).

March, C. J., Mosley, B., Larsen, A., Cerretti, D. P., Braedt, G., Price, V., Gillis, S., Henney, C. S., Kronheim, S. R., Grabstein, K., Conlon, P. J., Hopp, T. P., and Cosman, D. (1985). Cloning, sequence, and expression of two distinct human interleukin-1 complementary DNAs. *Nature (London)* **315**, 641–648.

Martin, M., and Resch, K. (1988). Interleukin 1: More than a mediator between lymphocytes. *Trends Pharmacol. Sci.* **9**, 171–177.

Matsushima, K., Kobayashi, Y., Copeland, T. D., Akahoshi, T., and Oppenheim, J. J. (1987). Phosphorylation of a cytosolic 65-kDa protein induced by interleukin-1 in glucocorticoid pretreated normal human peripheral blood mononuclear leukocytes. *J. Immunol.* **139**, 3367–3374.

Matsushima, K., Shiroo, M., Kung, H., and Copeland, T. D. (1988). Purification and characterization of a cystolic 65-kilodalton phosphoprotein in human leukocytes whose phosphorylation is augmented by stimulation with interleukin-1. *Biochemistry* **27**, 3765–3770.

Mayer, P., Lam, C., Obenhaus, H., Liehl, E., and Besemer, J. (1987). Recombinant human GM-CSF induces leukocytosis and activates peripheral blood polymorphonuclear neutrophils in nonhuman primates. *Blood* **70**, 206–213.

Metcalf, D. (1986). The molecular biology and functions of the granulocyte-macrophage colony-stimulating factors. *Blood* **67**, 257–267.

Metcalf, D., Begley, C. G., Williamson, D. J., Nice, E. C., DeLamarter, J., Mermod, J.-J., Thatcher, D., and Schmidt, A. (1987). Hemopoietic responses in mice injected with purified recombinant murine GM-CSF. *Exp. Hematol.* **15**, 1–9.

Mills, G. B., and May, C. (1987). Binding of interleukin 2 to its 75-kDa intermediate affinity receptor is sufficient to activate Na^+/H^+ exchange. *J. Immunol.* **139**, 4083–4087.

Miyajima, A., Miyatake, S., Schreurs, J., DeVries, J., Arai, N., Yokota, T., and Arai, K.-I. (1988). Coordinate regulation of immune and inflammatory responses by T cell-derived lymphokines. *FASEB J.* **2**, 2462–2473.

Mochizuki, D. Y., Eisenman, J. R., Conlon, P. J., Larsen, A. D., and Tushinski, R. J. (1987). Interleukin 1 regulates hematopoietic activity, a role previously ascribed to hemopoietin 1. *Proc. Natl. Acad. Sci. U.S.A.* **84**, 5267–5271.

Morla, A. D., Schreurs, J., Miyajima, A., and Wang, J. Y. J. (1988). Hematopoietic growth factors activate tyrosine phosphorylation of distinct sets of proteins in interleukin-3-dependent murine cell lines. *Mol. Cell. Biol.* **8**, 2214–2218.

Muraguchi, A., Kehrl, J. H., Longo, D. L., Volkman, D. J., Smith, K. A., and Fauci, A. S. (1985). Interleukin 2 receptors on human B cells. Implications for the role of interleukin 2 in B cell function. *J. Exp. Med.* **161**, 181–196.

Nakagawa, T., Hiramo, T., Nakagawa, N., Yoshizaki, K., and Kishimoto, T. (1985). Effect of recombinant IL2 and IFN-γ on proliferation and differentiation of human B cells. *J. Immunol.* **134**, 959–966.

Nathan, C. F., Murray, H. W., Wiebe, M. E., and Rubin, B. Y. (1983). Identification of interferon as the lymphokine that activates human macrophage oxidative metabolism and antimicrobial activity. *J. Exp. Med.* **158**, 670–689.

Park, L. S., Friend, D., Gillis, S., and Urdal, D. L. (1986). Characterization of the cell surface receptor for granulocyte-macrophage colony-stimulating factor. *J. Biol. Chem.* **261**, 4177–4183.

Pestka, S., Langer, J. A., Zoon, K. C., and Samuel, L. E. (1987). Interferons and their actions. *Annu. Rev. Biochem.* **56**, 727–777.

Price, V., Mochizuki, D., March, C., Cosman, D., Deeley, M., Klinke, R., Clevenger, W., Gillis, S., Baker, P., and Urdal, D. (1987). Expression, purification, and characterization of recombinant murine granulocyte-macrophage colony-stimulating factor and bovine interleukin-2. *Gene* **55**, 287–293.

Raines, E. W., Dower, S. K., and Ross, R. (1989). IL-1 mitogenic activity for fibroblasts and smooth muscle cells is due to PDGF-AA. *Science* **243**, 393–396.

Ramchaw, J. A., Andrew, M. E., Phillips, S. M., Boyle, D. B., and Coupor, B. E. H. (1987). Recovery of immunodeficient mice from a vaccinia virus/IL-2 recombinant infection. *Nature (London)* **329**, 545–546.

Raz, A., Wycke, A., Siegel, N., and Needleman, P. (1988). Regulation of fibroblast cyclooxygenase synthesis by interleukin-1. *J. Biol. Chem.* **263**, 3022–3028.

Reed, S. G., Pihl, D. L., Conlon, P. J., and Grabstein, K. H. (1989). IL-1 as adjuvant: Role of T cells in the augmentation of specific antibody production by human recombinant IL-1α. *J. Immunol.* **142**, 3129–3133.

Rosen, O. M. (1987). After insulin binds. *Science* **237**, 1452–1458.

Rosoff, P. M., Savage, N., and Dinarello, C. A. (1988). Interleukin-1 stimulates diacylglycerol production in T lymphocytes by a novel mechanism. *Cell (Cambridge, Mass.)* **54**, 73–81.

Rubenstein, M., Dorick, D., and Fischer, D. G. (1987). The human interferon-system. *Immunol. Rev.* **97**, 29–50.

Saltzman, E. M., Thorn, R. R., and Casnellie, J. E. (1988). Activation of a tyrosine protein kinase is an early event in the stimulation of T lymphocytes by interleukin-2. *J. Biol. Chem.* **263**, 6956–6959.

Schulman, H., and Lou, L. L. (1989). Multifunctional Ca^{++}/calmodulin-dependent protein kinase: Domain structure and regulation. *Trends Biochem. Sci.* **14**, 62–66.

Shaw, G., and Kamen, R. (1986). Conserved AU sequence from the untranslated region of GM-CSF mRNA mediates selective mRNA degradation. *Cell (Cambridge, Mass.)* **46**, 659–667.

Sims, J. E., March, C. J., Cosman, D. J., Widmer, M. B., MacDonald, H. R., McMahan, C. J., Grubin, C. E., Wignall, J. M., Jackson, J. L., Call, S. M., Friend, D., Alpert, A. A., Gillis, S., Urdal, D. L., and Dower, S. K. (1988). cDNA expression cloning of the IL-1 receptor, a member of the immunoglobulin superfamily. *Science* **241**, 585–589.

Smith, K. A. (1988). Interleukin 2: Inception, impact, and implication. *Science* **240**, 1169–1176.

Snapper, C. M., and Paul, W. E. (1987). Interferon-γ and B cell stimulatory factor-1 reciprocally regulate Ig isotype production. *Science* **236**, 944–947.

Staruch, M. J., and Wood, D. D. (1983). The adjuvanticity of interleukin 1 *in vivo*. *J. Immunol.* **130**, 191–2194.

Stralfors, P. (1988). Insulin stimulation of glucose uptake can be mediated by diacylglycerol in adipocytes. *Nature (London)* **335**, 554–556.

Sturgill, T. W., Ray, L. B., Erikson, E., and Maller, J. L. (1988). Insulin-stimulated MAP-2 kinase phosphorylates and activates ribosomal S6 kinase II. *Nature (London)* **334**, 715–718.

Sullivan, R., Griffin, J. D., Simons E. R., Schafer, A. I., Meshulum, T., Fredette, J. P., Maas, A. K., Gadenne, A. S., Leavitt, J. L., and Melnick, D. A. (1987). Effects of recombinant human granulocyte and macrophage colony-stimulating factors on signal transduction pathways in human granulocytes. *J. Immunol.* **139**, 3422–3430.

Taniguchi, T., Matsui, H., Fujita, T., Takaoka, C., Kashima, N., Yoshimo, R., and Hamuro, J. (1983). Structure and expression of a cloned cDNA for human interleukin 2. *Nature (London)* **302**, 305–310.

Trinchieri, G., and Perussia, B. (1985). Immune interferon: A pleiotropic lymphokine with multiple effects. *Immunol. Today* **6**, 131–136.

Urdal, D., Mochizuki, D., Conlon, P., March, C., Remerowski, M., Eisenman, J., Ramthun, C., and Gillis, S. (1984). Lymphokine purification by reverse-phase high-performance liquid chromatography. *J. Chromatogr.* **296**, 171–179.

Utsunomiya, N., Tsubori, M., and Nakanishi, M. (1986). Interleukin 2 increases T lymphocyte membrane mobility before the rise in cytosolic calcium concentration. *Biochemistry* **25**, 2582–2584.

Vadas, M. A., Nicola, N. A., and Metcalf, D. (1983). Activation of antibody dependent cell-mediated cytotoxicity of human neutrophils and eosinophils by separate colony-stimulating factors. *J. Immunol.* **130**, 795–799.

Vadhan-Raj, S., Buescher, S., Broxmeyer, H. E., LeMaistre, A., Lepe-Zuniga, J. L., Ventura, G., Jeha, S., Horwitz, L. J., Trujillo, J. M., Gillis, S., Hittelman, W. N., and Gutterman, J. U. (1988). Stimulation of myelopoiesis in patients with aplastic anemia by recombinant human granulocyte-macrophage colony-stimulating factor. *N. Engl. J. Med.* **319**, 1628–1334.

Wahl, M. I., Daniel, T. O., and Carpenter, G. (1988). Antiphosphotyrosine recovery of phospholipase C activity after EGF treatment of A-431 cells. *Science* **241**, 968–970.

Wahl, M. I., Nishibe, S., Suh, P.-G., Rhee, S. G., and Carpenter, G. (1989). Epidermal growth factor stimulates tyrosine phosphorylation of phospholopase C-II independently of receptor internalization and extracellular calcium. *Proc. Natl. Acad. Sci. U.S.A.* **86**, 1568–1572.

Weisbart, R. H., Golde, D. W., Clark, S. C., Wong, G. G., and Gasson, J. C. (1985). Human granulocyte-macrophage colony-stimulating factor is a neutrophil activator. *Nature (London)* **314**, 361–363.

Williams, L. T. (1989). Signal transduction by the platelet-derived growth factor receptor. *Science* **243,** 1564–1570.
Wong, G. G., Witek, J. S., Temple, P. A., Wilkens, K. M., Leary, A. C., Luxenberg, D. P., Jones, S. S., Brown, E. L., Kay, R. M., Orr, E. C., Shoemaker, C., Golde, D. W., Kaufman, R. J., Hewick, R. M., Wang, E. A., and Clark, S. C. (1985). Human GM-CSF: Molecular cloning of the complementary DNA and purification of the natural and recombinant proteins. *Science* **228,** 810–815.
Wong, G. H. W., Clark-Lewis, I., McKimm-Breschkin, J. L., Harris, A. W., and Schrader, J. W. (1983). Interferon-γ induces enhanced expression of Ia and H-2 antigens on B lymphoid, macrophage, and myeloid cell lines. *J. Immunol.* **131,** 788–793.
Zubler, R. H., Lowenthal, J. W., Errad, F., Hashimoto, N., Devos, R., and MacDonald, H. R. (1984). Activated B cells express receptor for and proliferate in response to pure interleukin-2. *J. Exp. Med.* **160,** 1170.

Interferon Immunomodulation in Domestic Food Animals

H. BIELEFELDT-OHMANN[*,1] AND S. R. MARTINOD[†]

Veterinary Infectious Disease Organization, University of Saskatchewan, Saskatoon, Saskatchewan, Canada S7N OWO, and
†*Biovet Unit, Ciba-Geigy Ltd., Centre de Recherches Agricoles, St. Aubin, Switzerland*

I. Introduction
II. Modulation of Nonspecific Antimicrobial Defense Mechanisms
III. Modulation of the Specific Cellular Immune Response
IV. Enhancement of Antimicrobial Mechanisms in the Gut
V. Immunoenhancement in Noninfectious Diseases
VI. Concluding Remarks
    References

I. Introduction

Although originally described as antiviral proteins (Isaacs and Lindenmann, 1957), it is now evident that the interferons (IFN) comprise a heterogeneous assembly of proteins and glycoproteins with a plethora of biologic functions, including cellular regulation and differentiation as well as potent immunoregulatory activities (DeMaeyer and DeMaeyer-Guignard, 1988). In recent years this latter capability has been the focus of intensive investigations, both in *in vitro* systems and *in vivo* including studies with clinical applications (DeMaeyer and DeMaeyer-Guignard, 1982, 1988; Kirchner, 1984; Bielefeldt-Ohmann *et al.*, 1987).

Within the veterinary field until very recently only the bovine IFN system had attracted attention to any substantial degree (Bielefeldt-Ohmann *et al.*, 1987). However, this situation is changing as work has now been initiated in the porcine, equine (Himmler *et al.*, 1986), and avian systems. In addition to the homologous factors, effects of heterolo-

---

[1] Present address: Menzies School of Health Research, Casuarina, Darwin, Australia

gous IFN, e.g., human, have been investigated in some large animal species (MacLachlan and Anderson, 1986; Schwers et al., 1988). Many of these aspects were recently reviewed (Bielefeldt-Ohmann et al., 1987; Lawman et al., 1989). To date, 4 of the more than 27 bovine IFN-α (BoIFN-α) genes, 2 of the 5 BoIFN-β genes and the only BoIFN-γ gene have been cloned and expressed in *Escherichia coli* by recombinant DNA technology (Leung et al., 1984; Capon et al., 1985; Cerretti et al., 1986). Large-scale production of rBoIFN-$α_I$1 and -γ has allowed clinical trials with cattle and swine to be conducted using these products for evaluation of their potential prophylactic and therapeutic value in viral and bacterial infections (Babiuk et al., 1986, 1987). Likewise, porcine IFN-α (PoIFN-α) (Lefevre and La Bonnardiere, 1986) and -γ (unpublished) have been cloned and expressed in a bacterial system.

None of the bovine or other animal lymphokines have yet been exploited solely for their immunomodulatory effects although work has now been initiated to study their adjuvanticity (see below). The primary interest of the clinical investigations conducted with rBoIFN-α and rHuIFN-α has been concerned with the antiviral effect of the compounds (Babiuk and Bielefeldt-Ohmann, 1984; Babiuk et al., 1986, 1987; Roney et al., 1985; Schwers et al., 1982, 1988).

II. Modulation of Nonspecific Antimicrobial Defense Mechanisms

One of the most extensively studied models of infectious diseases in domestic animals is the bovine respiratory disease complex (Yates, 1982; Bielefeldt-Ohmann and Babiuk, 1986c). This model involves viral–bacterial interactions with the primary respiratory viral infection being bovine herpesvirus-1 (BHV-1). This virus predisposes the animal, by as yet unresolved mechanisms, to a secondary, often fatal, bacterial pneumonia (Babiuk et al., 1989). The administration of rBoIFN-α or -γ markedly reduces severity of both clinical illness and mortality in BHV-1-infected calves (Babiuk and Bielefeldt-Ohmann, 1984; Babiuk et al., 1986, 1987). This effect apparently is due, in this model, to a reduced susceptibility to the secondary bacterial agent, most likely via an immunomodulatory mechanism, since pretreatment with rBoIFN-α (or -γ) does not significantly reduce BHV-1 replication in the nasal passages (Babiuk et al., 1986). However, since there are other viruses involved in bovine respiratory disease which are more susceptible to IFN *in vitro* (Anderson et al., 1985; Czarniecki et al., 1986; Trueblood and Manjara, 1972; Fulton et al., 1984), rBoIFN$α_I$1 may have a dual beneficial effect: antiviral and immunomodulatory. rBoIFN-$α_I$1 also significantly reduced the incidence of disease in field trials for enzootic calf pneumonia (Martinod et al., 1988; Table 1) and shipping fever (Lynn and Phillip, 1988).

In most organ systems, and prominently so in the respiratory tract, the first line of cellular defense against invading microorganisms is exerted by phagocytic cells, i.e., macrophages (Mø), and polymorphonuclear neutrophilic (PMN) and eosinophilic granulocytes. The cellular mechanisms involved in execution of the antimicrobial combat comprise migration from the blood into the infected foci, generation and release of hydrolytic enzymes, reactive oxygen species (ROS), IFN, prostaglandins and complement factors, phagocytosis, and cellular cytotoxicity. Most, if not all, of these functions can be modulated by

TABLE I

Effect of rBoIFN-α on Incidence of Respiratory Disease in Young Dairy Housed Calves

Study number	Treatment	% Incidence	% Advantage
1/87	Controls	84.2 (16/19)	—
	5 mg I.M.	61.9 (13/21)	+27
	0.5 mg I.M.	61.1 (11/18)	+28
2/87	Controls	83.3 (15/18)	—
	5 mg I.M. (1×)	71.4 (15/21)	+14
	5 mg I.M. (2×)	50.0 (10/20)[a]	+40
4/87	Controls	90.9 (20/22)	—
	5 mg	71.4 (18/25)	+21
7/87	Controls	75.0 (15/20)	—
	5 mg I.N.	84.0 (16/19)	−12
	5 mg I.M.	83.0 (15/18)	−11
10/87	Controls	90.0 (19/21)	—
	5 mg I.M. + 5 mg IN	83.0 (15/18)	+8
	5 mg I.M.	85.0 (17/20)	+8
40/87	Controls PI-3 vaccine	68.2 (15/22)	—
	PI-3 vaccine + 5 mg IFN I.M.	31.8 (7/22)[a]	+53
	5 mg IFN I.M.	36.4 (8/22)	+49

[a] Significantly different from control ($P < 0.05$), Fisher exact probability test.

$$\text{Incidence of BRD is} = \frac{\text{no. of animals ever diagnosed as sick during the study}}{\text{no. of healthy animals in the beginning of the study}}$$

Interferon was administered intramuscularly (I.M.) or intranasally (I.N.) on arrival at the farm after transportation. Each animal was checked daily and scored for the severity of clinical symptoms from day 0 up to and including day 21 of the study.

exposure to IFNs, but whether the result is an up- or a down-regulation depends on the particular function in question, the cellular environment (i.e., *in vitro* vs. *in vivo*), the IFN type, IFN dose and duration of exposure, as well as the health status of the recipient animal (or cell donor) (Bielefeldt-Ohmann and Babiuk, 1984, 1985a, 1986a,b; Bielefeldt-Ohmann et al., 1984, 1987; Steinbach et al., 1986; Roth and Frank, 1989; Brzoska and Obert, 1987). Especially the latter criterion appears to be very important, since contradicting results on PMN activities have been obtained in healthy and virus–bacteria-infected calves (Bielefeldt-Ohmann and Babiuk, 1985a). *In vivo* administration of rBoIFN-α_I1 to calves prior to BHV-1 and *Pasteurella hemolytica* challenge was shown to increase PMN functions as measured by cell migration and generation of ROS. This augmented activity of PMN appeared to correlate with reduction of overall clinical disease, i.e., number of sick days, lung lesions, and weight loss (Lawman et al., 1987; Bielefeldt-Ohmann and Babiuk, 1985a). In contrast, administration of rBoIFN-α_I1 or -γ to healthy calves suppresses PMN migration, but enhances ROS generation (Bielefeldt-Ohmann and Babiuk, 1985a, 1986b).

III. Modulation of the Specific Cellular Immune Response

In addition to the modulation of nonspecific defense mechanisms by IFNs, antigen-specific immune responses are amenable to regulation by IFN (DeMaeyer and DeMaeyer-Guignard, 1988). This effect may be indirect via activity of "bystander cells" and induction of other immunoregulatory factors, or it may be a direct modulation of lymphocyte functions by the IFN. As examples of either type of pathways it has been found that activation of PMN by rBoIFN-α_I1 leads to enhancement of their ability to suppress lymphocyte proliferation (Babiuk et al., 1987). In contrast, treatment of bovine Mø with rBoIFN-α or -γ causes enhanced MHC Class II antigen expression on the cell surface and increased IL-1 production, thereby enhancing the accessory cell potential of the Mø (Bielefeldt-Ohmann et al., 1986; Everlith and Splitter, 1986; Walrand et al., 1989).

During primary infection and hyperimmunization with BHV-1, increased non-MHC-restricted cellular cytotoxicity can be detected among peripheral blood mononuclear cells (PBMC). This enhancement of cell activity appears to be virus specific and occurs concomitantly with IFN-γ production (Campos et al., 1989). A scenario can be envisaged in which antigen-specific T helper cells are responding to the antigen exposure by producing, among an array of lymphokines, IFN-γ (DeMaeyer and DeMaeyer-Guignard, 1988). The IFN-γ activates the cytotoxic cells, which appear to reside in or be closely related to the Mø lineage (Bielefeldt-Ohmann et al., 1985; Campos et al., 1989). As in other species (Gidlund et al., 1978; Weigent et al., 1983; Belosevic et al., 1988) this cellular activity is highly responsive to in vitro and in vivo modulation by IFNs (Bielefeldt-Ohmann and Babiuk, 1985b), although recent results also suggest that other factors in addition to IFN-γ may be essential, at least, in the development of non-MHC-restricted cytotoxic responses during BHV-1 infection (Campos et al., 1989).

The rBoIFNs also have direct effects on lymphocyte functions. Following treatment of healthy calves with rBoIFN-$α_I$1 or -γ, a depression of the proliferative response of PBMC occurs (Bielefeldt-Ohmann and Babiuk, 1986b). This effect can partly be overcome by supplementing the cell cultures with interleukin-2 (IL-2), thus indicating at least partial suppression of T helper cell functions. However, another contributing factor to the decreased responsiveness appears to be a numerical deficit of responder cells (Griebel et al., 1989). Thus, the 24-hour lymphopenia seen in animals injected with rBoIFN-$α_I$1 appears to be due to a decrease in circulating T cells, especially of the $CD8^+$ phenotype, and in non-T/non-B lymphocytes (Griebel et al., 1989). These phenomena, i.e., depressed proliferative response and changes in cell trafficking, after rBoIFN$α_I$1 injection mimics what is seen in cattle infected with BHV-1 (Bielefeldt-Ohmann and Babiuk, 1985c; Griebel et al., 1988a,b). Thus, it seems likely that IFN-α plays a role in the acute-phase response to BHV-1 infection. It also has been shown that rBoIFN$α_I$1 inhibits the migration of lymphocytes from lymph nodes but not into lymph nodes (Kalaaji et al., 1988). This knowledge should help in establishing a treatment to circumvent the "immunosuppression" caused by BHV-1 and perhaps other viruses, and thus the enhanced susceptibility to secondary (bacterial) infections.

The mechanisms whereby IFN-γ affects lymphocyte functions may be different from those of IFN-α (Bielefeldt-Ohmann et al., 1987). Thus, IFN either enhances or suppresses lymphocyte proliferation depending on concentration and duration of exposure. This has led to speculations that IFN-γ may function in a feedback circuit, enhancing low cellular responses and suppressing high responses (Bielefeldt-Ohmann and Babiuk, 1986b; Bielefeldt-Ohmann et al., 1987; Brzoska and Obert, 1987). To further complicate this picture the indications also are that the relative concentrations at which IFN-γ exerts these pleiotropic effects depend on threshold sensitivities of each particular reaction chain, and that they vary depending on both the function and the general physiological status of the animal (Brzoska and Obert, 1987; J. A. Roth and D. E. Frank, unpublished). The implications of this, if correct, my be a limitation in the applicability of IFN-γ for therapeutic treatments. Furthermore, it becomes quite apparent that the effect of exogenous IFN-γ should be carefully evaluated for each particular therapeutic application. As an example of the disparity one may encounter, a comparison can be made of the effect of recombinant IFN-γ for prevention of respiratory disease in swine and in cattle. Treatment of piglets with rPoIFN-γ 24 hours prior to *Actinobacilus pleuropneumonia* challenge abolishes clinical disease; however, rBoIFN-γ cannot prevent clinical disease in cattle caused by *P. hemolytica* when rBoIFN-γ is given 24 hours prior to infection (i.e., 3 days after BHV-1 challenge). Rather the latter treatment regime seems to exacerbate the pneumonia, perhaps by enhancing rather than suppressing ongoing inflammation caused by the initial BHV-1 infection (Bielefeldt-Ohmann, 1990). Treatment with rBoIFN-γ also cannot prevent pneumonia in calves caused by *Haemophilus somnus* (Chiang et al., 1990).

Studies in humans and small laboratory animals have shown that IFN affects both *in vivo* and *in vitro* antibody production (DeMaeyer and DeMaeyer-Guignard, 1988). Its effect can be to increase or decrease the level of antibody. The up- or down-regulation of antibody production is dependent on many factors, some of which are IFN concentration, timing of administration, and the host system studied (Hooks et al., 1982). Thus, IFN-γ has greater modulating effects than both IFN-α and -β. IFN can depress antibody production if it is given early in the immune response (Chester et al., 1973) but will enhance it if low IFN concentrations are used and are added late (Gisler et al., 1974; Brodeur and Merigan, 1975). The depression of antibody production by IFN occurs with both T-dependent and T-independent antigens, whereas the increase occurs only with T-dependent antigens (Sonnenfeld et al., 1978). Other observations have shown that IFN, when added together with antigen or later, suppressed antibody production, whereas the addition of IFN prior to antigen enhanced the production of antibody (Parker et al., 1981).

Interferon has been shown to be able to substitute for a T cell replacement factor, which acts in concert with other factors to stimulate a B cell response (Leibson et al., 1984). Interferon can act as a B cell maturation factor, directly inducing resting B cells to exhibit cell-surface phenotype changes and to secrete antibody (Sidman et al., 1984). It seems, therefore, that IFNs can regulate B cells either by suppressing or augmenting the production of antibody. Furthermore, its effect occurs at both the proliferative and differentiation phases of B cell maturation (Mond et al., 1985).

Although no inhibitory effect of rBoIFN treatment on the antibody response to viral antigens, whether presented as intact virus or subunit entities, has been detected in cattle (Babiuk and Bielefeldt-Ohmann, 1984; H. Bielefeldt-Ohmann and M. Campos, unpublished data), both rBoIFN-α_I1 and -γ have profound effects on the *in vitro* secondary antibody response (Bielefeldt-Ohmann et al., 1987). In recent adjuvanticity/compatibility studies in cattle it was found that neither rBoIFN-γ nor rBoIFN-α_I1 given -24 hours, 0, or $+24$ hours relative to antigen injection had any effect on the immune response as measured by antibody production (H. Bielefeldt-Ohmann, M. Campos, and S. Martinod, unpublished data). These results seem to preclude an application for bovine IFNs as adjuvants in contrast to information presented by others (Playfair and de Souza, 1987; Mifune et al., 1987; Marcowitz et al., 1987; Anderson et al., 1988). However, it does indicate that the IFNs can be given simultaneously with a vaccine, for example when cattle enter a feedlot, without adversely affecting the vaccine response. This is important if rBoIFN-α_I1 (or -γ) is eventually to be used for prevention of bovine respiratory disease (Babiuk et al., 1988; Martinod et al., 1988).

IV. Enhancement of Antimicrobial Mechanisms in the Gut

Another serious disease complex in domestic food animals is infectious diarrhea in neonates and young calves. A multitude of different agents, viral, bacterial, and parasitic, can alone or in combination cause life-threatening and debilitating disease in the young. Active immunization is often not possible in these young animals and passive transfer of immunoglobulins have so far been the method of choice. Oral application of IFN is not feasible due to breakdown in the gut, unless special delivery systems are developed. It was recently reported that the intramuscular treatment of calves with human IFN-α decreased symptoms of rotavirus diarrhea although virus excretion was not altered (Werenne, 1985). Perhaps even more encouraging are the results obtained in salmonellosis in young calves. Septicemia with *S. typhimurium* was significantly reduced in calves given an intramuscular injection of rBoIFN-α_I1 prior to challenge with the bacteria (Fig. 1) when compared to calves receiving placebo (Peel et al., 1989). rBoIFN-α_I1 administered before challenge was beneficial only in severe infection: 90% of the calves survived a challenge with 10^8 CFU of bacteria.

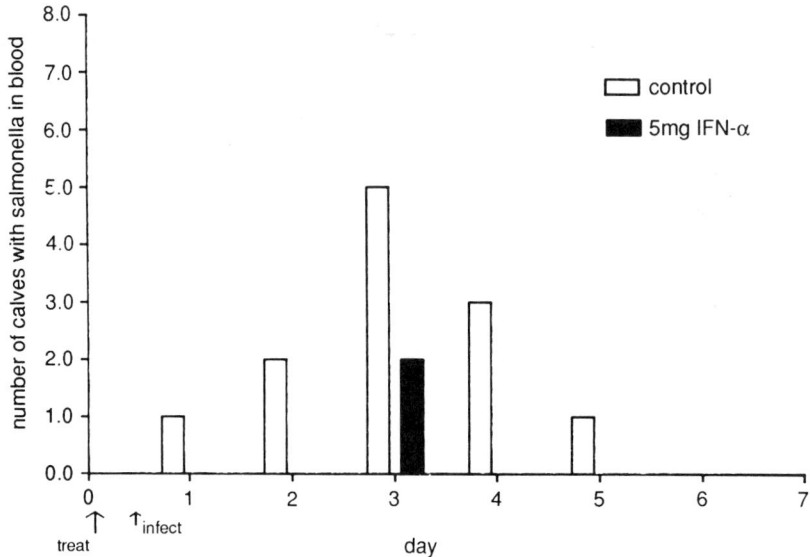

FIG. 1. Results of blood culture of calves. Two groups of calves were treated with either 5 mg rBoIFN-$\alpha_1$1 I.M. or a placebo 6 hours prior to a challenge with 10^7 colony-forming units of *Salmonella typhimurium*. Samples were taken daily for 7 days.

However, the same dose of rBoIFN-$\alpha_1$1 had no effect on the course of disease if the animals were infected with 10^7 CFU (Peel et al., 1990). Since IFN does not have a direct effect on bacterial growth the most likely mechanism for its effect is that of immunopotentiation. Gut leukocytes are responsive to IFNs in ways similar to those of leukocytes from other tissue environments (Nagi and Babiuk, 1988a,b) but until a better characterization of the anti-salmonella defense has been made, the exact mode of action of rBoIFN-$\alpha_1$1 can not be resolved. It is likely that the mechanism is comparable to that of rPoIFN-α or -γ against a bacterial infection with *A. pleuropneumonia* in the porcine lung (see above). The results reported here should, however, encourage the study of IFN treatment (pre- or post-) in diarrheal diseases caused by other bacterial, and perhaps also parasitic, agents.

V. Immunoenhancement in Noninfectious Diseases

A number of other disease groups in addition to infectious diseases may be potential candidates for an immunotherapeutic approach. These include cancer, malnutrition, autoimmunity, and allergy, as well as disturbances of hemopoiesis. The application of cytokines including IFNs in these areas within veterinary medicine was discussed in a recent review (Lawman et al., 1989) and will not be further discussed here. In many cases these diseases will be of limited interest in domestic food animals, partly for economic reasons and also because of the relative young age of this population. Exceptions may occur with animals of high genetic potential or personal and sentimental value. From a scientific viewpoint, however, much information of comparative value may be obtained through the application of cytokines, including the IFNs, in immunotherapeutic strategies against infectious and noninfectious diseases of domestic animals.

As an example, recent results have been obtained suggesting a physiological role for immunoregulatory cytokines in placental development and maternal-fetal allograft interaction. Ovine trophoblast protein (oTP-1), secreted by the embryonic trophectoderm, appears to possess a homology of more than 70% with bovine IFN-α_{II} and 37% with human IFN-α (Charpigny et al., 1988; Imakawa et al., 1987; Stewart et al., 1987). A secretory protein of the bovine trophoblast is immunologically related to oTP-1 (Helmer et al., 1987). One function of these two proteins is to prevent luteolysis and thus secure continued progesterone secretion from the ovary. The mechanism appears to be via inhibition of endometrial prostaglandin $F_2\alpha$ ($PGF_2\alpha$) release (Helmer et al., 1988a,b;

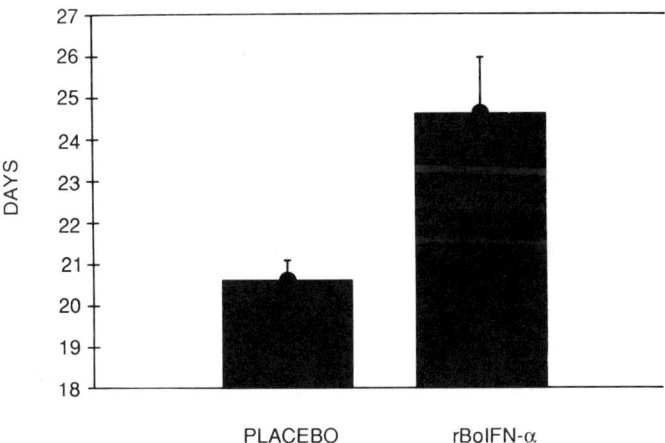

FIG. 2. Effect of intramuscular injection of rBoIFN-$\alpha_1$1 on estrus cycle lengths of dairy heifers (5 animals per group). Interestrus intervals were longer ($p < 0.01$) for heifers treated with 20 mg IFN twice daily from day 15 to 19 postestrus than for control heifers.

Thatcher et al., 1988). Very recently it was shown that a similar effect can be obtained in cattle by intrauterine infusion or intramuscular injection of rBoIFN-α_I1 (Plante et al., 1988, 1990). Furthermore, systemic treatment of cycling heifers with rBoIFNα_I1 can improve fertility (Martinod et al., 1990) (Fig. 2). This could prove useful as an approach in schemes to reduce embryonic mortality caused by aberrant secretion of embryonic IFNs.

VI. Concluding Remarks

The normal synthesis of IFNs is critical for the adequate functioning of the immune system and the maintenance of homeostasis. Disturbance of IFN synthesis can occur under the influence of endogenous or exogenous factors (e.g., viruses, bacteria, parasites, or physical and chemical agents) or can be genetically predetermined (i.e., by the presence of defective genes responsible for IFN synthesis and IFN repression).

In addition to the beneficial effects of IFNs in prevention of certain infectious diseases, there is now evidence indicating a negative action of IFN in some infections (Korngold and Doherty, 1985; Lairmore et al., 1988; Brzoska and Obert, 1987; Shurkovich et al., 1987; H. Bielefeldt-Ohmann, unpublished data) since a therapeutic effect can be obtained by administering anti-IFN antibodies (Wabuke-Bunoti et al., 1986; Breider et al., 1987).

This and the general lack of target specificity, as well as the variation in effects depending on doses, timing, and duration of target cell exposure, is of major concern for the clinical application of IFNs in immunotherapy. In addition, the complexity of the immune system may, in itself, be a formidable limitation to the clinical application. The cascade of cytokines involved in any particular immune function has still not been fully elucidated. However, from what is already known it has become clear that the administration of a single cytokine, such as an IFN, may not be adequate to produce the desired final immunomodulatory effect, but rather may exacerbate an already adverse situation (Shurkovich et al., 1987; Brzoska and Obert, 1987; Bielefeldt-Ohmann et al., 1990).

Many cytokines are rapidly inactivated or cleared from the body (Schrader et al., 1985). This may limit the duration and scope of cytokine immunotherapy. The use of "prolonged-release" carriers may partially circumvent this limitation. However, the timing of cytokine administration, relative to onset of an infection, may still be critical

(Babiuk et al., 1986). This careful timing may be difficult when dealing with a large population of susceptible animals. Moreover, repeated or prolonged-release treatment increases the risk of inducing antibodies to the cytokine (Itri et al., 1987; Hennes et al., 1987). This concern is now in focus in human medicine and should also be taken into account in the veterinary application of cytokines.

Despite these drawbacks, the positive results that have been obtained in certain viral and bacterial disease of cattle and swine do indicate that IFNs are applicable in veterinary medicine, although the range of applications may be more limited than those imagined in the initial years of IFN research. In this respect veterinary medicine is no worse off than its human counterpart (McCormick, 1988).

Acknowledgments

Research by the authors and their colleagues has been supported by CIBA-GEIGY Ltd., Switzerland, CIBA-GEIGY Canada Ltd., and the Natural Sciences and Engineering Research Council (NSERC) of Canada.

References

Anderson, K. P., Czarniecki, C., McCracken, J., Bielefeldt-Ohmann, H., and Babiuk, L. A. (1985). The potential uses of bovine interferon for bovine respiratory disease. *Proc. Vet. Respir. Symp., 4th, 1985.* pp. 39–54.

Anderson, K. P., Fennie, E. H., and Yilma, T. (1988). Enhancement of a secondary antibody response to vesicular stomatitis "G" protein by IFN-γ treatment at primary immunization. *J. Immunol.* **140,** 3599–3504.

Babiuk, L. A., and Bielefeldt-Ohmann, H. (1984). Effect of levamisole and bovine interferon-1 on bovine immune response and susceptibility to bovine herpesvirus 1. *Prog. Clin. Biol. Res.* **161,** 433–442.

Babiuk, L. A., Bielefeldt-Ohmann, H., Gifford, G., Czarniecki, C. W., Scialli, V. T., and Hamilton, E. B. (1986). Effect of bovine interferon on bovine herpesvirus type 1 induced respiratory disease. *J. Gen. Virol.* **66,** 2383–2394.

Babiuk, L. A., Lawman, M. J. P., and Gifford, G. (1987). Use of recombinant bovine alpha 1 interferon in reducing respiratory disease induced by bovine herpesvirus type 1. *Antimicrob. Agents Chemother.* **31,** 752–757.

Babiuk, L. A., Lawman, M. J. P., Gifford, G. A., Bielefeldt-Ohmann, H., and Campos, M. (1988). Use of recombinant bovine alpha$_1$ interferon in reducing respiratory disease induced by bovine herpesvirus type-1. *Proc. World Congr. Buiatr., 15th, 1988.*

Babiuk, L. A., Lawman, M. J. P., and Griebel, P. (1989). Immunosuppression by bovine herpesvirus-1 and other selected herpesviruses. *In* "Virus-Induced Immunosuppression" (S. Spector, M. Bendinelli, and H. Friedman, eds.), pp. 141–171. Plenum, New York.

Belosevic, M., Davis, C. E., Meltzer, M. S., and Nacy, C. A. (1988). Regulation of activated macrophage antimicrobial activities. Indentification of lymphokines that cooperate with IFN γ for induction of resistance to infection. *J. Immunol.* **141,** 890–896.

Bielefeldt-Ohmann, H., and Babiuk, L. A. (1984). Effect of bovine recombinant alpha-1 interferon on inflammatory responses of bovine phagocytes. *J. Interferon Res.* **4**, 249–263.

Bielefeldt-Ohmann, H., and Babiuk L. A. (1985a). Alteration of neutrophil function after *in vivo* and *in vitro* exposure to recombinant bovine interferon alpha or gamma. *J. Leukocyte Biol.* **24**, 165 (abstr.).

Bielefeldt-Ohmann, H., and Babiuk, L. A. (1985b). *In vitro* and systematic effects of recombinant bovine ineterferons on natural cell-mediated cytotoxicity in healthy and bovine herpesvirus-1 infected cattle. *J. Interferon Res.* **5**, 551–564.

Bielefeldt-Ohmann, H., and Babiuk, L. A. (1985c). Viral–bacterial pneumonia in calves: Effect of bovine herpesvirus-1 on immunological functions. *J. Infect. Dis.* **151**, 937–947.

Bielefeldt-Ohmann, H., and Babiuk, L. A. (1986a). Alteration of alveolar macrophage functions by *in vivo* treatment with recombinant interferons alpha-1 and gamma. *Proc. Int. Vet. Immunol. Symp., 1st, 1986.* p. 71.

Bielefeldt-Ohmann, H., and Babiuk, L. A. (1986b). Alteration of some leukocyte functions following *in vivo* and *in vitro* exposure to recombinant bovine alpha-1 and gamma. *J. Interferon Res.* **6**, 123–136.

Bielefeldt-Ohmann, H., and Babiuk, L. A. (1986c). Viral infections in domestic animals as models for studies of viral immunology and pathogenesis. *J. Gen. Virol.* **67**, 1–25.

Bielefeldt-Ohmann, H., Gilchrist, J. E., and Babiuk, L. A. (1984). Effect of recombinant DNA-produced bovine interferon alpha (BoIFN-α) on the interaction between bovine alveolar macrophages and bovine herpesvirus type 1. *J. Gen. Virol.* **65**, 1487–1495.

Bielefeldt-Ohmann, H., Davis, W. C., and Babiuk, L. A. (1985). Functinal and phenotypic characteristics of bovine natural cytotoxic cells. *Immunobiology* **169**, 503–519.

Bielefeldt-Ohmann, H., Davis, W. C., and Babiuk, L. A. (1986). Surface antigen expression by alveolar macrophages: Functional correlation and influence of interferons *in vivo* and *in vitro*. *Immunobiology* **171**, 125–142.

Bielefeldt-Ohmann, H., Lawman, M. J. P., and Babiuk, L. A. (1987). Bovine interferon: Its biology and application in veterinary medicine (review). *Antiviral Res.* **7**, 187–210.

Bielefeldt-Ohmann, H., Babiuk, L. A., and Harland, R. (1990). Cytokine synergy with viral cytopathic effects and bacterial products during pathogenesis of respiratory tract infection. *Clin. Immunol. Immunopathol.* In press.

Breider, M. A., Adams, L. G., and Womack, J. E. (1987). Influence of interferon in natural resistance of mice to Sendai virus pneumonia. *Am. J. Vet. Res.* **40**, 1746–1750.

Brodeur, B. R., and Merigan, T. C. (1975). Mechanisms of the suppressive effect of interferon on antibody synthesis *in vivo*. *J. Immunol.* **114**, 1323–1328.

Brzoska, V. J., and Öbert, H. J. (1987). Interferon gamma: Ein januskopfiger Mediator bei Entzundungen. *Arzneim-Forsch.* **37**, 1410–1416.

Campos, M., Bielefeldt-Ohmann, H., Hutchings, D., Rapin, N., Babiuk, L. A., and Lawman, M. J. P. (1989). Role of interferon gamma in inducing cytotoxicity of peripheral blood mononuclear leukocytes to bovine herpes virus type-1 (BHV-1)-infected cells. *Cell. Immunol.* **120**, 259–269.

Capon, D. J., Shepard, H. M., and Goeddel, D. V. (1985). Two distinct families of human and bovine interferon-α genes are coordinately expressed and encode functional polypeptides. *Mol. Cell. Biol.* **5**, 768–779.

Cerretti, D. P., McKerghau, K., Larsen, A., Cosman, D., Gillis, S., and Bailer, P. E. (1986). Cloning, sequence and expression of bovine interferon-γ. *J. Immunol.* **136**, 4561–4564.

Charpigny, G., Reinaud, P., Huet, J. C., Guillomot, M., Charlier, M., Pernollet, J. C., and Martal, J. (1988). High homology between a trophoblastic protein (trophoblastin) isolated from ovine embryo and alpha interferons. *FEBS Lett.* **228**, 12–16.

Chester, T. J., Pancher, K., and Merigan, T. C. (1973). Suppression of mouse antibody producing spleen cells by various interferon preparations. *Nature (London)* **246**, 92–94.

Chiang, Y. -W., Roth, J. A., and Andrews, J. J. (1990). Influence of recombinant bovine gamma interferon and dexamethasone on pneumonia in calves due to *Haemophilus somnus*. *Am. J. Vet. Res.* **51**, 759–762.

Czarniecki, C. W., Hamilton, E. B., Fennie, C. W., and Wolf, R. L. (1986). In vitro biological activities of *Escherichia coli*-derived bovine interferons-α -β and -γ. *J. Interferon Res.* **6**, 29–37.

DeMaeyer, E., and DeMaeyer-Guignard, J. (1982). Immunomodulating properties of interferons. *Philos. Trans. R. Soc. London, Ser. B* **299**, 77–90.

DeMaeyer, E., and DeMaeyer-Guignard, J. (1988). "Interferons and Other Regulatory Cytokines." Wiley, New York.

Everlith, K. M., and Splitter, G. A. (1986). Interleukin-1 regulates T cell response to *Brucella abortus* and gamma-interferon-activated macrophages. *Proc. Int. Vet. Immunol. Symp., 1st, 1986.* p. 77.

Fulton, R. W., Downing, M. M., and Cummins, J. M. (1984). Antiviral effects of bovine interferons on bovine repiratory tract viruses. *J. Clin. Microbiol.* **19**, 492–497.

Gidlund, M., Orn, A., Wigzell, H., Senik, A., and Gresser, I. (1978). Enhanced NK cell activity in mice injected with interferon and interferon inducers. *Nature (London)* **273**, 759–761.

Gisler, R. H., Lindahl, P., and Gresser, I. (1974). Effects of interferon on antibody synthesis *in vitro*. *J. Immunol.* **113**, 438–444.

Griebel, P. J., Qualtiere, L., Davis, W. C., Lawman, M. J. P., and Babiuk, L. A. (1988a). Bovine peripheral blood leukocyte subpopulation dynamics following a primary bovine herpesvirus-1 infection. *Viral Immunol.* **1**, 267–284.

Griebel, P. J., Qualtiere, L., Davis, W. C., Gee, A., Bielefeldt-Ohmann, H., Lawman, M. J. P., and Babiuk, L. A. (1988b). T lymphocyte population dynamics and function following a primary bovine herpesvirus type-1 infection. *Viral Immunol.* **1**, 287–304.

Griebel, P. J., Bielefeldt-Ohmann, H., Campos, M., Qualtiere, L., Davis, W. C., Lawman, M. J. P., and Babiuk, L. A. (1989). Bovine peripheral blood leukocyte population dynamics following treatment with recombinant bovine interferon-alpha$_I$. *J. Interferon Res.* **9**, 245–257.

Helmer, S. D., Hansen, P. J., Anthony, R. V., Thatcher, W. W., Bazer, F. W., and Roberts, R. M. (1987). Identification of bovine trophoblast protein-1, a secretory protein immunologically related to ovine trophoblat protein-1. *J. Reprod. Fertil.* **79**, 83–91.

Helmer, S. D., Gross, T. S., Hansen, P. J., and Thatcher, W. W. (1988a). Bovine conceptus secretory proteins (bCSP) and bovine trophoblast protein-1 (bTP-1), a component of bCSP, alter endometrial prostaglandin (PG) secretion and induce an intracellular inhibitor of PG synthesis *in vitro*. *Biol. Reprod.* **38**, Suppl. 1, 153 (abstr.).

Helmer, S. D., Hansen, P. J., Thatcher, W. W., Johnson, J. W., and Bazer, F. W. (1988b). Intrauterine infusion of purified bovine trophoblast protein-1 (bTP-1) extends corpus luteum (CL) lifespan in cyclic cattle. *J. Anim. Sci.* **67**, Suppl. 1, 415–416 (abstr.).

Hennes, U., Jucker, W., Fischer, E. A., Krummenacher, T., Palleroni, A. V., Trown, P. W., Linder-Ciccolunghi, S., and Rainisio, M. (1987). The detection of antibodies to recombinant alpha-2a in human serum. *J. Biol. Stand.* **15**, 231–244.

Himmler, A., Hauptmann, R., Adolf, G. R., and Swetly, P. (1986). Molecular cloning and expression in *Escherichia coli* of equine type I interferons. *J. Mol. Biol.* **5**, 345–349.

Hooks, J. J., Hooks, B. D., and Levinson, A. J. (1982). Interferons and immune reactivity. *Am. J. Vet. Res.* **181**, 1111–1114.

Imakawa, K., Anthony, R. V., Kazemi, M., Marotti, K. R., Pelites, H. G., and Roberts, R. M. (1987). Interferon-like sequence of ovine trophoblast protein secreted by embryonic trophectoderm. *Nature (London)* **33a,** 377–379.

Isaacs, A., and Lindenmann, J. (1957). Viral interference. I. The interferon. *Proc. R. Soc. London, Ser. B* **147,** 258–267.

Itri, L. M., Campion, M., Dennin, R. A., Palleroni, A. V., Gutterman, J. U., Groopman, J. E., and Trown, P. W. (1987). Incidence and clinical significance of neutralizing antibodies in patients receiving recombinant interferon alpha-2a by intramuscular injection. *Cancer (Philadelphia)* **59,** 668–674.

Kalaaji, A. M., Abernethy, N. J., McCullough, K., and Hay, J. B. (1988). Recombinant bovine interferon-$\alpha_I 1$ inhibits the migration of lymphocytes from lymph nodes but not into lymph nodes. *Reg. Immunol.* **1,** 56–61.

Kirchner, H. (1984). Interferons, a group of multiple lymphokines. *Springer Semin. Immunopathol.* **7,** 347–374.

Korngold, R., and Doherty, P. C. (1985). Treatment of mice with polyinosinic-polycytidilic polyribonucleotide reduces T-cell involvement in a localized inflammatory response to vaccinia virus challenge. *J. Virol.* **53,** 489–494.

Lairmore, M. D., Butera, S. T., Callaman, G. N., and DeMarini, J. C. (1988). Spontaneous interferon production by pulmonary leukocytes is associated with lentivirus-induced lymphoid interstitial pneumonia. *J. Immunol.* **140,** 779–785.

Lawman, M. J. P., Gifford, G., Gyongyossy-Issa, M., Dragann, R., Heise, J., and Babiuk, L. A. (1987). Activity of polymorphonuclear (PMN) leukocytes during bovine herpes virus-1 induced respiratory disease: Effect of recombinant bovine interferon alpha$_I$1. *Antiviral Res.* **8,** 225–237.

Lawman, M. J. P., Campos, M., Bielefeldt-Ohmann, H., Griebel, P., and Babiuk, L. A. (1989). Recombinant cytokines and their potential therapeutic value in veterinary medicine. *Compr. Biotechnol.* pp. 63–106.

Lefevre, F., and La Bonnardiere, C. (1986). Molecular cloning and sequencing of a gene encoding biologically active porcine α interferon. *J. Interferon Res.* **6,** 349–360.

Leibson, H. J., Gefter, M., Zlotnik, A., Marrack, P., and Kappler, J. W. (1984). Role of γ-interferon in antibody-producing responses. *Nature (London)* **309,** 799–801.

Leung, D. W., Capon, D. J., and Goeddel, D. V. (1984). The structure and bacterial expression of three bovine distinct β-interferon genes. *Bio Technology* **2,** 458–464.

Lynn, R. C., and Phillip, J. R. (1988). Recombinant bovine interferon alpha in the control of bovine respiratory disease. *Proc. World Congr. Buiatr., 15th, 1988,* pp. 145–149.

MacLachlan, N. J., and Anderson, K. P. (1986). Effect of recombinant DNA-derived bovine α-1 interferon on transmissible gastroenteritis virus infection in swine. *Am. J. Vet. Res.* **47,** 1149–1152.

Marcowitz, R., Germano, P. M. L., Rivere, Y., Tsiang, H., and Havanessan, A. G. (1987). The effect of interferon treatment in rabies prophylaxis in immunocompetent, immunosuppressed, and immunodeficient mice. *J. Interferon Res.* **7,** 17–28.

Martinod, S., McCullough, K., Miozzari, G., and Steiger, R. F. (1988). Potential use of recombinant bovine interferon alpha$_I$1 in the control of bovine respiratory disease in fattening calves. *Proc. World Congr. Buiatr., 15th, 1988,* pp. 150–154.

Martinod, S., Siegenthaler, B., and Gerber, C. (1990). Effect of recombinant bovine interferon alpha$_I$1 on the reproductive performance in dairy heifers. Submitted for publication.

McCormick, D. (1988). We happy few (editorial). *Bio Technology* **6,** 991.

Mifune, K., Mannen, K., Cho, S., and Narahara, H. (1987). Enhanced antibody responses in mice by combined administration of interferon with rabies vaccine. *Arch. Virol.* **94**, 287–295.

Mond, J. J., Sarma, C., O'Hara, J., Finkelman, F. D., and Serattis, S. (1985). Recombinant-inferferon (γ-IF) inhibits the B cell proliferation response stimulated by soluble but not by agarose bound anti-Ig antibodies. *Fed. Proc., Fed. Am. Soc. Exp. Biol.* **44**, 1296.

Nagi, A. M., and Babiuk, L. A. (1988a). Effects of recombinant bovine interferons-α and -γ on some *in vitro* immune functions of bovine intraepitheial and lamina propria leukocytes. *J. Interferon Res.* **8**, 494–505.

Nagi, A. M., and Babiuk, L. A. (1988b). Modulation of some Peyer's patch leukocyte functions following *in vitro* exposure to recombinant bovine alpha- and gamma-interferon. *Immunobiology* **177**, 329–338.

Parker, M. A., Mander, A. D., Wallace, H. T., and Sonnenfeld, G. (1981). Modulation of the human *in vitro* antibody response by human leukocyte interferon preparations. *Cell. Immunol.* **58**, 464–469.

Peel, J. E., Kolly, C., Siegenthaler, B., and Martinod, C. (1990). Effect of recombinant bovine interferon-$\alpha_1$1 (rBoIFNα) on the clinical course of severe systemic Salmonellosis caused by *S. thyphimurium* in calves. *Am. J. Vet. Res.* In press.

Plante, C., Hansen, P. J., and Thatcher, W. W. (1988). Prolongation of luteal lifespan in cows by intrauterine infusion of recombinant bovine alpha-interferon. *Endocrinology (Baltimore)* **122**, 2342–2344.

Plante, C., Hansen, P. J., Martinod, S., Siegenthaler, B., Thatcher, W. W., Pollard, J. W., and Leslie, J. (1989). Intrauterine and intramuscular administration of recombinant bovine interferon-alpha$_1$1 prolongs luteal lifespan in cattle. *J. Dairy Sci.* **72**, 1859–1865.

Playfair, J. H., and de Souza, J. B. (1987). Recombinant gamma interferon is a potent adjuvant for a malaria vaccine in mice. *Clin. Exp. Immunol.* **67**, 5–10.

Roney, C. S., Ross, C. R., Smith, P. C., Lauerman, L. C., Spano, J. S., Hanrahan, L. A., and William, J. C. (1985). Effect of human leukocyte A interferon on prevention of infectious bovine rhinotracheitis virus infection in cattle. *Am. J. Vet. Res.* **46**, 1251–1255.

Roth, J. A., and Frank, D. E. (1989). Recombinant bovine gamma interferon as an immunomodulator in dexamethasone-treated and non-treated cattle. *J. Interferon Res.* **9**, 143–151.

Schrader, J. W., Clark-Lewis, I., Crapper, R. M., Wong, G. H. W., and Schrader, S. (1985). *Contemp. Top. Mol. Immunol.* **1a**, 147–179.

Schwers, A., Vanden Broecke, C., Goossens, A., Maenhoudt, M., Bugyaki, L., Pastoret, P. P., and Werenne, J. (1982). Administration of human interferon to young calves: Circulating antiviral activity and biological response of the host. *Arch. Int. Physiol. Biochim.* **90**, B214–B215.

Schwers, A., Vanden Brocke, C., Maenhout, M., Coignoul, F., Devos, L., Kaeckenbeek, A., Jacquemin, E., Pastoret, P. P., and Werenne, J. (1988). Effect of bacterially produced HuIFNα_2C on rotavirus and/or enterotoxigenic *Escherichia coli* infection in colostrum deprived newborn calves. *Ann. Med. Vet.* **132**, 423–236.

Sidman, C. L., Marshall, J. D., Shultz, L. D., Gray P. W., and Johnson, H. M. (1984). Gamma interferon is one of several direct B cell maturing lymphokines. *Nature (London)* **309**, 801–804.

Skurkovich, S., Skurkovich, B., and Bellanti, J. A. (1987). A unifying model of the immunoregulatory role of the interferon system: Can interferon produce disease in humans? *Clin. Immunol. Immunopathol.* **43**, 362–373.

Sonnenfeld, G., Mandel, A. D., and Merigan, T. C. (1978). Time and dosage dependence of immuno-enhancement by ovine type II interferon preparations. *Cell. Immunol.* **40**, 285–293.

Steinbach, M. J., Roth, J. A., and Kaeberle, M. (1986). Activation of bovine neutrophils by recombinant interferon. *Cell. Immunol.* **98**, 137–144.

Stewart, H. J., McCann, S. H., Barker, P. J., Lee, K. E., Lamming, G. E., and Flint, A. P. (1987). Interferon sequence homology and receptor binding activity of ovine trophoblast antiluteolytic protein. *J. Endocrinol.* **115**, R13–R15.

Thatcher, W. W., Hansen, P. J., Gross, T. S., Helmer, S. D., Plante, C., and Baser, F. W. (1988). Antiluteolytic effects of bovine trophoblast protein-one. *J. Reprod. Fertil., Suppl.* **37**, 91.

Trueblood, M. S., and Manjara, J. (1972). Response of bovine viruses to interferon. *Cornell Vet.* **62**, 3–12.

Wabuke-Bunoti, M. A., Bennink, J. R., and Plotkin, S. A. (1986). Influenza virus-induced encephalopathy in mice: Interferon production and natural killer cell activity during acute infection. *J. Virol.* **60**, 1062–1067.

Warland, F., Picard, F., McCullough, K., Martinod, S., and Levy, D. (1989). Recombinant bovine interferon gamma enhances expression of class I and class II bovine lymphocyte antigen. *Vet. Immunol. Immunopathol.* **22**, 379–383.

Weigent, D. A., Stanton, G. J., and Johnson, H. M. (1983). Recombinant gamma interferon enhances natural killer cell activity similar to natural gamma interferon. *Biochem. Biophys. Res. Commun.* **111**, 525–259.

Werenne, J. (1985). Interferon in veterinary medicine: The present position and future prospects. *Outlook Agric.* **14**, 129–135.

Yates, W. D. G. (1982). A review of infectious bovine rhinotracheitis, shipping fever pneumonia and viral-bacterial synergism in respiratory disease of cattle. *Can. J. Comp. Med.* **46**, 225–263.

In Vivo Use of Interleukins in Domestic Food Animals

FRANK BLECHA

Department of Anatomy and Physiology, College of Veterinary Medicine, Kansas State University, Manhattan, Kansas 66506

I. Introduction
II. Rationale for Using Interleukins in Domestic Food Animals
   A. Defects in Immunoregulation
   B. *In Vitro* Studies
III. *In Vivo* Studies with Interleukins in Domestic Food Animals
   A. Recombinant Human IL-2 (rHuIL-2)
   B. Recombinant Bovine IL-2 (rBoIL-2)
   C. Recombinant Bovine IL-1β (rBoIL-1β)
IV. Conclusions and Prospects
   References

I. Introduction

Similar to other biological systems, proteins produced by cells of the immune system interact with cell receptors and regulate maturational processes and immune function. While today there is no question about the accuracy of this statement, it has not been that many years ago that the study of immune regulation was the science of "factorology."

During the 1960s, when much research was being conducted on antibody-mediated immune events and the structure and function of immunoglobulins, an intense research effort was begun on the regulation of cellular immune responses. These initial studies showed that cell-free soluble factors, produced *in vitro* when sensitized lymphocytes were incubated with antigen, could induce lymphocytes to proliferate. In 1969 the term lymphokine was introduced to describe "cell-free soluble factors, which are generated during interaction of sensitized lymphocytes with specific antigen, but which are expressed without reference to immunological specificity" (Dumonde et al., 1969). However, during this time there was much doubt concerning the role of lymphokines in immunoregulation; some even questioned their existence. This skepticism was understandable considering the many activities that were attributed to these lymphokines and the wide range of sources from which they were derived. However, by the late 1970s some of these lymphokines were purified to homogeneity and a new nomenclature was suggested to replace the traditional naming of lymphokines and monokines (monocyte/macrophage source), which had been based previously on their biologic activity (Aarden et al., 1979). Since most of these proteins seemed to act as communication signals between different populations of leukocytes, the term interleukin (between leukocytes) was proposed. Thus, lymphocyte activating factor (LAF) became interleukin-1 (IL-1) and thymocyte stimulating factor (TSF) became interleukin-2 (IL-2).

At present there are nine proteins that are designated interleukins, interleukin-1 through interleukin-8 (two different proteins exist as interleukin-1, IL-1α and IL-1β; Table I). While there is little reason to

TABLE I

INTERLEUKINS THAT HAVE BEEN CLONED, INCLUDING SYNONYMS, CELL SOURCE, AND CELL TARGETS

Name	Acronym	Synonyms	Cell source	Cell targets
Interleukin-1α	IL-1α	Lymphocyte activating factor (LAF)	Activated monocytes or macrophages, endothelial cells, dendritic cells, natural killer cells, Langerhans's cells, astrocytes, glioma cells, microglial cells, fibroblasts, epithelial cells, B cell lines	Thymocytes, T cells, B cells, neutrophils, hepatocytes, condrocytes, muscle cells, endothelial cells, osteocytes, macrophages
Interleukin-1β	IL-1β	Endogenous pyrogen (EP), mitogenic protein (MP), T cell replacing factor III (TRF III), B cell activating factor (BAF), B cell differentiation factor (BCDF)		
Interleukin-2	IL-2	Thymocyte stimulating factor (TSF), T cell growth factor (TCGF), thymocyte mitogenic factor	T cells, large granular lymphocytes	T cells, B cells, macrophages

(continued)

TABLE I (*Continued*)

Name	Acronym	Synonyms	Cell source	Cell targets
Interleukin-3	IL-3	Colony forming unit-stimulating activity (CFU-SA), multicolony stimulating factor (Multi-CSF), burst promoting activity (BP), mast cell growth factor (MCGF)	T cells	Multipotential stem cells, mast cells
Interleukin-4	IL-4	B cell growth factor (BCGF), B cell stimulating factor 1 (BSF-1), T cell growth factor II (TCGF II), mast cell growth factor II (MCGF II)	T cells	T cells, B cells, macrophages, myeloid progenitors
Interleukin-5	IL-5	Eosinophil differentiating factor (EDF), T cell replacing factor (TRF), B cell growth factor II (BCGF II), eosinophil colony stimulating factor (EO-CSF)	T cells	Eosinophils, B cells (mouse)
Interleukin-6	IL-6	Interferon β_2, B cell stimulating factor II (BSF II), plasmacytoma growth factor (PCT-GF), interleukin hybridoma/plasmacytoma-1 (IL-HP1)	Fibroblasts, activated monocytes or macrophages, T cells	T cells, B cells, fibroblasts, myeloid progenitors
Interleukin-7	IL-7	Lymphopoietin-1	Stromal cells	T and B cell precursors
Interleukin-8	IL-8	Monocyte-derived neutrophil chemotactic factor (MDNCF)	T cells, fibroblasts, keratinocytes, endothelial cells	Neutrophils, T cells

think that more interleukins will not be discovered and cloned, the current system of assigning numbers to the cloned proteins (IL-40?) may soon be revised. At the Sixth International Lymphokine Workshop (Evian-Les-Bains, France, October 23–28, 1988) it was suggested that the current system of interleukin naming should be reconsidered. One can imagine the obscurity and frustration of learning and dealing with IL-1 through IL-n. However, in domestic food animals IL-1 and IL-2 are the only interleukins that have been cloned, sequenced, and expressed (Table II). While work is progressing on the cloning of porcine IL-2, only bovine recombinant interleukins are presently available.

Interleukin-1 is a predominantly macrophage/monocyte-derived protein that modulates many of the responses involved in the process of host defense to infection. Two biochemically distinct but functionally related IL-1 proteins have been cloned; IL-1α (Lomedico et al., 1984; Maliszewski et al., 1987; Leong et al., 1988a) and IL-1β (Auron et al., 1984; Maliszewski et al., 1987; Leong et al., 1988b). Additionally, a considerable amount of work has been done on the characterization of the two porcine IL-1 proteins (Saklatvala et al., 1983; 1985a,b). Interleukin-1β is the predominantly secreted form of IL-1; mRNA ratios of IL-1β to IL-α are 10:1 in activated human monocytes (March et al., 1985) and 15:1 in activated U937 myeloid cells (Nishida et al., 1987). Interleukin-2 is secreted by a subset of T cells (Morgan et al., 1976) and

TABLE II

Bovine and Porcine Cloned Interleukins and Interleukin Receptors

Name	Species	Reference
Interleukin-1α	Bovine	Maliszewski et al. (1987); Leong et al. (1988a)
Interleukin-1β	Bovine	Maliszewski et al. (1987); Leong et al. (1988b)
Interleukin-1α	Porcine	Maliszewski et al. (1990)
Interleukin-2	Bovine	Cerretti et al. (1986); Reeves et al. (1986)
Interleukin-2 receptor	Bovine	Weinberg et al. (1988b)

large granular lymphocytes (Kasahara *et al.*, 1983) after stimulation with mitogen or antigen. This lymphokine induces the clonal expansion of activated T cells (Gillis and Smith, 1977) and B cells (Mittler *et al.*, 1985; Boyd *et al.*, 1985) and activates natural killer (NK) cells (Lanier *et al.*, 1985). The very important regulatory role that these two interleukins have in the immune response have made them prime candidates to use in immunomodulation studies.

II. Rationale for Using Interleukins in Domestic Food Animals

The availability of recombinant interleukins has generated much interest and many studies with these proteins in laboratory animals and humans. Augmentation of immunity with IL-2 and/or adoptive transfer of lymphokine-activated killer (LAK) cells have shown the therapeutic use of IL-2 in the treatment of cancer in humans (Grimm *et al.*, 1982; Rosenberg *et al.*, 1985). However, since most domestic food animals do not live long enough for tumors to present much of a health problem, what then is the rationale for using these proteins in farm animals? Simply stated, the rationale for using interleukins in domestic food animals is the same rationale for using any immunomodulator in domestic food animals, namely to augment host immunity in the hope of decreasing disease susceptibility. Chapter 1 of this volume contains a thorough discussion of the rationale for using immunomodulators in domestic food animals; a brief review of that discussion will be presented here.

A. Defects in Immunoregulation

Several economically important diseases of domestic food animals, such as bovine respiratory disease in feedlot calves (Babiuk *et al.*, 1987) and mastitis in dairy cattle, still cause enormous economic losses. Some of the problems in susceptibility to disease have been associated with problems in immunoregulation. For example, immaturity of the neonatal immune system, stress-associated immunosuppression, and pathogen-induced immunosuppression have been linked to increased disease susceptibility (for review see Chapter 1 of this volume). Thus, there exists a need to provide complementary or alternative therapeutic strategies for these diseases. Augmentation of the host's immune response, perhaps by using interleukins, as will be discussed later, may decrease the financial loss caused by disease in domestic food animals.

Stress-associated changes in endocrine function have been related to alterations in host immunity (Blecha, 1988; Kelley, 1988; Griffin, 1989). Although not all stress-associated changes in immune function are caused by glucocorticoids (Keller *et al.*, 1983, 1988; Dantzer and Kelley, 1989), increased concentrations of cortisol or corticosterone are considered to be hallmarks of stress exposure. Similarly, virus-induced immunosuppression has been associated with disease susceptibility (Babiuk and Ohmann, 1985). Does stress- and/or virus-induced immunosuppression involve problems with interleukin regulation? Will administration of interleukins restore immune function in immunosuppressed animals? A few studies have provided answers to both of these questions.

One of the first observations made with IL-2 was that, in an *in vitro* system, the synthetic glucocorticoid, dexamethasone, decreased the production of this lymphokine from mitogen-stimulated lymphocytes (Gillis *et al.*, 1979a,b). Furthermore, exogenous IL-2 added to dexamethasone-treated mitogen-stimulated lymphocytes restored the proliferative capability of these cells. Similarly, interleukin-1 production is decreased also by treatment with synthetic glucocorticoids (Knudsen *et al.*, 1987; Roberta *et al.*, 1987; Lew *et al.*, 1988). Glucocorticoid-induced immunosuppression has been studied extensively in cattle (Roth, 1985). Importantly, in an *in vitro* study that used concentrations of cortisol that are attainable in stressed cattle, mitogen-stimulated lymphocyte proliferation and bovine IL-2 production were decreased by cortisol (Blecha and Baker, 1986). When concanavalin A-generated lymphocyte supernatants were added to those cortisol-treated, mitogen-stimulated bovine lymphocytes, the lymphocyte proliferative responses were restored. Other studies with cattle (Murray and Chenault, 1982; Ojo-Amaize *et al.*, 1988) and pigs (Westly and Kelley, 1984) have also found decreases in lymphocyte proliferative responses at physiologically high concentrations of cortisol. Similarly, when concentrations of cortisol were increased in cattle by injections of adrenocorticotropic hormone (ACTH) (Blecha and Baker, 1986) or by ACTH injections or restraint in pigs (Klemcke *et al.*, 1987), IL-2 production from the ACTH-treated or restrained animals was lower when compared to values from control animals. These studies imply that IL-2 regulation is altered in stressed animals and suggest that administration of IL-2 to stressed animals may restore immune function. Indeed, Ezine and Papiernik (1984) and Conlon *et al.* (1985) found that *in vivo* injections of IL-2 could restore the immune responsiveness of mice that had been immunosuppressed by injecting hydrocortisone, and Thoman and Weigle (1985) reconstituted cytotoxic responses of aged mice with *in vivo* IL-2 administration. Similarly, *in vivo* injections of human IL-1β

or a synthetic nonapeptide of human IL-1β restored the immunodepressed state of mice that had been induced by sublethal irradiation, aging, or both (Frasca et al., 1988).

Problems in interleukin regulation have also been related to infections with several different pathogens, including viruses (Wainberg et al., 1983; Orsz et al., 1985; Flaming et al., 1989), bacteria (Mohagheghour et al., 1985), and parasites (Tarleton, 1988). Immunodeficiency induced by the parasite *Trypanosoma cruzi* can be restored by *in vivo* treatment of IL-2 (Reed et al., 1984) or IL-1 (Reed et al., 1989ab). These examples illustrate some of the immune defects that may occur via stress- or pathogen-induced immunosuppression and provide encouraging results that suggest that interleukin treatment may provide potential therapeutic benefits.

B. *In Vitro* Studies

Several laboratories have produced and characterized IL-1 or IL-2 from domestic food animals, including: cattle (Baker and Knoblock, 1982a,b; Namen and Magnuson, 1984; Oldham and Williams, 1984; Miller-Edge and Splitter, 1984; Brown and Grab, 1985; Mastro et al., 1986; Bielefeldt-Ohmann and Babiuk, 1986; Zelarney and Belden, 1988; Sambhara and Belden, 1988; Weinberg et al., 1988a; Carter et al., 1989); pigs (Saklatvala et al., 1983, 1985a,b; Gasbarre et al., 1984; Charley et al., 1985; English et al., 1985); sheep (English and Whitehurst, 1984; Ellis and DeMartini, 1985; Knisley and Pearson, 1987); and chickens (Kromer et al., 1986; Vainio et al., 1986). Similarly, several studies have evaluated the *in vitro* influence of the recombinant interleukins, IL-1 or IL-2, on different immune functions in cattle and pigs (Anderson et al., 1986; Fong and Doyle, 1986; Stott et al., 1986; Hopfner-Topliff and Blecha, 1987; Charley and Fradelizi, 1987; Bhagyam et al., 1988; Nagi and Babiuk, 1989). However, it was the availability of large quantities of the recombinant interleukins (see Tables I and II) that allowed *in vivo* studies with IL-1 and IL-2 to be conducted in domestic food animals.

III. *In Vivo* Studies with Interleukins in Domestic Food Animals

A. Recombinant Human IL-2 (rHuIL-2)

1. *Actinobacillus (Haemophilus) pleuropneumoniae*

Anderson et al. (1987) conducted one of the first experiments evaluating the use of IL-2 in domestic food animals. Twenty-four pigs (10–15 kg each) were vaccinated on days 0 and 21 with a formalin-inactivated

A. *pleuropneumoniae* bacterin. At each vaccination pigs were injected intramuscularly with either 10^3 or 10^5 units of rHuIL-2/kg body weight (IL-2 units were defined by the manufacturer as the reciprocal of the dilution of IL-2 that induced a proliferative response equal to 50% of the maximum response on an IL-2-dependent murine cell line; units/mg of protein were not provided). The two dosages of rHuIL-2 were evaluated in a single injection at each vaccination and in a regimen of daily injections for 5 consecutive days beginning at each vaccination day. Additionally, one control group of pigs received only the *A. pleuropneumoniae* bacterin and another control group was not vaccinated with the bacterin or injected with rHuIL-2. On day 42 of the study all pigs were challenged intranasally with virulent *A. pleuropneumoniae* serotype 1. Pigs that received the bacterin and 5 daily injections of rHuIL-2 at each vaccination were the least severely affected by the bacterial challenge; there did not appear to be a difference between the two dosages of HrIl-2 when administered in multiple injections. Pigs that were not vaccinated and did not receive rHuIL-2 and pigs that only received the bacterin were the most severely affected by the bacterial challenge. Necropsy findings collected on day 71 of the study indicated that pigs that received the multiple injections of rHuIL-2 (at both dosages) had the least amount of lung affected by the bacterial challenge. However, a single injection of 10^5 units/kg also produced protection comparable to the multiple-injected pigs. Additionally, antibody titers to *A. pleuropneumoniae* were higher in those pigs that received the high dose of rHuIL-2. These findings were confirmed by Nunberg *et al.* (1988) in a similar experiment that evaluated multiple daily injections of rHuIL-2 (10^4 or 10^5 units/kg) in *A. pleuropneumoniae*-vaccinated and challenged pigs. Adverse side effects of the rHuIL-2 administration were noted during the period of injection (moderate diarrhea and lack of appetite), but these initial *in vivo* studies demonstrated the potential of IL-2 as an adjuvant in pigs.

2. *Pseudorabies Virus*

The efficacy of rHuIL-2 as an adjuvant to pseudorabies virus vaccination has been recently evaluated (Kawashima and Platt, 1989). Twelve weanling crossbred pigs were used in a 2 × 2 factorial arrangement of vaccination with a pseudorabies virus subunit vaccine and rHuIL-2 administration. Pigs were vaccinated two times (3 weeks apart) with either 5 or 25 μg of the subunit vaccine. At each vaccination, pigs that received rHuIL-2 were injected subcutaneously with 10^5 units of rHuIL-2/kg body weight daily for 5 consecutive days. Three weeks after the second vaccination all pigs were challenged intranasally with

10^5 PFU of the virus. Pigs that were vaccinated with 25 μg of the pseudorabies subunit vaccine and injected with rHuIL-2 had modest but significantly higher serum neutralizing antibody titers than pigs that did not receive rHuIL-2 injections. Virus excretion, lymphocyte proliferative responses to pseudorabies virus antigen, and body weight changes were not influenced by rHuIL-2 treatment. Although a limited number of animals were used in this study, the data imply that rHuIL-2 may augment humoral immunity to pseudorabies virus subunit vaccines.

3. Natural Killer Cells

In vitro studies have shown that rHuIL-2 augments mitogen-stimulated lymphocyte proliferation in cattle and pigs (Anderson *et al.,* 1986; Stott *et al.,* 1986; Fong and Doyle, 1986; Bhagyam *et al.,* 1988). Additionally, Fong and Doyle (1986), Charley and Fradelizi (1987), and Bhagyam *et al.* (1988) demonstrated that porcine NK cell cytotoxicity was enhanced by incubating peripheral blood mononuclear cells with rHuIL-2. We were interested in determining if *in vivo* injections of rHuIL-2 would augment porcine immune functions including NK cell cytotoxicity (Hennessy *et al.,* 1990). Eighteen pigs (6 pigs/group) were injected with either 10^4 or 10^5 units/kg body weight of rHuIL-2 or an equivalent volume of sterile physiological saline (control) on days 0 through 4. The activity of the rHuIL-2 was 1.3×10^7 units/mg and corresponded to 0.77 and 7.7 μg/kg/day for the 10^4 and 10^5 units/kg treatment groups, respectively. All pigs were immunized with an *Escherichia coli* J5 bacterin on day 0. Cytolytic activity to porcine fibroblasts (PK-15) was increased in pigs treated with rHuIL-2 when compared to control animals. Cytotoxicity to K-562 cells also showed a tendency of increased cytolytic activity in the rHuIL-2-treated pigs. Mitogen-stimulated lymphocyte blastogenesis, IL-2 production, and concentrations of serum iron were not different between treatment groups. Antibody concentrations to *E. coli* J5 antigens increased significantly in all groups after immunization, but there were no differences between treatment groups. These data suggest that *in vivo* injections of rHuIL-2 increase NK cell activity in pigs without influencing other immune activities (Table III).

4. Dexamethasone-Induced Immunosuppression

Roth *et al.* (1990) have investigated the capability of rHuIL-2 to influence neutrophil and lymphocyte responses and to reverse dexamethasone-induced immunosuppression in cattle. Holstein steers were administered a single subcutaneous injection of rHuIL-2 (2.5×10^7

TABLE III

SUMMARY OF THE *IN VIVO* EFFECTS OF rHuIL-2 IN PIGS

Item	Observation	Reference
Cellular immune responses	Increased NK cell cytotoxicity	Hennessy et al. (1990)
	No change in mitogen-stimulated lymphocyte blastogenesis or IL-2 production	Hennessy et al. (1990)
Antibody-mediated immunity	Increased antibody titers to *Haemophilus pleuropneumoniae*	Anderson et al. (1987)
	Increased antibody titers to pseudorabies virus	Kawashima and Platt (1989)
	No change in antibody titer to an *E. coli* J5 bacterin	Hennessy et al. (1990)
Clinical signs and susceptibility to disease	Moderate diarrhea and inappetence during IL-2 administration	Anderson et al. (1987)
	No change in serum iron concentrations	Hennessy et al. (1990)
	Increased protection, including: lower extent of clinical disease, less affected lung, and greater increase in body weight after challenge with *Haemophilus pleuropneumoniae*	Anderson et al. (1987); Nunberg et al. (1988)
	No difference in body weight response after a pseudorabies virus challenge	Kawashima and Platt (1989)

units) mixed in a gelatin solution. In calves that received injections of dexamethasone, rHuIL-2 was injected 8 hours after the administration of the glucocorticoid. A single injection of rHuIL-2 did not influence total or differential leukocyte numbers or neutrophil functions, such as *Staphylococcus aureus* ingestion, cytochrome c reduction, iodination, and antibody-dependent cell-mediated cytotoxicity. Interleukin-2 injection did cause an inhibition of neutrophil random migration. Lymphocyte proliferative responses to mitogens were not influenced by rHuIL-2 administration. Immunosuppression induced by dexamethasone was not abrogated by administration of a single injection of rHuIL-2. These data imply that a single injection of rHuIL-2 has limited biological activity in cattle.

B. Recombinant Bovine IL-2 (rBoIL-2)

1. Bovine Herpesvirus-1 (BHV-1)

One of the main pathogens involved in the multifactorial etiology of bovine respiratory disease is BHV-1. Since *in vivo* use of IL-2 in mice had been shown to enhance immunity to herpes simplex virus (Rouse *et al.*, 1985), we were very interested in determining if rBoIL-2 could enhance immunity and protection in BHV-1-vaccinated and challenged calves (Reddy *et al.*, 1989).

Our initial experiment was designed to determine if rBoIL-2 alone augmented immunity and protection in BHV-1-challenged calves and if the lymphokine had any adjuvant effect when used in conjunction with a BHV-1 vaccine. The dosage of rBoIL-2 that we used was based on an extrapolation, on a body-weight basis, of the dose of rHuIL-2 that had induced protection in *A. pleuropneumoniae*-vaccinated and challenged pigs (Anderson *et al.*, 1987). Twenty-four Hereford or Hereford × Longhorn heifers (185 kg each and seronegative for BHV-1) were assigned randomly to one of four treatments: (1) no rBoIL-2 and no BHV-1 vaccine; (2) rBoIL-2; (3) BHV-1 vaccine; and (4) rBoIL-2 and BHV-1 vaccine. Calves were vaccinated with a modified-live BHV-1 vaccine (Norden Laboratories, Lincoln, NE) at the beginning and at day 18 of the study and were injected intramuscularly with rBoIL-2 (25 μg/kg/day) for 5 consecutive days at each vaccination. Calves that were not injected with rBoIL-2 received an equivalent volume of sterile physiologic saline. On day 28 of the study, all calves were challenged intranasally (1 ml) and conjunctivally (1 ml) with 10^8 PFU/ml of BHV-1.

Peripheral blood mononuclear cell cytotoxicity against BHV-1-infected bovine fibroblasts was increased by rBoIL-2 treatment (Fig. 1A). Cells from calves that received only rBoIL-2 developed the same capability to lyse virus-infected target cells as cells from calves that received the vaccine in addition to the BHV-1 vaccine. Additionally, serum neutralizing antibody titers to BHV-1 were increased sixfold and the amount of virus shed in nasal secretion was fourfold less in calves vaccinated and treated with rBoIL-2 when compared to calves that received the vaccine but no rBoIL-2. Importantly, calves that were vaccinated with BHV-1 and injected with rBoIL-2 had less severe clinical signs of BHV-1 infection, including lower rectal temperatures after challenge (Fig. 2A). Unfortunately, treatment of calves with rBoIL-2 at 25 μg/kg resulted in adverse side effects in the animals during the period of lymphokine injection including diarrhea and mild fever. While some degree of adverse clinical effects of immunotherapy can be tolerated in human patients undergoing cancer treatment, it is doubt-

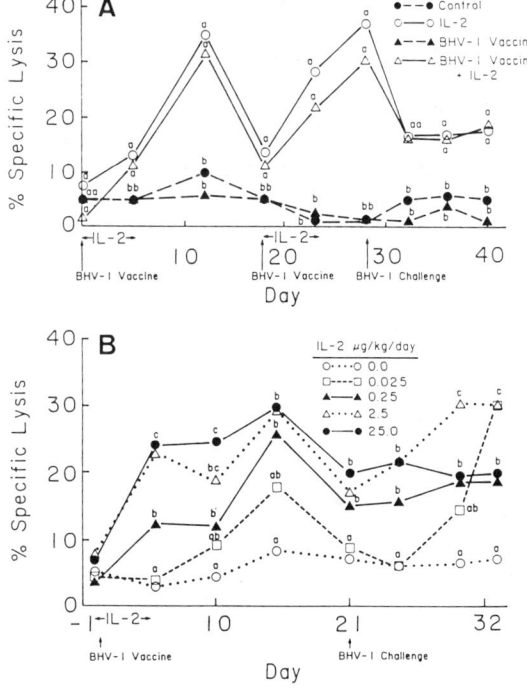

FIG. 1. Bovine peripheral blood mononuclear cell (PBMC) cytotoxicity against bovine herpesvirus-1 (BHV-1)-infected bovine fibroblasts. (A) Experiment 1. (B) Experiment 2. Means within each day with different superscripts are different ($p < 0.05$). From Reddy et al., 1989, with permission.

ful if immunomodulators will be used in domestic food animal medicine if illness is produced during administration of the immunomodulator. However, since Baker (1987) found that rBoIL-2 was approximately 3 times more effective than rHuIL-2 when both lymphokines were evaluated on bovine lymphocytes, it seemed reasonable to hypothesize that a lower dose of rBoIL-2 might still enhance resistance to BHV-1 infection without causing illness during administration of the lymphokine.

Our second rBoIL-2 and BHV-1 experiment was designed to determine a dose of rBoIL-2 that would enhance immunity to BHV-1 without causing adverse side effects (Reddy et al., 1989). Twenty-five Holstein or crossbred beef calves (4–6 months old and seronegative for BHV-1) were allotted by weight to 5 groups: 25.0, 2.5, 0.25, or 0.025 µg/kg/day

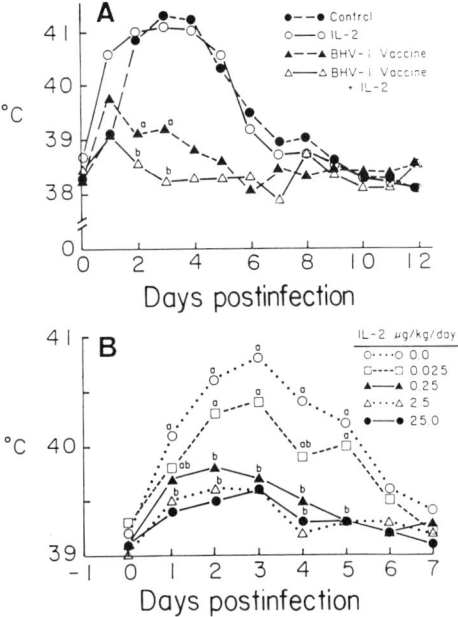

FIG. 2. Rectal temperatures of calves following challenge with bovine herpesvirus-1. (A) Experiment 1. (B) Experiment 2. Means within each day with different superscripts are different ($p < 0.05$). From Reddy et al., 1989, with permission.

of rBoIL-2 for 5 days, and controls that received an equivalent volume of sterile physiologic saline. At the start of the experiment, all calves received a modified-live BHV-1 vaccine and respective doses of rBoIL-2 or placebo. All calves were challenged with 10^7 PFU of BHV-1 on day 21. Cytotoxicity of peripheral blood mononuclear cells against BHV-1-infected bovine fibroblasts was increased in rBoIL-2-treated calves in a dose-dependent manner (Fig. 1B). Calves treated with 25.0, 2.5, and 0.25 µg/kg/day of rBoIL-2 had higher serum neutralizing titers to BHV-1, and after challenge lower BHV-1 titers in nasal secretions when compared to values from control calves. Additionally, clinical disease was less severe in the calves that received rBoIL-2 at the 3 higher dosages (Fig. 2B). Importantly, while rBoIL-2 at 25.0 µg/kg/day caused adverse side effects similar to those observed in our first experiment, calves that received doses of rBoIL-2 less than 25 µg/kg/day remained healthy and normal during the period of rBoIL-2 administration.

Several important conclusions can be made from these data obtained using rBoIL-2 in BHV-1-vaccinated and challenged calves. First, rBoIL-2 augments protection against a BHV-1 challenge beyond the protection afforded by vaccination alone. Second, while rBoIL-2 used in nonvaccinated calves increased some immune functions, protection against the viral challenge was only observed when rBoIL-2 was used as an adjuvant to vaccination. Finally, dosages of rBoIL-2 that do not induce illness during the injection period enhance immunity and protection to BHV-1. Similar to other studies that have shown a beneficial adjuvant effect of IL-2 (Perrin *et al.*, 1988; Nunberg *et al.*, 1989), these studies with rBoIL-2 in cattle clearly indicate the potential value of using this lymphokine in domestic food animal medicine.

2. *Mastitis*

Since mastitis is the most devastating disease affecting dairy cows, it is important to find more effective ways to minimize the impact of this disease on milk production. The capability of rBoIL-2 to enhance immune responses in mastitic cows has been evaluated recently by Nickerson *et al.* (1989). Jersey cows were selected that had 2 udder quarters that had chronic, subclinical *Staphylococcus aureus* mastitis and 2 quarters from which *S. aureus* had never been isolated. When the cows were dried off, miniosmostic pumps that were designed to release 1.0, 10.0, or 100.0 μg of rBoIL-2 or a placebo over a 1- or 3-week period were surgically inserted into teat cisterns. Histological evaluation of the mammary tissue indicated that total lymphoid cell numbers and IgG_1- and IgG_2-secreting plasma cells were similar in quarters that had subclinical mastitis and in quarters that were treated with rBoIL-2. The greatest response in lymphoid cell numbers and IgG_1 and IgG_2 plasma cells was found in quarters that had subclinical *S. aureus* mastitis and were implanted with miniosmotic pumps containing rBoIL-2. Secretions from rBoIL-2-treated quarters had higher numbers of lymphocytes and macrophages when compared to values from the placebo-treated quarters. These results suggest that rBoIL-2-induced stimulation of mammary gland immune defenses may be a possible means of enhancing protection against mastitis.

C. RECOMBINANT BOVINE IL-1β (rBoIL-1β)

The encouraging data that we had obtained with rBoIL-2 in a BHV-1 vaccination and challenge protocol prompted us to evaluate other cytokines that also may be effective in enhancing immunity in cattle. Because of the well-documented adjuvant effect of IL-1 (Staruch and

Wood, 1983; Nencioni *et al.*, 1987; Frasca *et al.*, 1988; Reed *et al.*, 1989b), including its use in viral and bacterial infections in mice (Damme *et al.*, 1987; Czuprynski and Brown, 1987), and because of the availability of rBoIL-1β (Maliszewski *et al.*, 1987), we conducted a study that was designed to determine the capability of rBoIL-1β to augment immunity in BHV-1-vaccinated and challenged calves (Reddy *et al.*, 1990).

Twenty-four Holstein bull calves (150 kg each and seronegative for BHV-1) were assigned randomly to four groups. All calves received a modified-live BHV-1 vaccination on days 1 and 15 of the study. At each vaccination, calves received one intramuscular injection of rBoIL-1β at 33, 100, or 330 ng/kg. Control calves received an equivalent volume of physiologic sterile saline. On day 22, all calves were challenged (1 ml intranasally and 1 ml intratracheally) with 10^7 PFU/ml of BHV-1. To determine if rBoIL-1β influenced the reactivation of BHV-1 from infected calves, dexamethasone was injected (0.04 mg/kg) on days 58 and 59 of the study and virus excretion in nasal secretions was determined.

Serum neutralizing antibody titers to BHV-1 tended to be higher and cytotoxic responses against BHV-1-infected fibroblasts were increased in rBoIL-1β-treated calves. Calves treated with rBoIL-1β at 100 ng/kg shed less virus in nasal secretions during the postchallenge period when compared to values from control calves and calves that had been injected with rBoIL-1β at 330 ng/kg. Calves treated with rBoIL-1β had a tendency to have increased BoT4/BoT8 cell ratios. During the prechallenge period the increase in BoT4/BoT8 was caused by an increase in the BoT4 subset. The postchallenge increase in BoT4/BoT8 was due to a decrease in the BoT8 subset. Severity of clinical signs was not different between rBoIL-1β-treated calves and control calves. However, calves that had been treated with 100 ng/kg of rBoIL-1β excreted less BHV-1 in nasal secretions after injection with dexamethasone 35 days after viral challenge. Importantly, no adverse side effects were observed in the calves during treatment with rBoIL-1β.

IV. Conclusions and Prospects

While the data generated using interleukins in domestic food animals allows much speculation about the possible modes of protection induced by these proteins, i.e., increased antibody titers, increased cellular cytotoxic responses, and altered cell trafficking, several conclusions relative to the *in vivo* use of interleukins in cattle and pigs can be made:

1. IL-1 and IL-2 can be administered to cattle and pigs at dosages that augment immune responses and provide protection against disease, but which do not induce adverse clinical effects during the period of administration.
2. Natural cytotoxic cell responses are increased by *in vivo* treatment of rBoIL-1β and rBoIL-2 in cattle and rHuIL-2 in pigs. However, protection against a BHV-1 challenge in cattle was only afforded when rBoIL-2 was used as an adjuvant to vaccination. It is not known if rBoIL-1β has any nonspecific immune augmenting influences in cattle.
3. Immunocyte numbers in the mammary gland are increased by local administration of rBoIL-2. Augmentation of local immune responses such as in the mammary gland, may be possible by using interleukin therapy.
4. Dexamethasone-induced reactivation of BHV-1 was reduced in calves that were administered rBoIL-1β as an adjuvant to vaccination.

Collectively, the data that have been collected using IL-1 and IL-2 in cattle and pigs are very encouraging and may portend a new era in domestic food animal medicine; a day perhaps, when immunotherapy with interleukins and other cytokines may be as common as antibiotic therapy is today.

REFERENCES

Aarden, L. A., *et al.* (1979). Letter to the Editor. Revised nomenclature for antigen-nonspecific T cell proliferation and helper factors. *J. Immunol.* **123**, 2928–2929.

Anderson. G., Johnson, J., and Baker, P. (1986). Bovine neonatal lymphocyte stimulation with human recombinant interleukin-2. *Conf. Res. Workers Anim. Dis.*, p. 62.

Anderson, G., Urban, O., Fedorka-Cray, P., Newell, A., Nunberg, J., and Doyle M. (1987). Interleukin-2 and protective immunity in *Haemophilus pleuropneumoniae:* Preliminary studies. *In* "Vaccines '87. Modern Approaches to New Vaccines: Prevention of AIDS and Other Viral Bacterial and Parasitic Disease" (R. M. Chanock, R. A. Lerner, F. Brown, and H. Ginsberg, eds.), pp. 22–25. Cold Spring Harbor Lab., Cold Spring Harbor, New York.

Auron, P. E. Webb, A. C., Rosenwasser, L. J., Mucci, S. F., Rich, A., Wolf, S. M., and Dinarello, C. A. (1984). Nucleotide sequence of human monocyte interleukin-1 precursor cDNA. *Proc. Natl. Acad. Sci. U.S.A.* **81**, 7907–7911.

Babiuk, L. A., and Ohmann, H. B. (1985). Bovine herpesvirus-1 (BHV-1) infection in cattle as a model for viral induced immunosuppression. *Prog. Leukocyte Biol.* **1**, 99–104.

Babiuk, L. A., Lawman, M. J. P., and Gifford, G. A. (1987). Bovine respiratory disease. Pathogenesis and control by interferon. *In* "A Seminar in Bovine Immunology", pp. 12–23. Veterinary Learning Systems Co., Lawrenceville, New Jersey.

Baker, P. E. (1987). Bovine interleukin 2: Cloning, high level expression, and purification. *Vet. Immunol. Immunopathol.* **17**, 193–209.

Baker, P. E., and Knoblock, K. F. (1982a). Bovine costimulator. I. Production kinetics, partial purification, and quantification in serum-free Iscove's medium. *Vet. Immunol. Immunopathol.* **3**, 365–379.

Baker, P. E., and Knoblock, K. F. (1982b). Bovine costimulator. II. Generation and maintenance of a bovine costimulator-dependent bovine lymphoblastoid cell line. *Vet. Immunol. Immunopathol.* **3**, 381–397.

Bhagyam, R. C., Jarret–Zaczek, D., and Ferguson, F. G. (1988). Activation of swine peripheral blood lymphocytes with human recombinant interleukin-2. *Immunol.* **64**, 607–613.

Bielefeldt-Ohmann, H., and Babiuk, L. (1986). Bovine alveolar macrophages: Phenotypic and functional properties of subpopulations obtained by Percoll density gradient centrifugation. *J. Leukocyte Biol.* **39**, 167–181.

Blecha, F. (1988). Immunomodulation: A means of disease prevention in stressed livestock. *J. Anim. Sci.* **66**, 2084–2090.

Blecha, F., and Baker, P. E. (1986). Effect of cortisol *in vitro* and *in vivo* on production of bovine interleukin-2. *Am. J. Vet. Res.* **47**, 841–845.

Boyd, A. W., Fisher, D. C., Fox, D. A., Scholssman, S. F., and Nadler, L. M. (1985). Structural and functional characterization of IL 2 receptors on activated human B cells. *J. Immunol.* **134**, 2387–2392.

Brown, W. C., and Grab, D. J. (1985). Biological and biochemical characterization of bovine interleukin 2. Studies with cloned bovine T cells. *J. Immunol.* **133**, 3184–3190.

Carter, J. J., Weinberg, A. D., Pollard, A., Reeves, R., Magnuson, J. A., and Magnuson, N. S. (1989). Inhibition of T-lymphocyte mitogenic responses and effects on cell functions by bovine herpesvirus 1. *J. Virol.* **63**, 1525–1530.

Cerretti, D. P., McKereghan, K., Larsen, A., Cantrell, M. A., Anderson, D., Gillis, S., Cosman, D., and Baker, P. E. (1986). Cloning, sequence, and expression of bovine interleukin 2. *Proc. Natl. Acad. Sci. U.S.A.* **83**, 3223–3227.

Charley, B., and Fradelizi, D. (1987). Differential effects of human and porcine interleukin 2 on natural killing (NK) activity of newborn piglets and adult pigs lymphocytes. *Ann. Rech. Vet.* **18**, 227–232.

Charley, B., Petit, E., LeClerc, C., and Stefanos, S. (1985). Production of porcine interleukin-2 and its biological and antigenic relationships with human interleukin-2. *Immunol. Lett.* **10**, 121–126.

Conlon, P. J., Washkewicz, T. L., Mochizuki, D. Y., Urdal, D. L., Gillis, S., and Henney, C. S. (1985). The treatment of induced immune deficiency with interleukin-2. *Immunol. Lett.* **10**, 307–314.

Czuprynski, C. J., and Brown, J. F. (1987). Recombinant murine interleukin-1α enhancement of nonspecific antibacterial resistance. *Infect. Immun.* **55**, 2061–2065.

Damme, J. V., Ley, M. D., Snick, J. V., Dinarello, C. A., and Billiau, A. (1987). The role of interferon-β1 and the 26-Da interleukin-1 and tumor necrosis factor. *J. Immunol.* **139**, 1867–1872.

Dantzer, R., and Kelley, K. W. (1989). Stress and immunity: An integrated view of relationships between the brain and the immune system. *Life Sci.* **44**, 1995–2008.

Dumonde, D. C., Wolstencroft, R. A. Panayi, G. S., Matthew, M., Morley, J., and Howson, W. T. (1969). "Lymphokines": Non-antibody mediators of cellular immunity generated by lymphocyte activation. *Nature (London)* **224**, 38–42.

Ellis, J. A., and DeMartini, J. C. (1985). Ovine interleukin 2: Partial purification and assay in normal sheep and sheep with ovine progressive pneumonia. *Vet. Immunol. Immunopathol.* **8**, 15–25.

English, L. S., and Whitehurst, M. (1984). The production of T cell growth factor (TCGF) in vivo in sheep. *Cell. Immunol.* **85,** 364–372.

English, L. S., Binns, R. M., and Licence, S. T. (1985). Characterization of pig T cell growth factor and its species-restricted activity on human, mouse and sheep cells. *Vet. Immunol. Immunopathol.* **9,** 59–69.

Ezine, S., and Papiernik, M. (1984). Abnormal T-lymphocyte proliferation and cytotoxic responses induced by a neonatal injection of hydrocortisone: Normalization by interleukin-2 addition. *Int. J. Immunopharmacol.* **6,** 125–132.

Flaming, K. P., Blecha, F., and Anderson, G. A. (1989). Influence of isoprinosine on lymphocyte function in virus-infected feeder pigs. *Am. J. Vet. Res.* **50,** 1653–1657.

Fong, S., and Doyle, M. V. (1986). Response of bovine and porcine peripheral blood mononuclear cells to human recombinant interleukin 2_{125}. *Vet. Immunol. Immunopathol.* **11,** 91–100.

Frasca, D., Boraschi, D., Baschieri, S., Bossu, P., Tagliabue, A., Adorini, L., and Doria, G. (1988). In vivo restoration of T cell functions by human IL-1β or its 163–171 nonapeptide in immunodepressed mice. *J. Immunol.* **141,** 2651–2655.

Gasbarre, L. C., Urban, J. F., and Romanowski, R. D. (1984). Porcine interleukin 2: Parameters of production and biochemical characterization. *Vet. Immunol. Immunopathol.* **5,** 221–236.

Gillis, S., and Smith, K. A. (1977). Long-term culture of tumor-specific cytotoxic T-cells. *Nature (London)* **268,** 154–156.

Gillis, S., Crabtree, G. R., and Smith, K. A. (1979a). Glucocorticoid-induced inhibition of T cell growth factor production. I. The effect on mitogen-induced lymphocyte proliferation. *J. Immunol.* **123,** 1624–1631.

Gillis, S., Crabtree, G. R., and Smith, K. A. (1979b). Glucocorticoid-induced inhibition of T cell growth factor production. II. The effect on the *in vitro* generation of cytolytic T cells. *J. Immunol.* **123,** 1632–1638.

Griffin, J. F. T. (1989). Stress and immunity: A unifying concept. *Vet. Immunol. Immunopathol.* **20,** 263–312.

Grimm, E. A., Mazumder, A., Zhang, H. Z., and Rosenberg, S. A. (1982). Lymphokine-activated killer cell phenomenon. Lysis of natural kill-resistant fresh solid tumor cells by interleukin 2-activated autologous human peripheral blood lymphocytes. *J. Exp. Med.* **155,** 1823–1841.

Hennessy, K. J., Blecha, F., Fenwick, B. W., Thaler, R. C., and Nelssen, J. L. (1990). Human recombinant interleukin-2 augments porcine natural killer cell cytotoxicity *in vivo*. *Ann. Rech. Vét.* **21,** 101–109.

Hopfner-Topliff, D., and Blecha, F. (1987). Bovine recombinant interleukin-2 (IL-2) induces lymphokine-activated bovine killer cells. *J. Anim. Sci.* **65,** Suppl. 1, 359.

Kasahara, T., Djeu, J. Y., Dougherty, S. F., and Oppenheim, J. J. (1983). Capacity of human large granular lymphocytes (LGL) to produce multiple lymphokines: Interleukin 2, interferon, and colony stimulating factor. *J. Immunol.* **131,** 2379–2385.

Kawashima, K., and Platt, K. B. (1989). The effect of human recombinant interleukin-2 on the porcine immune response to a pseudorabies virus sub-unit vaccine. *Vet. Immunol. Immunopathol.* **22,** 345–353.

Keller, S. E., Weiss, J. M., Scheifer, S. J., Miller, N. E., and Stein, M. (1983). Stress-induced supression of immunity in adrenalectomized rats. *Science* **113,** 1301–1304.

Keller, S. E., Schleifer, S. J., Liotta, A. S., Bond, R. N., Farhoody, N., and Stein, M. (1988). Stress-induced alteration of immunity in hypophysectomized rats. *Proc. Natl. Acad. Sci. U.S.A.* **85,** 9297–9301.

Kelley, K. W. (1988). Cross-talk between the immune and endocrine systems. *J. Anim. Sci.* **66,** 2095–2108.

Klemcke, H., Blecha, F., and Nienaber, J. (1987). Rapid effects of adrenocorticotropic hormone (ACTH) and restraint stressor on porcine lymphocyte function. *J. Anim. Sci.* **65,** Suppl. 1, 224.

Knisley, K. A., and Pearson, L. D. (1987). Production and assay of ovine T cell growth factor by concanavalin A stimulated peripheral blood leukocytes. *Vet. Immunol. Immunopathol.* **16,** 37–46.

Knudsen, P. J., Dinarello, C. A., and Storm, T. B. (1987). Glucocorticoids inhibit transcriptional and post-transcriptional expression of interleukin-1 in U937 cells. *J. Immunol.* **139,** 4129–4134.

Kromer, G., Schauenstein, K., and Wick, G. (1986). Avian lymphokines: An improved method for chicken IL-2 production and assay. A ConA-erythrocyte complex induces higher T cell proliferation and IL-2 production than does free mitogen. *J. Immunol. Methods* **73,** 273–281.

Lanier, L. L., Benike, C. J., Phillips, J. H., and Engleman, E. G. (1985). Recombinant interleukin 2 enhanced natural killer cell-mediated cytotoxicity in human lymphocyte subpopulations expressing the Leu 7 and Leu 11 antigens. *J. Immunol.* **134,** 794–801.

Leong, S. R., Flaggs, G. M., Lawman, M., and Gray, P. W. (1988a). The nucleotide sequence for the cDNA of bovine interleukin-1 alpha. *Nucleic Acids Res.* **16,** 9053.

Leong, S. R., Flaggs, G. M., Lawman, M., and Gray, P. W. (1988b). The nucleotide sequence for the cDNA of bovine interleukin-1 beta. *Nucleic Acids Res.* **16,** 9054.

Lew, W., Oppenheim, J., and Matsushima, K. (1988). Analysis of the suppression of IL-α and IL-1β production in human peripheral blood mononuclear adherent cells by a glucocorticoid hormone. *J. Immunol.* **140,** 1895–1902.

Lomedico, P. T., Gubler, U., Hellman, C. P., Dukovich, M., Giri, J. G., Pan, Y. E., Collier, K., Semionow, R., Chua, A. O., and Mizel, S. B. (1984). Cloning and expression of murine interleukin-1 in *E. coli*. *Nature (London)* **312,** 458–462.

Maliszewski, C. R., Baker, P. E., Schoenborn, M. A., Davis, B. S., Cosman, D., Gillis, S., and Cerretti, D. P. (1987). Cloning, sequence and expression of bovine interleukin-1α and interleukin-1β complementary DNAs. *Mol. Immunol.* **25,** 429–437.

Maliszewski, C. R., Gallis, B., and Baker, P. E. (1990). The molecular biology of large animal cytokines. *In* "Immunomodulation in Domestic Food Animals" (F. Blecha and B. Charley, eds.). Academic Press, San Diego, California.

March, C. J., Mosely, B., Larsen, A., Cerretti, D. P., Braedt, G., Price, V., Gillis, S., Henney, C. S., Kronheim, S. R., Grabstein, K., Conlon, P. J., Hopp, T. P., and Cosman, D. (1985). Cloning, sequence and expression of two distinct human interleukin-1 complementary DNAs. *Nature (London)* **315,** 641–648.

Mastro, A. M., Bortner, D. M., and Pishak, S. A. (1986). DNA synthesis and production of interleukin 1 by lymph node macrophages in culture. *J. Leukocyte Biol.* **39,** 63–75.

Miller-Edge, M., and Splitter, G. A. (1984). Bovine interleukin 2 (IL2) production and activity on bovine and murine cell lines. *Vet. Immunol. Immunopathol.* **7,** 119–130.

Mittler, E., Rao, P., Olini, G., Westberg, E., Newman, W., Hoffman, M., and Goldstein, G. (1985). Activated human B cells display a functional IL-2 receptor. *J. Immunol.* **134,** 2393–2399.

Mohagheghour, N., Gelber, R. H., Larrick, J. W., Sasake, O. T., Brennan, F. J., and Engleman, E. G. (1985). Defective cell-mediated immunity in leprosy: Failure of T cells from lepromatous leprosy patients to respond to *Mycobacterium leprae*. *Immunol. Rev.* **80,** 77–86.

Morgan, D. A., Ruscetti, F. W., and Gallo, R. C. (1976). Selective *in vitro* growth of T lymphocytes from normal human bone marrows. *Science* **193,** 1007–1008.

Murray, F. A., and Chenault, J. R. (1982). Effects of steroids on bovine T-lymphocyte blastogenesis *in vitro*. *J. Anim. Sci.* **55**, 1132–1138.

Nagi, A. M., and Babiuk, L. A. (1989). Recombinant human interleukin-2-induced mitogenic proliferation of *in vitro* unstimulated bovine intestinal lymphocytes. *Can. J. Vet. Res.* **53**, 68–75.

Namen, A. E., and Magnuson, J. A. (1984). Production and characterization of bovine interleukin-2. *Immunology* **52**, 469–475.

Nencioni, L., Villa, L., Tagliabue, A., Antoni, G., Presentini, R., Perin, F., Silvestri, S., and Boraschi, D. (1987). *In vivo* immunostimulating activity of the 163-171 peptide of human IL-1β. *J. Immunol.* **139**, 800–804.

Nickerson, S. C., Baker, P. E., and Trinidad, P. (1989). Local immunostimulation of the bovine mammary gland with interleukin-2. *J. Dairy Sci.* **72**, 1764–1773.

Nishida, R., Nishino, N., Takano, M., Kawai, K., Bando, K., Masue, Y., Nakai, S., and Hirai, Y. (1987). cDNA cloning of IL-1α and IL-1β mRNA of U937 cell line. *Biochem. Biophys. Res. Commun.* **143**, 345–352.

Nunberg, J. H., Doyle, M. V., Newell, A. D., Anderson, G. A., and York, C. J. (1988). Interleukin-2 as an adjuvant to vaccination. *In* "Vaccines '88. New Chemical and Genetic Approaches to Vaccination: Prevention of AIDS and Other Viral, Bacterial, and Parasitic Diseases" (H. Ginsberg, F. Brown, R. A. Lerner, and R. M. Chanock, eds.), pp. 247–251. Cold Spring Harbor Lab., Cold Spring Harbor, New York.

Nunberg, J. H., Doyle, M. V., York, S. M., and York, C. J. (1989). Interleukin 2 acts as an adjuvant to increase the potency of inactivated rabies virus vaccine. *Proc. Natl. Acad. Sci. U.S.A.* **86**, 4240–4243.

Ojo-Amaize, E., Guidry, A., Paape, M., and Mayer, H. (1988). *In vitro* depression on bovine lymphocyte function by treatment of cultured bovine lymphocytes with physiologic concentrations of hydrocortisone. *Am. J. Vet. Res.* **49**, 851–856.

Oldham, G., and Williams, L. (1984). Interleukin 2 (IL2) production by mitogen stimulated bovine peripheral blood lymphocytes and its assay. *Vet. Immunol. Immunopathol.* **7**, 201–212.

Orsz, C. G., Zimm, N. E., Olsen, R. G., and Mathes, L. E. (1985). Retrovirus-mediated immunosuppression. I. FeLV-UV and specific FeLV proteins alter T Lymphocyte behaviour by inducing hyporesponsiveness to lymphokines. *J. Immunol.* **134**, 3396–3403.

Perrin, P., Joffret, M. L., LeClerc, C., Oth, D., Sureau, P., and Thibodeau, L. (1988). Interleukin 2 increases protection against experimental rabies. *Immunobiology* **177**, 199–209.

Reddy, P. G., Blecha, F., Minocha, H. C., Anderson, G. A., Morrill, J. L., Fedorka-Cray, P. J., and Baker, P. E. (1989). Bovine recombinant interleukin-2 augments immunity and resistance to bovine herpesvirus infection. *Vet. Immunol. Immunopathol.* **23**, 61–74.

Reddy, D. N., Reddy, P. G., Minocha, H. C., Baker, P. E., Davis, W. C., and Blecha, F. (1990). Adjuvanticity of recombinant bovine interleukin-1β: Influence on immunity, infection, and latency in a bovine herpesvirus-1 infection. *Lymphokine Res.* (in press).

Reed, S. G., Inverso, J. A., and Roters, S. B. (1984). Suppressed antibody responses to sheep erythrocytes in mice with chronic *Trypanosoma cruzi* infections are restored with interleukin 2. *J. Immunol.* **133**, 3333–3337.

Reed, S. G., Pihl, D. L., and Grabstein, K. H. (1989a). Immune deficiency in chronic *Trypanosoma cruzi* infection: Recombinant IL-1 restores Th function for antibody production. *J. Immunol.* **142**, 2067–2071.

Reed, S. G., Pihl, D. L., Conlon, P. J., and Grabstein, K. H. (1989b). IL-1 as adjuvant: Role of T cells in the augmentation of specific antibody production by recombinant human IL-1α. *J. Immunol.* **142,** 3129–3133.

Reeves, R., Spies, A. G., Nissen, M. S., Buck, C. D., Weinberg, A. D., Barr, P. J., Magnuson, N. S., and Magnuson, J. A. (1986). Molecular cloning of a functional bovine interleukin 2 cDNA. *Proc. Natl. Acad. Sci. U.S.A.* **83,** 3228–3232.

Roberta, J. A., Lamb, R. J., Reed, J. C., Daniele, R. P., and Nowell, P. C. (1987). Dexamethasone inhibition of interleukin-1β by human monocytes. *J. Clin. Invest.* **81,** 237–244.

Rosenberg, S. A., Lotze, M. T., Muul, L. M., Leitman, S., Chang, A. E., Ettinghausen, S. E., Matory, Y. L., Skibber, J. M., Shiloni, E., Vetto, J. T., Seipp, C. A., Simpson, C., and Reichert, C. M. (1985). Observations on the systemic administration of autologous lymphokine-activated killer cells and recombinant interleukin-2 to patients with metastatic cancer. *N. Engl. J. Med.* **313,** 1485–1492.

Roth, J. A. (1985). Cortisol as mediator of stress-associated immunosuppression in cattle. *In* "Animal Stress" (G. P. Moberg, ed.), pp. 225–243. Am. Physiol. Soc., Bethesda, Maryland.

Roth, J. A., Abruzzini, A. F., and Frank, D. E. (1990). Influence of recombinant human interleukin-2 administration on lymphocyte and neutrophil function in clinically normal and dexamethasone-treated cattle. *Am. J. Vet. Res.* **51,** 546–549.

Rouse, B. T., Miller, L. S., Turtinen, L., and Morré, R. N. (1985). Augmentation of immunity to herpes simplex virus by *in vivo* administration of interleukin 2. *J. Immunol.* **134,** 926–930.

Saklatvala, J., Curry, V. A., and Sarsfield, S. J. (1983). Purification to homogeneity of pig leucocyte catabolin, a protein that causes cartilage resportion *in vitro*. *Biochem. J.* **215,** 385–392.

Saklatvala, J., Sarsfield, S. J., and Townsend, Y. (1985a). Pig interleukin 1. Purification of two immunologically different leukocyte proteins that cause cartilage resorption, lymphocyte activation and fever. *J. Exp. Med.* **162,** 1208–1222.

Saklatvala, J., Sarsfield, S. J., and Wood, D. D. (1985b). An antiserum to pig IL1 (catabolin) reacts with the acidic but not the neutral form of human IL1. *Br. J. Rheumatol.* **24,** Suppl. 1, 68–71.

Sambhara, S. R., and Belden, E. L. (1988). Bovine interleukin 2: Production and characterization. *Vet. Immunol. Immunopathol.* **18,** 165–172.

Staruch, M. J., and Wood, D. D. (1983). The adjuvanticity of interleukin 1 *in vivo*. *J. Immunol.* **130,** 2191–2194.

Stott, J. L., Fenwick, B. W., and Osburn, B. I. (1986). Human recombinant interleukin-2 augments *in vitro* blastogenesis of bovine and porcine lymphocytes. *Vet. Immunol. Immunopathol.* **13,** 31–38.

Tarleton, R. L. (1988). *Trypanosoma cruzi*-induced suppression of IL-2 production. Evidence for a role for suppressor cells. *J. Immunol.* **140,** 2769–2773.

Thoman, M., and Weigle, W. O. (1985). Reconstitution of *in vivo* cell-mediated lympholysis responses in aged mice with interleukin 2. *J. Immunol.* **134,** 949–952.

Vainio, O., Ratcliffe, M. J. H., and Leanderson, T. (1986). Chicken T-cell growth factor: Use in the generation of a long term cultured T-cell line and biochemical characterization. *Scand. J. Immunol.* **23,** 135–142.

Wainberg, M. A., Vydelingum, S., and Margoleswe, R. G. (1983). Viral inhibition of lymphocyte mitogenesis: Interference with the synthesis of functionally active T cell growth factor (TCGF) activity and reversal of inhibition by addition of the same. *J. Immunol.* **130,** 2372–2378.

Weinberg, A. D., Magnuson, N. S., Reeves, R., Wyatt, C. R., and Magnuson, J. A. (1988a). Evidence for two discrete phases of IL-2 production in bovine lymphocytes. *J. Immunol.* **141,** 1174–1179.

Weinberg, A. D., Shaw, J., Paetkau, V., Bleakley, R. C., Magnuson, N. S., Reeves, R., and Magnuson, J. A. (1988b). Cloning of cDNA for the bovine IL-2 receptor (bovine Tac antigen). *Immunology* **63,** 603–610.

Westey, H. J., and Kelley, K. W. (1984). Physiologic concentrations of cortisol suppress cell-mediated immune events in the domestic pig. *Proc. Soc. Exp. Biol. Med.* **177,** 156–164.

Zelarney, P. T., and Belden, E. L. (1988). Bovine interleukin 2: Production by an E-rosette-defined lymphocyte subpopulation. *Vet. Immunol. Immunopathol.* **18,** 297–305.

Part IV
Physiologically Regulated Immunomodulation

Nutritional Modulation of Immunity in Domestic Food Animals

P. G. REDDY* AND R. A. FREY†

*Department of Microbiology, School of Veterinary Medicine,
Tuskegee University, Tuskegee, Alabama 36088, and
†Department of Anatomy and Physiology, College of Veterinary Medicine
Kansas State University, Manhattan, Kansas 66506*

I. Introduction
II. Protein and Energy
III. Fat-Soluble Vitamins
   A. Vitamin A
   B. Vitamin D
   C. Vitamin E
IV. Water-Soluble Vitamins
   A. B-Complex Vitamins
   B. Vitamin C
V. Minerals
   A. Selenium
   B. Iron
   C. Zinc
   D. Copper
   E. Cobalt
VI. Conclusion
   References

Introduction

Experimental evidence for the effect of single nutrients on the ability of domestic food animals to mount an immune response against infectious agents, or on the outcome of an infection is very sparse. However, there is a growing interest now to study the interactions of nutrition and disease resistance because modern management systems have evolved towards high-density confinement-rearing of livestock. Under such conditions, animals are subjected to more stress and increased incidence of diseases. Continued high morbidity and mortality of livestock warrants research emphasis on optimizing the immune response and necessitates improving our understanding of the role of nutrition in disease resistance. The present recommendations for nutrient requirements of various species of livestock are based entirely on their growth and production responses and are not assessed to maximize their immune response. Changes in nutrient recommendations designed to optimize immune responses and disease resistance mechanisms may be cost effective when reduced morbidity and mortality can be demonstrated.

Although some attempts have been made in the past few years to understand the role of single nutrients in the immune responses of various species of livestock, many more studies are needed to bring into perspective the synergistic interactions between nutritional factors and functions of immunocompetent cells. Resistance against infectious agents is controlled by an array of factors in the host. These include the physical barriers of skin and mucus membranes, mucus and cilia on epithelial surfaces, phagocytes, including neutrophils and macrophages, the complement system, immunoglobulins, cell-mediated immune responses, and secretion of various cytokines that regulate both cell-mediated and humoral immune responses. Host defenses also depend upon several other humoral factors that influence immunity and disease resistance. These are generally grouped as nonspecific factors of resistance, and include many substances such as C-reactive protein, lysozymes, and hormones. Many of these specific and nonspecific factors may be affected by alterations in the status of particular nutrients. For example, chronic mild-to-moderate vitamin and mineral deficiencies, even in the absence of clinical malnutrition, may have a negative effect on the immune system. Rapidly growing neonatal animals are likely to be affected worst by marginal deficiencies of nutrients. Even though mortality is uncommon, marginal deficiencies may result in permanent damage to the immune system.

Nutrients may affect host response to disease-causing organisms either directly by acting on the immunocompetent cells or indirectly by altering metabolic, neurological, or endocrine parameters. Single nutrients, for example, may affect stability and integrity of cellular and subcellular membranes and expression of cell surface receptors on immunocompetent cells or may even alter the circulating subsets of T cells. Indeed, nutritional factors may regulate the ontogeny and maintenance of disease-resistance mechanisms of livestock through a variety of pathways. Further, the nutritional status of an animal also may influence the outcome of an infection.

While considering immunopotentiation through nutritional modulation, it is also appropriate to consider various means to avoid harmful immunological responses to dietary antigens. Replacement of milk protein in the diets of neonatal calves and pigs with conventionally processed soy protein has been found to inhibit the performance of animals; part of this problem has been attributed to an immunological reaction to soy protein. If the inferior performance of animals fed soybean products can be related to hypersensitivity responses, then it may be necessary to apply some immunological criteria to the processing of soybean products. Products that are processed by alternate methods in order to denature the antigenic proteins may lead to more efficient utilization by the animals.

The purpose of this chapter is to review existing literature on the role of various nutrients on the immune response in domestic food animals and to consider the potential for nutritional modulation in immune dysfunctions and suggest some directions for future research. A summary on the effect of nutrients on immunity in different species is given in Table I.

II. Protein and Energy

Specific experiments delineating the effects of protein-energy malnutrition (PEM) on the immune response of various classes of livestock are limited.

Protein-energy malnutrition during pregnancy or during the neonatal period may have profound effects on the ontogeny of the immune system of newborn animals. Neonatal calves fed a diet resulting in PEM were found to have lower lymphocyte interleukin-2 (IL-2) activity and proliferative responses to mitogens as compared to calves fed normal diets (Griebel *et al.*, 1987). However, in adult cattle, prolonged PEM was not found to compromise humoral or cell-mediated immunity (Friske and Adams, 1985). Protein deficiency during pregnancy may adversely affect neonatal survival and weight gain. This may be due to a decrease in the secretion of immunoglobulin in milk or decreased development of absorptive cells in the intestine of the newborn. Blecha *et al.* (1981) observed no significant correlations between immunoglobulins in the sera or colostrum of first-calf beef heifers and protein consumption during the prenatal period. However, absorption of colos-

TABLE I

SUMMARY OF THE EFFECT OF NUTRIENTS ON IMMUNITY IN DOMESTIC FOOD ANIMALS

Nutrient	Species	Influence on Immunity	Reference
Protein and energy	Cattle	Deficiency ↓ IL-2 activity and lymphocyte proliferative responses to mitogens in neonatal calves	Griebel et al. (1987)
		Deficiency has no effect on humoral or cell-mediated immunity in adult cattle	Friske and Adams (1985)
		Deficiency ↓ absorption of colostral Ig by the offspring	Blecha et al. (1981)
	Pigs	Deficiency has no effect on piglet's ability to synthesize antibody	Haye et al. (1981); Corley et al. (1983)
		Deficiency ↓ antibody synthesis	McGillivray (1967)
Vitamin A	Cattle	Positive correlation with serum concentration and lymphocyte blastogenesis in calves	Stern et al. (1981)
		Low plasma levels correlated with ↑ California Mastitis Test Scores	Chew et al. (1982)
	Pigs	Deficiency causes tenfold decrease in antibody synthesis	Harmon et al. (1963)
Vitamin D	Cattle	↓ lymphocyte proliferative response to mitogens, however, at higher doses ↑ Con A-induced proliferation	Reinhardt and Hustmyer (1987)
Vitamin E	Cattle	Supplementation ↑ lymphocyte proliferative responses and ↑ antibody synthesis in calves	Cipriano et al. (1982); Reddy et al. (1986, 1987b)
		Supplementation ↑ resistance against mastitis	Smith et al. (1984, 1985)
	Sheep	Supplementation ↑ antibody synthesis following secondary challenge with parainfluenza-3	Reffett et al. (1988)
		Supplementation ↑ resistance against Chlamydia	Stephens et al. (1979)
		Adjuvant effect when given along with bacterial vaccines	Tengerdy et al. (1983); Afzal et al. (1984)
	Pigs	Supplementation ↑ lymphocyte blastogenesis	Larsen and Tollersrud (1981)

B-complex vitamins	Cattle	Supplementation ↓ morbidity in shipping-stressed calves	Cole et al. (1982); Zinn et al. (1987)
	Pigs	Deficiency causes ↓ antibody synthesis	Miller et al. (1962)
		Supplementation ↑ antibody production	Harmon et al. (1963)
Vitamin C	Cattle	Supplementation ↑ bronchopneumonia from 50 to 22.5% in young calves	Itze (1984)
		Supplementation ↑ antibody production in calves deprived of colostrum	Cummins and Brunner (1989)
		Supplementation has no effect on neutrophil-mediated phagocytosis, ADCC, and lymphocyte proliferative responses	Pruiett et al. (1989)
		Supplementation ↑ neutrophil oxidative metabolism and ADCC	Roth and Kaeberle (1985)
	Pigs	Supplementation has no effect on cell-mediated and humoral immune response	Yen and Pond (1987); Kornegay et al. (1986)
		Supplementation ↑ antibody production in immunosuppressed chicken; no effect in healthy chicken	Pardue and Thaxton (1984); Pardue et al. (1985); McCorkle et al. (1980)
	Chickens	Supplementation ↑ resistance against infectious bursal disease	Pardue (1987)
Selenium	Cattle	Deficiency ↓ antibody production	Reffett et al. (1987)
		Supplementation ↑ antibody titers	Reffett et al. (1988)
	Pigs	Supplementation ↑ lymphocyte proliferative responses	Larsen and Tollersrud (1981)
		Supplementation ↑ antibody response	Peplowski et al. (1981)
		Weaning stress ↑ mortality in selenium-deficient pigs	Meyer et al. (1981); Mahan and Moxon (1980)
	Sheep	Deficiency ↓ lymphocyte proliferative responses in lambs from selenium-deficient ewes	Turner et al. (1985)
		Supplementation ↑ lymphocyte blastogenesis and antibody response	Jelinek et al. (1988)

(continued)

TABLE I (*Continued*)

Nutrient	Species	Influence on Immunity	Reference
	Goats	Deficiency ↓ neutrophil phagocytosis, random and chemotactic migration, and leukotriene B_4 production	Aziz *et al.* (1984)
Iron	Pigs	Large dose ↑ mortality in baby pigs challenged with *E. coli*	Kadis *et al.* (1984); Klasing *et al.* (1980); Knight *et al.* (1983)
		Supplementation ↓ susceptibility to bacterial endotoxin	Osborne and Davis (1968)
	Chicks	Deficiency ↑ susceptibility to *S. gallinarum* and excess survival rate	Hill and Smith (1974); Smith *et al.* (1977a,b); Harry (1979)
Zinc	Cattle	Deficiency ↑ susceptibility to bacterial infections	Miller (1970)
		Supplementation ↑ resistance to BHV-1 and ↓ number of treatments for morbid steers	Hutcheson (1989)
	Pigs	Deficiency causes thymic atrophy and supplementation ↑ resistance to *S. pullorum*	Miller *et al.* (1968)
Copper	Cattle	Deficiency ↓ phagocytosis by neutrophils	Jones and Suttle (1981)
	Sheep	↑ mortality due to ataxia and infections in lambs from copper-deficient ewes	Wiener and Field (1969); Wiener *et al.* (1985); Whitelaw *et al.* (1979); Yeoman (1983)
		Deficiency ↓ phagocytosis by neutrophils	Jones and Suttle (1981)
		↓ lymphocyte proliferative responses in hypocupremic animals and supplementation restores the response	Suttle and Jones (1986)
Cobalt	Cattle	Deficiency ↓ immunity in calves	Wright *et al.* (1982)
		Deficiency ↓ neutrophil functions	MacPherson *et al.* (1987)
	Sheep	Deficiency ↑ susceptibility to infections	MacPherson *et al.* (1976); Downey (1966)

tral immunoglobulins (IgG1 and IgG2) by their calves was positively correlated to maternal crude protein consumption. Loh et al. (1971) observed that protein restriction of rat dams decreased the development of absorptive cells in the pup's jejunum and, in turn, resulted in reduced absorption of protein. Moderate restriction of protein in the sow's diet does not seem to affect passive transfer of immunoglobulins or the piglet's ability to synthesize antibodies. Feeding a 9% crude protein (CP) diet during gestation and an 18% CP diet during lactation had no effect on the piglet's ability to synthesize antibody (Haye et al., 1981). Similar results were reported by Corley et al. (1983).

Early weaning may impose both a nutritional and psychological stress and adversely affect the immune response at least for a short period of time. Gwazdauskas et al. (1978) observed a decreased synthesis of antibody to heterologous erythrocytes injected at the time when calves were weaned. Pigs weaned at 2–3 weeks of age have lower lymphocyte blastogenic and delayed-type hypersensitivity responses compared to nonweaned littermates (Blecha et al., 1983). Early weaning was also found to adversely affect the ability of pigs to synthesize antibodies (Miller et al., 1962; Blecha and Kelley, 1981; Haye and Kornegay, 1979). However, Crenshaw et al. (1986) observed no differences in humoral or cell-mediated immune responses in pigs weaned onto either simple or complex weaning diets. Cell-mediated immune response of calves weaned at 2 weeks on an early weaning program were similar to those of calves on a conventional program and weaned at 6 weeks of age (Reddy et al., 1985a). Calves weaned at 2 weeks of age in this experiment had access to a highly palatable, all milk-protein, pelleted diet right from birth.

Protein-deficient diets also may adversely affect immune responses of young growing animals. When the CP content in the diet of young pigs ranged from 0 to 35%, there was a linear increase in antibody titers to heat-killed *Salmonella pullorum* (McGillivray, 1967).

Inclusion of conventionally processed soybean products in the diets of young calves and baby pigs has been found to cause immediate-type hypersensitivity reactions (Kilshaw and Sissons, 1979a,b; Barrat et al., 1978; Sissons, 1982; Sissons and Thurston, 1984; Dawson et al., 1988; Kelley and Easter, 1987; Li et al., 1989). Major structural proteins of soybean products, i.e., glycinin and β-conglycinin, have been implicated as the major antigenic proteins, although information about the antigenic nature of other minor proteins of soybean products is lacking. This hypersensitivity is characterized by a serum antibody response specific to glycinin and β-conglycinin and generally coincides with abnormal villous morphology and crypt elongation in the small intestine, diarrhea, and decreased weight gains (Barrat et al., 1978; Sissons and Thurston, 1984; Dawson et al., 1988; Li et al., 1989). Blood and intestinal lymphocytes were found to not proliferate when cultured in the presence of purified soybean proteins (Dawson et al., 1988; Li et al., 1989). These studies have suggested that alternate processing methods may need to be explored for more efficient utilization of soybean products and to avoid deleterious effects because of hypersensitivity responses. A simple enzyme-linked immunosorbent assay has been developed (Reddy et al., 1989) to test for residual antigenic proteins and to predict the suitability of soybean products before their inclusion in the diets of neonatal animals.

III. Fat-Soluble Vitamins

A. Vitamin A

Vitamin A is well known for its role in the differentiation of epithelial cells and inhibition of keratinization and thus is essential in maintaining the stability and integrity of mucosal surfaces. Vitamin A deficiency leads to keratinization of the secretory epithelia of the respiratory tract and salivary and prostate glands, thereby increasing the susceptibility to infectious agents. A decrease in the number of goblet cells with an accompanying decrease in mucus production, which disrupts the nonspecific defense mechanisms of the intestines, is another common observation of vitamin A deficiency. The role of vitamin A and β-carotene on host defense mechanisms has been reviewed recently (Chew, 1987).

Very little is known about the regulatory role of vitamin A on the functional activities of immunocompetent cells in food animals. In a preliminary study with calves from birth to 5 weeks of age, Stern et al. (1981) reported a positive correlation between mitogen-stimulated lymphocyte blastogenesis and serum vitamin A levels in calves. Calves were fed colostrum and then milk replacer containing deficient, normal, or high levels of vitamin A as retinyl palmitate. Similar results were obtained when vitamin A was added to lymphocyte cultures in vitro. Chew et al. (1982) have investigated the relationship between vitamin A and β-carotene in blood and milk and severity of mammary gland infections in the lactating dairy cow. They observed a highly significant, independent effect for concentrations of plasma vitamin A, β-carotene, and total vitamin A equivalent on California Mastitis Test scores; cows with lower plasma vitamin A, β-carotene, and total vitamin A equivalent had higher test scores than cows with higher vitamin A and β-carotene. Concentrations of plasma β-carotene less than 200 μg/dl and vitamin A less than 80 μg/dl were considered to reflect a deficiency status in relation to udder health in Holsteins (Chew et al., 1984). Vitamin A deficiency in pigs was found to result in a tenfold decrease in the synthesis of antibody. With baby pigs fed semisynthetic diets deficient in vitamin A, the correlation coefficient between serum vitamin A and agglutination antibody titer to *Salmonella pullorum* was 0.70 and highly significant (Harmon et al., 1963). Although the importance of vitamin A in the diets of food animals is well recognized, specific studies to determine the requirements to maximize the functions of immunocompetent cells are clearly lacking.

B. Vitamin D

The concept that 1,25-dihydroxyvitamin-D (1,25-$(OH)_2D$) does have an immunoregulatory function in the body arises from the finding that certain cells of the immune system, such as cells of calf thymus gland and lymph nodes, exhibit receptors for 1,25-$(OH)_2D$ (Reinhardt et al., 1982). Receptors for 1,25-$(OH)_2D$ are also present on peripheral blood monocytes. Resting T and B lymphocytes, per se, do not have receptors for 1,25-$(OH)_2D$ but do express receptors when activated by mitogens or viruses (Bhalla et al., 1983; Provvedini et al., 1983). Vitamin D deficiency, severe enough to cause rickets in children, was found to inhibit certain functions of monocytes and neutrophils (Stroder and Kasal, 1970; Lorente et al., 1976), which could be corrected by vitamin D therapy. Vitamin D deficiency also was found to inhibit macrophage functions, which can be reversed by treatment with vitamin D (Bar-Shavit et al., 1987). Vitamin D also augments the expression of Class II major histocompatibility antigens (Morel et al., 1986). Contrary to the enhancement of monocyte and neutrophil functions, vitamin D was found to inhibit lymphocyte proliferation and IL-2 secretion (Manolagas et al., 1985). An inhibitory effect of vitamin D on mitogen-induced proliferation of lymphocytes also was observed in bovine cells; however, at higher doses vitamin D was found to enhance Con A-induced proliferation of bovine lymphocytes (Reinhardt and Hustmyer, 1987). Vitamin D also was found to inhibit immunoglobulin production by B cells (Lemire et al., 1984, 1985). Thus, growing evidence shows the immunoregulatory properties of vitamin D. However, little is known about its role in the immune system of domestic food animals. It may be useful to determine what concentrations of vitamin D in the blood will maximize the functions of macrophages and neutrophils, without adversely affecting the functions of T and B lymphocytes.

C. Vitamin E

Vitamin E is an excellent free-radical scavenger in a lipid environment and is nontoxic even at high levels of intake. The C-4 and C-8 methyl groups of tocopherol's phytol side chain are in close association with the C-15 double bonds of arachidonic acid (Diplock and Lucy, 1973). This interaction probably reduces the membrane fluidity created by larger amounts of membrane polyunsaturated fatty acids (PUFA), which are subject to free-radical attack in the absence of a suitable antioxidant. The regulatory role played by vitamin E in the biosynthesis of prostaglandin, thromboxane, leukotriene, and cortisol has been documented (Afzal et al., 1986; Machlin, 1978; Goetzl, 1980; Chan et al., 1980; Reddy et al., 1987b; Lim et al., 1981; Watson and Petro, 1982); this may partly explain its immunoregulatory property.

Calves and pigs are usually born with low levels of blood vitamin E and are particularly vulnerable to deficiency. If these rapidly growing animals are fed diets limited in vitamin E, the rate of deposition in newly formed membranes may be insufficient to prevent peroxidative damage, especially if the diets are rich in PUFA. An increase in serum concentrations of certain lysosomal enzymes, such as serum glutamic oxalacetic transaminase (SGOT), lactic dehydrogenase (LDH), and creatine kinase (CK), generally indicates damage to cell membranes. Calves fed conventional diets were found to have higher SGOT and LDH activities (Reddy et al., 1987a) and higher CK activity (Reddy et al., 1985b) than calves receiving supplemental vitamin E. Immunocompetent cells such as lymphocytes may be more prone to peroxidative damage than other cells in the body, because they usually have higher concentrations of free fatty acids (FFA). For example, Kigoshi and Ito (1973) observed that Guinea pig spleen cells contain 14–17% FFA, whereas cells from viscera contain only 2–3% FFA. Lipid peroxidation and free-radical attack may alter the membrane fluidity and result in changes in cell–cell and cell–substrate interaction and subsequent metabolic process in lymphoid tissue, and thus, may be responsible for observed immunosuppression.

Vitamin E has been shown to enhance humoral immune (HI) responses as a dietary supplement or an immunoadjuvant to both living and nonliving agents in several species of animals, including cattle, chickens, sheep, and swine (Tengerdy et al., 1984). Calves supplemented with vitamin E had higher antibody titers (Fig. 1) to bovine herpesvirus-1 (BHV-1) following a booster vaccination with modified-live intranasal vaccine (Reddy et al., 1987b). Lambs supplemented with vitamin E were found to produce more antibodies following a secondary

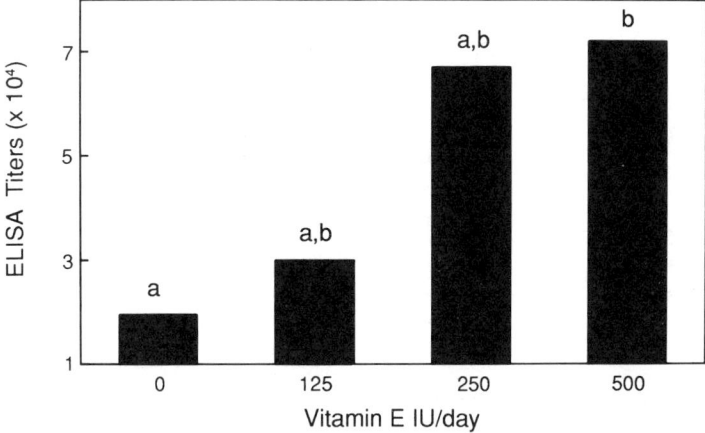

FIG. 1. Serum antibody titers to BHV-1 in calves at 24 weeks of age. Calves received supplemental vitamin E from birth to 24 weeks of age and were vaccinated (modified-live intranasal) at the age of 7 and 21 weeks. a, b: Means with different superscripts differ ($p < 0.05$). Adopted from Reddy et al. (1987b).

challenge with parainfluenza-3 virus (Reffett et al., 1988). The adjuvant effect of vitamin E in enhancing the protection provided by bacterial vaccines has been documented (Tengerdy et al., 1983; Afzal et al., 1984). Supplemental vitamin E has been shown to enhance resistance against E. coli in chicks and against chlamydia in lambs (Heinzerling et al., 1974; Stephens et al., 1979). The role of vitamin E on the viability and immune response of poultry has been reviewed recently (El Boushy, 1988). Supplemental vitamin E also was found to reduce the incidence of clinical mastitis in dairy cows (Smith et al., 1984, 1985). In one study (Smith et al., 1984), supplemental vitamin E (1.0 g/cow/day during prepartum) was found to reduce the incidence of mastitis by 37%. In a second trial, the same group of workers observed a 42.2% reduction in new intramammary infections at calving in heifers supplemented with vitamin E and selenium both during pre- and postpartum periods (Smith et al., 1985). However, no attempt was made to determine the specific mechanisms of action of vitamin E in protecting the mammary gland against infection. Plasma and vitamin E levels also were found to be low in mastitic cows in another study reported by Atroshi et al. (1986).

A beneficial role of vitamin E in enhancing cell-mediated immune responses has been well documented in pigs (Larsen and Tollersrud,

TABLE II

Effect of Supplemental Vitamin E on Lymphocyte Stimulation Indices with Different T and B Cell Mitogens

Mitogen	Supplemental vitamim E (IU/calf/day)				SEM
	0	125	250	500	
Phytohemagglutinin	31.6^a	$39.5^{a,b}$	$39.9^{a,b}$	$35.2^{a,b}$	2.9
Concanavalin A	29.2^a	37.2^b	$34.5^{a,b}$	36.3^b	2.2
Pokeweed mitogen	20.3^a	$24.5^{a,b}$	$23.2^{a,b}$	26.9^b	1.5
Lipopolysaccharide	3.7^a	5.8^b	$5.0^{a,b}$	5.9^b	.6

Notes: Reprinted with permission from Reddy et al. (1987b). Least square means averaged across weeks.

a,b Means within a row with different superscripts differ ($p < 0.05$).

1981) and in calves (Cipriano et al., 1982; Reddy et al., 1986, 1987b). In one experiment, calves were supplemented with 125, 250, and 500 mg of dl-tocopheryl acetate/calf/day from birth to 24 weeks of age. Overall lymphocyte proliferative responses to concanavalin A or lipopolysaccharide were significantly higher for calves given 125 and 500 mg/day than for control calves (Table II). However, responses did not increase linearly with increased supplementation, and also the overall growth performance of calves given 125 mg/day was superior to that of calves supplemented with 500 mg/day. Although optimum concentrations of vitamin E may protect neutrophils from peroxidative damage, a high level of supplementation may compromise bactericidal potency of neutrophils because of an impairment of H_2O_2 release (Baehner et al., 1982; Johnson et al., 1985; Boxer, 1986).

Further research is needed to refine the estimates of vitamin E requirements of various classes of livestock, identify factors that affect requirements, and further elucidate the biochemical functions of vitamin E in the animal body.

IV. Water-Soluble Vitamins

A. B-Complex Vitamins

All animals require B-complex vitamins because animal cells are incapable of their synthesis except for niacin and choline. Ruminants do not require these vitamins in the diet, because rumen microorganisms are capable of synthesizing them. All other animals including preruminant calves, especially those reared on milk replacers, do require preformed B-complex vitamins in their diet. Very little is known about the role of these vitamins in the immune system of domestic food animals, except for studies with pantothenic acid, pyridoxine, or riboflavin in pigs conducted at Michigan State University (Miller et al., 1962; Harmon et al., 1963).

Four-week-old baby pigs produced significantly lower serum antibody titers when they were fed a diet deficient in pantothenic acid, pyridoxine, or riboflavin (Miller et al., 1962). In another study (Harmon et al., 1963), two trials were conducted with 48 Yorkshire-Hampshire crossbred pigs that were fed semisynthetic diets with or without pantothenic acid, pyridoxine, and riboflavin. In the first trial, pigs were given a series of *Salmonella pullorum* injections, and in the second trial human erythrocytes were injected. In both trials, supplemented pigs produced a significantly higher amount of antibody titers than control pigs. A paired feeding study revealed that inhibition of antibody synthesis was attributable to deficiency of B vitamins, without the influence of inanition that invariably follows when pigs are fed diets deficient in B-complex vitamins.

Supplementation of diets of shipping-stressed feedlot calves with B vitamins was found to reduce the number of animals clinically diagnosed as sick during the first 10 days of a trail (Zinn et al., 1987), although it had no influence on weight gain or feed conversion. Similar results were reported earlier by Cole et al. (1982).

B. Vitamin C

Considerable work has been done to elucidate the immunoregulatory role of vitamin C in normal and immunosuppressed subjects and also during the course of infection. This has been investigated to some extent in the case of chickens (Pardue, 1987) but not with other domestic food animals. Leukocytes contain higher concentrations of vitamin C than serum or other body tissues (DeChatelet et al., 1974). Stress and viral infections were found to deplete vitamin C concentrations in leukocytes (Wilson and Loh, 1973; Hume and Weyers, 1973). Vitamin C appears to exert its regulatory role in antigen clearance (Wilson, 1975), interferon production (Siegel, 1975), and lymphocyte proliferation (Anderson et al., 1980). Dietary supplementation with vitamin C has been reported to augment immunity in a variety of laboratory animals and human beings; nevertheless, controversy exists on the beneficial effects of high levels of supplementation. However, based on the evidence available so far, it is reasonable to assume that a deficiency of vitamin C could lead to immunosuppression.

The effect of supplemental vitamin C in chicken diets has been reviewed (Pardue, 1987). Although vitamin C supplementation of diets does not appear to augment antibody production in healthy chickens (McCorkle et al., 1980), it was found to increase antibody production in the immunosuppressed chickens (Pardue and Thaxton, 1984; Pardue et al., 1985). Additionally, supplemental vitamin C was found to enhance disease resistance against infectious bursal disease (Pardue, 1987).

Neonatal calves below the age of 4 months may not be able to synthesize their own vitamin C (Itze, 1984), and supplementation may be necessary especially when calves are reared on milk replacer diets. Supplemental vitamin C (two injections of 500 mg ascorbic acid) was found to reduce the incidence of bronchopneumonia from 50 to 22.5% in young calves (Itze, 1984). Vitamin C also may be of some benefit to neonatal calves deprived of colostrum (Cummins and Brunner, 1989). In terms of neutrophil-mediated phagocytosis or ADCC and lymphocyte proliferative responses to mitogens, no beneficial effects of supplemental vitamin C were observed in neonatal calves fed milk replacers (Pruiett et al., 1989). However, Roth and Kaeberle (1985) observed an increased neutrophil oxidative metabolism and neutrophil-mediated ADCC when cattle were injected with vitamin C (20 mg/kg). Additionally, vitamin C tended to reverse the immunosuppressive effects of dexamethasone on some neutrophil functions.

In pigs, Yen and Pond (1987) and Kornegay et al. (1986) observed no significant influence of supplemental vitamin C on cellular and humoral immune responses.

Present evidence suggests that supplemental vitamin C may be beneficial to stressed livestock in restoring compromised functions of immunocompetent cells. More work is needed to substantiate the benefits to normal healthy animals and to animals that are particularly prone to respiratory diseases.

V. Minerals

A. SELENIUM

In the last few years, a substantial number of reports have shown the immunoregulatory role of selenium in different food animals. A review of the literature reveals overwhelming evidence for immunosuppression in various species of animals on selenium-deficient diets. A few of these studies also indicate that immunosuppression because of selenium deficiency can be corrected by selenium supplementation, and a few others show that immunity can be enhanced with additional supplementation in normal, healthy subjects otherwise on adequate selenium nutrition. Selenium is a component of the enzyme, glutathione peroxidase (GSH_{px}), which catalyzes the two-electron reduction of both organic and inorganic hydroperoxides using glutathione as the electron donor (Shamberger, 1983) and thus is considered a very good antioxidant.

In addition to protecting body tissues from oxidative damage, selenium is also considered to protect neutrophils from antotoxic damage (Fletcher et al., 1988). Neutrophils from selenium-deficient animals show decreased killing ability (Boyne and Arthur, 1979, 1981, 1986; Gyang et al., 1984). This impaired neutrophil function with selenium deficiency is associated with decreased GSH_{px} (Boyne and Arthur, 1979). The reactive oxygen products produced by neutrophils during phagocytosis may escape the membrane-bound phagocytic vacuoles and cause damage to the neutrophils, thereby impairing neutrophil functions.

In goats, selenium deficiency reduces neutrophil phagocytosis and random and chemotactic migration (Aziz et al., 1984). Selenium deficiency also was found to inhibit neutrophil leukotriene B_4 production (Aziz and Klesius, 1986). Selenium deficiency was reported to adversely affect lymphocyte proliferative responses to mitogens in pigs (Larsen and Tollersrud, 1981) and in lambs from selenium-deficient ewes (Turner et al., 1985). Supplemental selenium was found to enhance phytohemagglutinin-induced lymphocyte proliferative responses in Merino sheep (Jelinek et al., 1988). However, no significant depression in lymphocyte proliferative responses was observed in selenium-deficient young lambs not suffering from muscular dystrophy (Turner et al., 1984).

Selenium appears to have a more profound effect on humoral immune responses of several animal species. Weanling pigs receiving supplemental selenium (0.5 ppm) produced significantly higher antibody when challenged with sheep red blood cells than pigs fed an unsupplemented basal diet containing 0.2 ppm of selenium (Peplowski et al., 1981). Merino sheep fed a high selenium diet had higher antibody titers to B. abortus during a primary immune response phase and higher titers to rabbit red blood cells (Jelinek et al., 1988). Similar results were observed in 2-week-old chicks (Marsh et al., 1981). Selenium deficiency was found to inhibit specific antibody production when calves were challenged with infectious bovine rhinotracheitis virus (Reffett et al.,

1987). In another study, supplemental selenium (0.2 mg/kg of diet) was found to enhance antibody titers in calves challenged with parainfluenza-3 virus (Reffett et al., 1988). This response was more apparent after primary challenge than after the secondary challenge. Stressful conditions may influence the interaction of selenium and disease resistance. Stress from weaning in selenium-deficient pigs not only increases the concentration of selenium required in the diet to prevent selenium depletion but also increases mortality (Meyer et al., 1981; Mahan and Moxon, 1980; Peplowski et al., 1981).

B. Iron

Many studies, predominantly with laboratory animals, have revealed a pattern suggesting that both iron deficiency and iron excess can alter host resistance (Sherman, 1984). The necessity of iron for bacterial growth and the ability of the host to sequestrate iron and make it unavailable for the bacteria are well recognized as factors that largely determine the final outcome of an infection (for review, see Griffiths and Bullen, 1987). Susceptibility to a bacterial infection increases, unless iron in the body is bound by transferrin or lactoferrin (Weinberg, 1978). Apart from this, iron status also may have a direct influence on the functional activities of immunocompetent cells.

The role of iron in various aspects of immune function and disease resistance has been studied to some extent in chickens and pigs. Large oral doses of iron (200 mg) given through the sow's milk increases mortality in baby pigs challenged with *E. coli* (Kadis et al., 1984). Even parenteral administration of large amounts of iron was found to have a similar effect (Klasing et al., 1980; Knight et al., 1983). However, the effect of route of administration of iron on the outcome of infection needs to be further examined in food animals. Parenteral administration may increase the severity of disease as compared to oral administration of iron to infected animals (Sussman, 1974). However, there was an increased incidence of diarrhea in baby pigs when supplemental iron was given orally rather than intramuscularly (Kadis et al., 1984). Unlike the pigs, chicks fed diets containing excess iron do not appear to be more susceptible when challenged with a pathogenic organism. Chicks fed a diet deficient in iron were more susceptible to *S. gallinarum*, whereas excess supplemental iron in an iron-sufficient diet increased survival rate (Hill and Smith, 1974). These workers also observed an increased survival in chicks injected with iron. Similar results were observed in several other studies (Smith et al., 1977a,b; Harry, 1979). Thus, iron deficiency appears to be more critical in chickens.

Moderate iron supplementation may be necessary to prevent anemia in baby pigs and also to increase their immunocompetence. Osborne and Davis (1968) observed increased susceptibility to bacterial endotoxin in baby pigs that did not receive supplemental iron for 4 weeks after birth, when compared, to their iron-supplemented littermates. Similar results were reported by Parsons et al. (1977).

Specific studies to define a direct role of iron in the functional activities of various immunocompetent cells are generally lacking. Also, the effect of iron on immune responses against nonbacterial pathogens such as fungi and protozoans, and especially viruses, has not been studied.

C. Zinc

Zinc is one of the essential trace elements that play a key role in carbohydrate metabolism, protein synthesis, nucleic acid metabolism, and many other biochemical reactions in the body. In recent years, zinc has been shown to have a beneficial effect on the immune system of humans and laboratory animals. Zinc deficiency in experimental animals results in atrophy of thymic and lymphoid tissue and lymphopenia (Prasad, 1966). Zinc deficiency adversely affects phytohemagglutinin (PHA)-induced transformation of lymphocytes (Fernandes et al., 1979), delayed-type hypersensitivity reactions (Golden et al., 1978), and thymocyte maturation (Iwata et al., 1979). Oral zinc supplementation significantly increased lymphocyte proliferative responses to PHA and concanavalin A in normal human subjects (Duchateau et al., 1981). Zinc also appears to modify cell membranes. The observations of Bettger and O'Dell (1981) support the hypothesis that zinc plays a role analogous to that of vitamin E by stabilizing membrane structure, and thus reducing peroxidative damage to the cell.

Zinc-deficient calves are highly susceptible to nonspecific secondary infections, which often result in death (Miller, 1970). Calves are lethargic and their wounds heal slowly (Miller, 1970). Requirement of cows for dietary zinc may vary considerably under different conditions. Although severe zinc deficiency is not a major problem, mild deficiencies appear to exist, which may be economically important. Borderline deficiencies may be accentuated by high levels of calcium in the diet (Miller, 1970). Cows in early lactation are usually provided with high calcium diets.

Following experimental infection of cattle with BHV-1 virus, serum zinc levels were found to decrease dramatically (Hutcheson, 1989) (Fig. 2). Cattle receiving supplemental zinc methionine at 220 mg/kg of diet had significantly lower rectal temperatures than control unsupple-

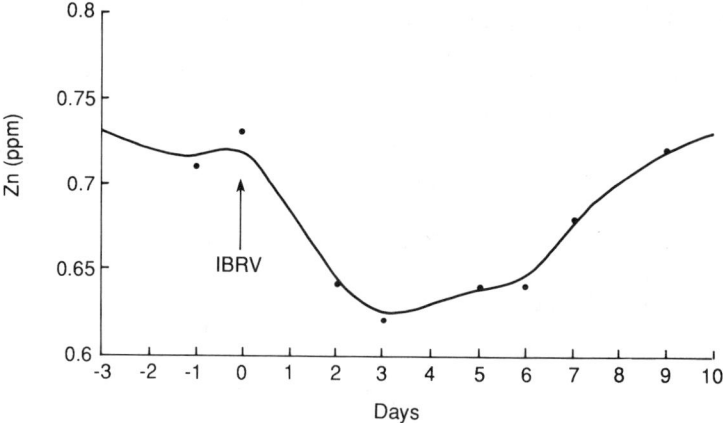

FIG. 2. Serum zinc concentrations following infection with BHV-1 (IBRV). Reprinted with permission from Hutcheson (1989).

mented cattle, when they were challenged with BHV-1 virus. Supplementation (350 mg zinc/head daily) was found to increase weight gains in morbid steers and also reduce the number of treatments required (Hutcheson, 1989).

Thymic atrophy in zinc deficiency also has been demonstrated in pigs (Miller *et al.*, 1968). Thymic atrophy was accompanied by lymphopenia and an increase in the percentage of band neutrophils. When challenged with *S. pullorum*, all zinc-deficient pigs died, whereas there was no mortality of pigs that received zinc supplementation.

Because of zinc's key role in several enzyme systems and its positive role in wound healing and proper functioning of the immune system, careful evaluations of the zinc requirement of various food animals is essential.

D. Copper

The relationship between copper status and disease resistance has not been well studied. The critical role of copper in several metabolic functions as a component of various metalloenzymes and as a cofactor is well known (Fletcher *et al.*, 1988). As a component of superoxide dismutase, it may also play a key role in the prevention of lipid peroxidation.

Copper deficiency was found to inhibit microbicidal activity of peripheral blood leukocytes in cattle and sheep (Jones and Suttle, 1981).

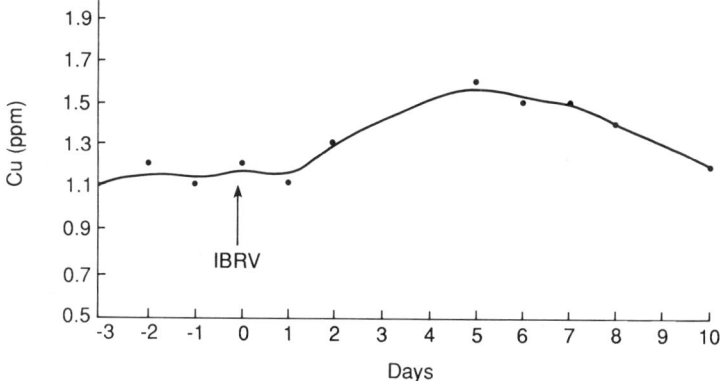

FIG. 3. Serum copper concentrations following infection with BHV-1 (IBRV). Reprinted with permission from Hutcheson (1989).

This functional deficit coincided with a decreased intracellular superoxide dismutase activity, probably resulting in autotoxic damage to the cells from the reactive oxygen products.

Contrary to the decrease in serum iron and zinc, serum copper was found to increase during the course of an infection (Biesel, 1976). This also has been observed by Hutcheson (1989) in cattle infected with BHV-1 (Fig. 3). Mortality from ataxia and infection was high in lambs from Scottish Blackface ewes (traditionally hypocupremic) compared to lambs from Welsh Mountain ewes when both were on a marginally copper-deficient diet (Wiener and Field, 1969; Wiener et al., 1985). Similar results were reported by Whitelaw et al. (1979) and Yeoman (1983). Proliferative responses of lymphocytes to mitogens were found to be depressed in hypocupremic animals, and copper supplementation was found to restore the proliferative responses in these animals (Suttle and Jones, 1986).

E. Cobalt

The importance of cobalt as a component of vitamin B_{12} is well known. It also may have some other functions in the body, especially as an activating ion in certain enzyme reactions (McDonald et al., 1969). However, these functions of cobalt are not clearly defined. Rumen microorganisms synthesize vitamin B_{12}, and cobalt is required for this process. Consequently, on a cobalt-deficient diet, not enough vitamin B_{12} will be synthesized in the rumen to meet the animal's requirement.

A diet deficient in cobalt was found to enhance the susceptibility to disease in sheep (MacPherson *et al.*, 1976). Cobalt deficiency also was found to compromise immunity in calves (Wright *et al.*, 1982). Lambs reared on a cobalt-deficient diet had higher worm egg counts when challenged with *Ostertagia circumcinata* compared to lambs on a cobalt-sufficient diet (Downey, 1966). In a more recent experiment, MacPherson *et al.* (1987) observed an impaired neutrophil function in cobalt-deficient cattle. These animals also had significantly higher worm egg counts and shorter prepatent periods than cobalt-sufficient calves, when they were challenged with *Ostertagia ostertagi*.

VI. Conclusion

The nutritional status of the domestic food animal plays an important role in resistance mechanisms against disease causing agents. It also may influence the outcome of disease in infected animals. Complex interrelationships between single nutrients and host resistance factors pose problems in interpreting the results of a limited number of studies with domestic food animals. The stress from highly intensive farming conditions coupled with the use of highly processed and stored feeds and lack of access to pastures puts additional burdens on host resistance against infectious agents. Many more studies are needed to delineate the interactions between single nutrients and immunity at the cellular and molecular level. The design of these studies should keep in view the explosive growth in our understanding of the immune system in the last decade. Specifically, it may be necessary to identify nutritional factors that influence the changes in the subsets of various immunocompetent cells in the circulation, production of various lymphokines and monokines, and expression of receptors for these immunoregulatory factors. It may be necessary to stress that any future evaluations of the requirements of particular nutrients should include not only growth and production criteria but also immunological criteria.

Acknowledgment

This chapter was previously published as contribution No. 90-270-B from the Kansas Agricultural Experiment Station, Manhattan, Kansas 66506.

References

Afzal, M., Tengerdy, R. P., Ellis, R. P., Kimberling, C. V., and Morris, C. J. (1984). Protection of rams against epididymitis by a *B. ovis*-vitamin E adjuvant vaccine. *Vet. Immunol. Immunopathol.* **7,** 293–304.

Afzal, M., Tengerdy, R. P., Brodie, S. J., DeMartini, J. C., Ellis, R. P., Jones, R. L., and Kimberling, C. V. (1986). The imune responses in rams experimentally infected with *Brucella ovis*. *Res. Vet. Sci.* **41,** 85–89.

Anderson, R., Oosthuizen, R., Maritz, R., Theron, A., and Van Rensburg, A. J. (1980). The effects of increasing weekly doses of ascorbate on certain cellular and humoral immune functions in normal volunteers. *Am. J. Clin. Nutr.* **33,** 71–76.

Atroshi, F., Tyopponen, J., Sankari, S., Kangasniemi, R., and Parantainen, J. (1986). Possible roles of vitamin E and glutathione metabolism in bovine mastitis. *Int. J. Vitam. Nutr. Res.* **57,** 37–43.

Aziz, E. S., and Klesius, P. H. (1986). Effects of selenium deficiency on caprine polymorphonuclear leukocyte production of leukotriene B_4 and its neutrophil chemotactic activity. *Am. J. Vet. Res.* **47,** 426–428.

Aziz, E. S., Klesius, P. H., and Frandsen, J. C. (1984). Effects of selenium on polymorphonuclear leukocyte functions in goats. *Am. J. Vet. Res.* **45,** 1715–1718.

Baehner, R. L., Boxer, L. A., and Ingraham, L. M. (1982). The influence of vitamin E on human polymorphonuclear cell metabolism and function. *Ann. N.Y. Acad. Sci.* **393,** 237–250.

Barrat, M. E. J., Strachan, P. J., and Porter, P. (1978). Antibody mechanisms implicated in digestive disturbances following ingestion of soya protein in calves and piglets. *Clin. Exp. Immunol.* **31,** 305–312.

Bar-Shavit, Z., Moff, D., Edelstein, S., Meyer, M., Shibolet, S., and Goldman, R. (1987). 1, 25-$(OH)_2$ D_3 and the regulation of macrophage function. *Calcif. Tissue Int.* **33,** 673–676.

Bettger, W., and O'Dell, B. L. (1981). A critical physiological role of zinc in the structure and function of biomembranes. *Life Sci.* **28,** 1425–1438.

Bhalla, A. K., Amento, E. P., Clements, T. R., Holick, M. P., and Krane, S. M. (1983). Specific high affinity receptors for 1, 25-dihydroxyvitamin D_3 in human peripheral blood mononuclear cells: Presence in monocytes and induction in T lymphocytes following activation. *J. Clin. Endocrinol. Metab.* **57,** 1302–1310.

Biesel, W. R. (1976). Trace elements in infectious processes. *Med. Clin. North Am.* **60,** 831–849.

Blecha, F., and Kelley, K. W. (1981). Effects of cold and weaning stressors on the antibody-mediated immune response of pigs. *J. Anim. Sci.* **53,** 439–447.

Blecha, F., Bull, R. C., Olson, D. P., Ross, R. H., and Curtis, S. (1981). Effects of prepartum protein restriction in the beef cow on immunoglobulin content in blood and colostral whey and subsequent immunoglobulin absorption by the neonatal calf. *J. Anim. Sci.* **53,** 1174–1180.

Blecha, F., Pollmann, D. S., and Nichols, D. A. (1983). Weaning pigs at an early age decreases cellular immunity. *J. Anim. Sci.* **56,** 396–400.

Boxer, L. A. (1986). Regulation of phagocyte function by α-tocopherol. *Proc. Nutr. Soc.* **45,** 333–344.

Boyne, R. and Arthur, J. R. (1979). Alterations of neutrophil function in selenium-deficient cattle. *J. Comp. Pathol.* **89,** 151–158.

Boyne, R., and Arthur, J. R. (1981). Effects of selenium and copper deficiency on neutrophil function in cattle. *J. Comp. Pathol.* **91,** 271–276.

Boyne, R., and Arthur, J. R. (1986). The response of selenium-deficient mice to *Candida albicans* infection. *J. Nutr.* **116,** 816–822.

Chan, A. C., Allen, C. E., and Hegarty, P. V. J. (1980). The effects of vitamin E depletion and repletion on PG synthesis in semitendinosus muscle of young rabbits. *J. Nutr.* **110,** 66–81.

Chew, B. P. (1987). Vitamin A and B-carotene on host defense. *J. Dairy Sci.* **70,** 2732–2743.

Chew, B. P., Hollen, L. L., Hillers, J. K., and Herlugson, M. L. (1982). Relationship between vitamin A and B-carotene in blood plasma and milk and mastitis in Holsteins. *J. Dairy Sci.* **65,** 2111–2118.

Chew, B. P., Holpuch, D. M., and O'Fallon, J. V. (1984). Relative concentration of vitamin A and B-carotene in bovine and porcine plasma, liver, corpora lutea and follicular fluid. *J. Dairy Sci.* **67,** 1316–1322.

Cipriano, J. E., Morrill, J. L., and Anderson, N. V. (1982). Effect of dietary vitamin E on immune response of calves. *J. Dairy Sci.* **65,** 2357–2365.

Cole, N. A., McLaren, J. B., and Hutcheson, D. P. (1982). Influence of preweaning and B-vitamin supplementation of the feedlot receiving diet on calves subjected to marketing and transit steers. *J. Anim. Sci.* **54,** 911–917.

Corley, J. R., Esch, M. W., Bahr, J. M., and Easter, R. A. (1983). Amino acid supplementation of low protein diets for swine: Effects of gestation treatment on reproductive performance of gilts and sows. *J. Anim. Sci.* **56,** 108–117.

Crenshaw, T. D., Cook, M. E., Odle, J., and Martin, R. E. (1986). Effect of nutritional status, age at weaning and room temperature on growth and systemic immune response of weanling pigs. *J. Anim. Sci.* **63,** 1845–1853.

Cummins, K. A., and Brunner, C. J. (1989). Dietary ascorbic acid and immune response in dairy calves. *J. Dairy Sci.* **72,** 129–134.

Dawson, D. P., Morrill, J. L., Reddy, P. G., and Minocha, H. C. (1988). Soy protein concentrate and heated soy flours as protein sources in milk replacer for preruminant calves. *J. Dairy Sci.* **71,** 1301–1309.

DeChatelet, L. R., McCall, C. E., and Cooper, M. R., and Shirley, P. S. (1974). Ascorbic acid levels in phagocytic cells. *Proc. Soc. Exp. Biol. Med.* **145,** 1170–1173.

Diplock, A. T., and Lucy, J. A. (1973). The biochemical modes of action of vitamin E and selenium: A hypothesis. *FEBS Lett.* **29,** 205–210.

Downey, N. E. (1966). Some relationship between trichostrongylid infestation and cobalt status in lambs. III. *Trichostrongylus axei* and *Ostertagia circumcinata* infestation. *Br. Vet. J.* **122,** 316–324.

Duchateau, J., Delespesse, G., and Vereccke, P. (1981). Influence of oral zinc supplementation on the lymphocyte response to mitogens of normal subjects. *Am. J. Clin. Nutr.* **34,** 88–93.

El Boushy, A. R. (1988). Vitamin E affects viability, immune response of poultry. *Feedstuffs* **60**(44), 20–26.

Fernandes, C., Nair, M., Onoe, K., Tanaka, T., Floyd, R., and Good, R. A. (1979). Impairment of cell-mediated immunity functions by dietary zinc deficiency in mice. *Proc. Natl. Acad. Sci. U.S.A.* **76,** 457–461.

Fletcher, M. P., Gershwin, M. E., Keen, C. L., and Hurley, L. (1988). Trace element deficiencies and immune responsiveness in humans and animal models. *In* "Nutrition and Immunology" (R. K. Chandra, ed.), pp. 215–239. Alan R. Liss, New York.

Friske, R. A., and Adams, L. G. (1985). Immune responsiveness and lymphoreticular morphology in cattle fed hypo- and hyperalimentation diets. *Vet. Immunol. Immunopathol.* **8,** 225–244.

Goetzl, E. J. (1980). Vitamin E modulates the lypoxygenation of arachidonic acid in leukocytes. *Nature (London)* **288,** 183–185.

Golden, M. H. N., Golden, B. E., and Harland, P. S. E. G. (1978). Zinc and immunocompetence in protein-energy malnutrition. *Lancet* **1,** 1226–1228.

Griebel, P. J., Schoonderwoerd, M., and Babiuk, L. A. (1987). Ontogeny of the immune response: Effect of protein-energy malnutrition in neonatal calves. *Can. J. Vet. Res.* **51,** 428–435.

Griffiths, E., and Bullen, J. J. (1987). Iron and infection: Future prospects. *In* "Iron and Infection" (J. J. Bullen and E. Griffiths, eds.), pp. 283–317. Wiley, New York.

Gwazdauskas, F. C., Gross, W. B., Bibb, T. L., and McGilliard, M. L. (1978). Antibody titers and corticoids near weaning in steer and heifer calves. *Can. Vet. J.* **19,** 150–154.

Gyang, E. O., Stevens, J. B., Olson, W. G., Tsitsamis, S. D., and Usenik, E. A. (1984). Effects of selenium–vitamin E injection on bovine polymorphonucleated leukocytes phagocytosis and killing of *Staphylococcus aureus*. *Am. J. Vet. Res.* **45,** 175–177.

Harmon, B. G., Miller, E. R., Hoefer, J. A., Ullrey, D. E., and Luecke, R. W. (1963). Relationship of specific nutrient deficiencies to antibody production in swine. II. Pantothenic acid, pyridoxine or riboflavin. *J. Nutr.* **79,** 269–275.

Harry, E. G. (1979). Increase in resistance to acute experimental coli-septicaemia in chicks given high levels of ferrous sulphate in the diet. *Res. Vet. Sci.* **27,** 175–179.

Haye, S. N., and Kornegay, E. T. (1979). Immunoglobulin G, A and M and antibody response in sow reared and artificially-reared pigs. *J. Anim. Sci.* **48,** 1116–1122.

Haye, S. N., Kornegay, E. T., and Mahan, D. C. (1981). Antibody response and serum protein and immunoglobulin in pigs from sows fed different protein sequences during gestation and lactation. *J. Anim. Sci.* **53,** 1262–1268.

Heinzerling, R. H., Tengerdy, R. P., Wick, L. L., and Lueker, D. C. (1974). Vitamin E protects mice against *Diplococcus pneumoniae* type I infection. *Infect. Immun.* **10,** 1292–1295.

Hill, R., and Smith, I. M. (1974). *In* "Trace Element Metabolism in Animals-2" (W. G. Hoekstra, J. W. Suttie, H. E. Ganther, and W. Mertz, eds.), pp. 641–643. University Park Press, Baltimore, Maryland.

Hume, R., and Weyers, E. (1973). Changes in leukocyte ascorbic acid during the common cold. *Scott. Med. J.* **18,** 3–7.

Hutcheson, D. P. (1989). Nutritional factors affect immune response in cattle. *Feedstuffs* **61**(15), 16–24.

Itze, L. (1984). Ascorbic acid metabolism in ruminants. *In* "Ascorbic Acid in Domestic Animals" (I., Wegger, F. J., Tagwerker, and J. Moustgaard, eds.), pp. 120–130. Royal Danish Agricultural Society, Copenhagen.

Iwata, T., Incefy, G. S., Tanaka, T., Fernandes, G., Botet, C. J., Pih, K., and Good, R. A. (1979). Circulating thymic hormone levels in zinc deficiency. *Cell. Immunol.* **47,** 100–105.

Jelinek, P. D., Ellis, T., Worth, R. H., Sutherland, S. S., Masters, H. G., and Peterson, D. S. (1988). The effect of selenium supplementation on immunity, and the establishment of an experimental *Hemonchus contortus* infection, in weaner Merino sheep fed a low selenium diet. *Aust. Vet. J.* **65,** 214–217.

Johnson, L., Bowen, F., Soraya, A., Herrmann, N., Weston, M., Sacks, L., Porat, R., Stahl, G., Peckman, G., Papadopoulas, M. D., Quinn, G., and Schaffer, D. (1985). Relationship of vitamin E to incidence of sepsis and necrotizing enterocolitis. *Pediatrics* **75,** 619–638.

Jones, D. G., and Suttle, N. F. (1981). Some effects of copper deficiency on leukocyte function in sheep and cattle. *Res. Vet. Sci.* **31,** 151–156.

Kadis, S., Udeze, F. A., Polanco, J., and Dreesen, D. W. (1984). Relationship of iron administration to susceptibility of newborn pigs to enterotoxic colibacillosis. *Am. J. Vet. Res.* **45,** 255–259.

Kelley, K. W., and Easter, R. (1987). Nutritional factors can influence immune response of swine. *Feedstuffs* **59**(22), 14–16.

Kigoshi, S., and Ito, R. (1973). High levels of free fatty acids in lymphoid cells with special reference to their cytotoxicity. *Experientia* **29,** 1408–1410.

Kilshaw, P. J., and Sissons, J. W. (1979a). Gastro-intestinal allergy to soybean protein in preruminant calves. Antibody production and digestive disturbances in calves fed heated soybean flour. *Res. Vet. Sci.* **27,** 361–365.

Kilshaw, P. J., and Sissons, J. W. (1979b). Gastro-intestinal allergy to soybean protein in preruminant calves. Allergenic constituents of soybean products. *Res. Vet. Sci.* **27,** 366–371.

Klasing, K. C., Knight, C. D., and Forsyth, D. M. (1980). Effects of iron on the anti-coli capacity of sow's milk *in vitro* and in ligated intestinal segments. *J. Nutr.* **110,** 1914–1921.

Knight, C. D., Klasing, K. C., and Forsyth, D. M. (1983). *E. coli* growth in serum of iron dextran-supplemented pigs. *J. Anim. Sci.* **57,** 387–395.

Kornegay, E. T., Meldrum, J. B., Schurig, G., Lindemann, M. D., and Gwazdauskas, F. C. (1986). Lack of influence of nursery temperature on the response of weanling pigs to supplemental vitamins C and E. *J. Anim. Sci.* **63,** 484–491.

Larsen, H. J., and Tollersrud, S. (1981). Effect of dietary vitamin E and selenium on the phytohemagglutinin response of pig lymphocytes. *Res. Vet. Sci.* **31,** 301–305.

Lemire, J. M., Adams, J. S., Sakai, R., and Jordan, S. C. (1984). 1, 25-$(OH)_2$ D_3 suppresses proliferation and immunoglobulin production by normal human peripheral blood mononuclear cells. *J. Clin. Invest.* **74,** 657–661.

Lemire, J. M., Adams, J. S., Kerncani-Arab, V., Bakke, A. C., Sakai, R., and Jordan, S. C. (1985). 1, 25-$(OH)_2$ D_3 suppresses human T helper/inducer lymphocyte activity *in vitro. J. Immunol.* **134,** 3032–3035.

Li, D. F., Nelssen, J. L., Reddy, P. G., Blecha, F., Hancock, J. D., Allee, G. L., and Goodband, R. D. (1990). Transient hypersensitivity to soybean meal in the early-weaned pig. *J. Anim. Sci.* (in press).

Lim, T. S., Putt, N., Safranski, D., Chung, C., and Watson, R. R. (1981). Effect of vitamin E on cell-mediated immune responses and serum corticosterone in young and maturing mice. *Immunology* **44,** 289–295.

Loh, K. W., Shrader, R. E., and Zeman, F. J. (1971). Effect of maternal protein deprivation on neonatal absorption in rats. *J. Nutr.* **101,** 1663–1672.

Lorente, F., Fontan, G., Jara, P., Cosa McGarcia-Rodriquez, C., and Ojida, J. A. (1976). Defective neutrophil motility in hypovitaminosis D rickets. *Acta Paediatr. Scand.* **65,** 695–699.

Machlin, L. (1978). Vitamin E and prostaglandins. *In* "Tocopherol, Oxygen and Biomembranes" (C. deDuve, and O. Hayashi, eds.), pp. 179–189. Am. Elsevier, New York.

MacPherson, A., Moon, F. E., and Voss, R. C. (1976). Biochemical aspects of cobalt deficiency in sheep with special reference to vitamin status and a possible involvement in the aetiology of cerbrocortical necrosis. *Br. Vet. J.* **132,** 294–308.

MacPherson, A., Gray, D., Mitchell, G. B. B., and Taylor, C. N. (1987). Ostertagia infection and neutrophil function in cobalt-deficient and cobalt-supplemented cattle. *Br. Vet. J.* **143,** 348–353.

Mahan, D. C., and Moxon, A. L. (1980). Effect of dietary selenium and injectable vitamin E-selenium for weanling swine. *Nutr. Rep. Int.* **21,** 829–832.

Manolagas, S. C., Provvedini, D. M., and Tsoukas, C. D. (1985). Interactions of 1, 25-dihydroxyvitamin D_3 and the immune system. *Mol. Cell. Endocrinol.* **43**, 113–122.

Marsh, J. A., Dietert, R. R., and Combs, G. F., Jr. (1981). Influence of dietary selenium and vitamin E on the humoral immune responses of the chick. *Proc. Soc. Exp. Biol. Med.* **166**, 228–236.

McCorkle, F., Taylor, R., Stinson, R., Day, E. J., and Glick, G. (1980). The effects of megalevel of vitamin C on the immune response of the chicken. *Poult. Sci.* **59**, 1324–1327.

McDonald, P., Edwards, R. A., and Greenhalgh, J. F. D. (1969). "Animal Nutrition," pp. 88–89, Oliver & Boyd, Edinburgh.

McGillivray, H. (1967). Immunological response of the pig as affected by amino acid nutrition. Ph.D. Dissertation, University of Illinois at Urbana-Champaign.

Meyer, W. R., Mahan, D. C., and Moxon, A. L. (1981). Value of dietary selenium and vitamin E for weanling swine as measured by performance and tissue selenium and glutathione peroxidase activities. *J. Anim. Sci.* **52**, 302–311.

Miller, E. R., Harmon, B. G., Ullrey, D. E., Schmidt, D. A., Luecke, R. W., and Hoefer, J. A. (1962). Antibody absorption, retention and production by the baby pig. *J. Anim. Sci.* **21**, 309–314.

Miller, E. R., Luecke, R. W., Ullrey, D. E., Baltzer, B. V., Bradley, B. L., and Hoeffer, J. A. (1968). Biochemical, skeletal and allometric changes due to zinc deficiency in the baby pig. *J. Nutr.* **95**, 278–286.

Miller, W. J. (1970). Zinc nutrition of cattle: A review. *J. Dairy Sci.* **53**, 1123–1135.

Morel, P. A., Manolagas, S. C., Provvedini, D. M., Wagmann, D. R., and Chiller, J. M. (1986). Interferon-Y-induced IA expression in WEHF cells is enhanced by the presence of 1, 25-dihydroxyvitamin D_3. *J. Immunol.* **136**, 2181–2186.

Osborne, J. C., and Davis, J. W. (1968). Increased susceptibility to bacterial endotoxin of pigs with iron-deficiency anemia. *J. Am. Vet. Med. Assoc.* **152**, 1630–1632.

Pardue, S. L. (1987). Recent findings on vitamin C supplementation in poultry. In "The Role of Vitamins on Animal Performance and Immune Response," Proc. Roche Tech. Symp. pp. 18–33. Hoffman-La Roche Inc., Nutley, New Jersey.

Pardue, S. L., and Thaxton, J. P. (1984). Evidence for amelioration of steroid-mediated immunosuppression by ascorbic acid. *Poult. Sci.* **63**, 1262–1268.

Pardue, S. L., Thaxton, J. P., and Brake, J. (1985). Role of ascorbic acid in chicks exposed to high environmental temperature. *J. Appl. Physiol.* **58**, 1511–1516.

Parsons, M. P., Miller, E. R., Bebiak, D. M., Erickson, J. P., Hogberg, M. G., Ellis, D. J., and Ullrey, D. E. (1977). Influence of iron status of weanling pigs when exposed to TGE. *Mich., Agric. Exp. Stn., Res. Rep.* **343**, 10.

Peplowski, M. A., Mahan, D. C., Murray, F. A., Moxon, A. L., Cantor, A. H., and Ekström, K. E. (1981). Effect of dietary and injectable vitamin E and selenium in weanling swine antigenically challenged with sheep red blood cells. *J. Anim. Sci.* **51**, 344–351.

Prasad, A. S., ed. (1966). "Zinc Metabolism." Thomas, Springfield, Ilinois.

Provvedini, D. M., Tsoukas, C. D., Deftos, L. J., and Manolagas, S. C. (1983). 1, 25-dihydroxyvitamin D_3 receptors in human leukocytes. *Science* **221**, 1181–1183.

Pruiett, S. D., Morrill, J. L., Blecha, F., Reddy, P. G., Higgins, J., and Anderson, N. V. (1989). Effect of supplemental vitamins C and E in milk replacer on lymphocyte and neutrophil function in bull calves. *J. Dairy Sci.* **67**, Suppl. 1, 243.

Reddy, P. G., Morrill, J. L., and Minocha, H. C. (1985a). Effect of early weaning on the cell-mediated immune response of dairy calves. *Nutr. Rep. Int.* **31**, 501–503.

Reddy, P. G., Morrill, J. L., Frey, R. A., Morrill, M. B., Minocha, H. C., and Galitzer, S. J. (1985b). Effects of supplemental vitamin E on the performance and metabolic profiles of calves. *J. Dairy Sci.* **68**, 2259–2266.

Reddy, P. G., Morrill, J. L., Minocha, H. C., Morrill, M. B., Dayton, A. D., and Frey, R. A. (1986). Effect of supplemental vitamin E on the immune system of calves. *J. Dairy Sci.* **69**, 164–171.

Reddy, P. G., Morrill, J. L., and Frey, R. A. (1987a). Vitamin E requirements of dairy calves. *J. Dairy Sci.* **70**, 123–129.

Reddy, P. G., Morrill, J. L., Minocha, H. C., and Stevenson, J. S. (1987b). Vitamin E is immunostimulatory in calves. *J. Dairy Sci.* **70**, 993–999.

Reddy, P. G., Blecha, F., Minocha, H. C., and Morrill, J. L. (1990). A comparison of hemagglutination inhibition assay and enzyme-linked immunosorbent assay for detecting residual antigens in soybean products. *J. Dairy Sci.* (in preparation).

Reffett, J. K., Spears, J. W., and Brown, T. T., Jr. (1987). Effect of dietary selenium on the primary and secondary immune response in calves challenged with infectious bovine rhinotracheitis virus. *J. Nutr.* **118**, 229–235.

Reffett, J. K., Spears, J. W., and Brown, T. T., Jr. (1988). Effect of dietary selenium and vitamin E on the primary and secondary immune response in lambs challenged with parainfluenza-3 virus. *J. Anim. Sci.* **66**, 1520–1528.

Reinhardt, T. A., and Hustmyer, F. G. (1987). Role of vitamin D in the immune system. *J. Dairy Sci.* **70**, 952–962.

Reinhardt, T. A., Horst, R. L., Littledike, E. T., and Beitz, D. C. (1982). 1, 25-Dihydroxyvitamin D_3 receptor in bovine thymus gland. *Biochem. Biophys. Res. Commun.* **106**(3), 1012–1018.

Roth, J. A., and Kaeberle, M. L. (1985). *In vivo* effect of ascorbic acid on neutrophil function in healthy and dexamethasone-treated cattle. *Am. J. Vet. Res.* **46**, 434–2436.

Shamberger, R. J. (1983). "Biochemistry of Selenium." Plenum, New York.

Sherman, A. R. (1984). Iron, infection, and immunity. *In* "Nutrition, Disease Resistance and Immune Function" (R. R. Watson, ed.), pp. 251–266. Dekker, New York.

Siegel, B. V. (1975). Enhanced interferon production by poly (rI) poly (rC) in mouse cell cultures by ascorbic acid. *Nature (London)* **254**, 531–532.

Sissons, J. W. (1982). Effects of soya-bean products on digestive processes in the gastrointestinal tract of preruminant calves. *Proc. Nutr. Soc.* **41**, 53–61.

Sissons, J. W., and Thurston, S. M. (1984). Survival of dietary antigens in the digetive tract of calves intolerant to soybean products. *Res. Vet. Sci.* **37**, 242–246.

Smith, K. L., Harrison, J. H., Hancock, D. D., Todhunter, D. A., and Conrad, H. R. (1984). Effect of vitamin E and selenium supplementation on incidence of clinical mastitis and duration of clinical symptoms. *J. Dairy Sci.* **67**, 1293–1300.

Smith, K. L., Conrad, H. R., Amiet, B. A., Schoenberger, P. S., and Todhunter, D. A. (1985). Effect of vitamin E and selenium dietary supplementation on mastitis in first lactation dairy cows. *J. Dairy Sci.* **68**, Suppl. 1, 190.

Smith, L. M., Hill, R., and Licence, S. T. (1977a). Enhancement of survival in acute experimental fowl typhoid in chicks by the administration of iron dextran. *Res. Vet. Sci.* **22**, 151–157.

Smith, L. M., Hill, R., and Licence, S. T. (1977b). Increased survival from acute *Salmonella gallinarum* infection in chicks given diets with high levels of some forms of iron. *Res. Vet. Sci.* **23**, 263–268.

Stephens, L. C., McChesney, A. E., and Nockels, C. F. (1979). Improved recovery of vitamin E-treated lambs that have been experimentally infected with intratracheal *Chlamydia. Br. Vet. J.* **135**, 291–293.

Stern, L. T., Stowe, H. D., Kaneene, J. B., and Marteniuk, J. V. (1981). *In vivo* and *in vitro* influence of vitamin A on bovine lymphocyte blastogenesis. *J. Anim. Sci.* **53**, Suppl. 1, 433.

Stroder, J., and Kasal, P. (1970). Evaluation of phagocytosis in rickets. *Acta. Paediatr. Scand.* **59,** 288–292.

Sussman, M. (1974). Iron and infection. *In* "Iron in Biochemistry and Medicine" (A. Jacobs and W. Worwood, eds.), pp. 649–679. Academic Press, New York.

Suttle, N. F., and Jones, D. G. (1986). Copper and disease resistance in sheep: a rare natural confirmation of interaction between a specific nutrient and infection. *Proc. Nutr. Soc.* **45,** 317–325.

Tengerdy, R. P., Meyer, D. L., Lauerman, L. H., Lueker, D. C., and Nockels, C. F. (1983). Vitamin E enhances humoral antibody response to *Clostridium perfringens* type D in sheep. *Br. Vet. J.* **139,** 147–152.

Tengerdy, R. P., Mathias, M. M., and Nockels, C. F. (1984). Effect of vitamin E on immunity and disease resistance. *In* "Vitamins, Nutrition and Cancer" (K. Prasad, ed.), pp. 123–133. Karger, Basel.

Turner, R. J., L. E. Wheaty, L. E., and Beck, N. F. G. (1984). Impaired mitogen response in lambs with white muscle disease. *Res. Vet. Sci.* **37,** 357–358.

Turner, R. J., Wheaty, L. E., and Beck, F. G. (1985). Stimulatory effects of selenium on mitogen responses in lambs. *Vet. Immunol. Immunopathol.* **8,** 119–124.

Watson, R. R., and Petro, T. M. (1982). Cellular immune response, corticosteroid levels, and resistance to *Listeria monocytogenes* and murine leukemia in mice fed a high vitamin E diet. *Ann. N. Y. Acad. Sci.* **393,** 205–208.

Weinberg, E. D. (1978). Iron and infection. *Microbiol. Res.* **42,** 45–66.

Whitelaw, A., Armstrong, R. H., Evans, C. C., and Fawcett, A. R. (1979). A study of the effects of copper deficiency in Scottish blackface lambs on improved hill pasture. *Vet. Rec.* **104,** 455–460.

Wiener, G., and Field, A. C. (1969). Copper concentrations in the liver and blood of sheep of different breeds in relation to swayback history. *J. Comp. Pathol.* **79,** 7–14.

Wiener, G., Wooliams, J. A., Suttle, N. F., and Jones, D. G. (1985). Genetic selection for Cu status in the sheep and its consequences for performance. *Trace Elem. Man. Anim.—TEMA 5, Proc. Int. Symp., 5th, 1984,* p. 48.

Wilson, C. W. M. (1975). Clinical pharmacological aspects of ascorbic acid. *Ann. N. Y. Acad. Sci.* **258,** 355–376.

Wilson, C. W. M., and Loh, H. S. (1973). Vitamin C and colds. *Lancet* **1,** 1058–1059.

Wright, C. L., MacPherson, A., and Taylor, C. N. (1982). *Proc. World Congr. Dis. Cattle, 12th,* p. 1315.

Yen, J. T., and Pond, W. G. (1987). Effect of dietary supplementation with vitamin C or carbadox on weanling pigs subjected to crowding stress. *J. Anim. Sci.* **64,** 1672–1681.

Yeoman, G. H. (1983). Copper in relation to lamb losses. *Vet. Rec.* **113,** 547.

Zinn, R. A., Owens, F. N., Stuart, R. L., Dunbar, J. R., and Norman, B. B. (1987). B-vitamin supplementation of diets for feedlot calves. *J. Anim. Sci.* **65,** 267–277.

Neuroendocrine-Immune Interactions

KEITH W. KELLEY* AND ROBERT DANTZER†

*Laboratory of Immunophysiology, Department of Animal Sciences,
University of Illinois, Urbana, Illinois 61801, and
† Psychobiologie des Comportements Adaptatifs, Institut National de la
Recherche Agronomique and Institut National de la Santé et de la Recherche
Médicale, Unité 259, Domain de Carreire, 33077 Bordeaux, France*

I. Introduction
II. Characteristics of the Neuroendocrine-Immune System
   A. Innervation of the Immune System
   B. Receptors for Hormones and Neuropeptides on Lymphoid Cells
   C. Hormones and Neuropeptides Affect Cells of the Immune System
   D. Hormones are Synthesized by Leukocytes
   E. Brain Lesions Affect the Immune Response
   F. Cytokines Affect the Central Nervous System
III. Conclusions
   References

I. Introduction

The concept that myeloid and lymphoid cells are regulated by neuropeptides and hormones[1] has gained substantial support during recent years. In the past, immunologists have concentrated on identifying the types of cells within the immune system, the major factors that control their differentiation from progenitor stem cells, and the molecular mechanisms that mediate important activities of lymphocytes, such as gene rearrangement during the course of antibody synthesis and ex-

---

[1] Neuropeptides are peptides that are elaborated by nerve cells and which allow communication within the nervous system (neurotransmitter) or between the nervous system and other endocrine glands (hormone).

pression of T cell receptors within the thymus gland. An enormous amount of knowledge about the immune system has accumulated within the past thirty years, and advances that have been made in applying techniques of molecular biology to immunological problems have greatly accelerated the rate of progress during the past ten years.

This fundamental information that now forms the basis of essential concepts in immunology sets the stage for a new era in immunological research, namely, understanding the complex interactions that exist between the immune system and other physiologic systems. Several recent reviews have been written on the topic of immunophysiology (Blalock, 1989; Kelley, 1988; Dantzer and Kelley, 1989). Indeed, the 100th issue of *Immunological Reviews* was entirely devoted to the topic of neuroimmunomodulation (Möller, 1987).

The challenges in this new field are great, but the rewards could be enormous. This type of research will most likely lead to a more complete understanding of intractable maladies such as allergies, endocrine-associated autoimmune diseases (e.g., diabetes, thyroiditis), and perhaps even mental diseases that are so important in human health. Animal scientists and veterinarians may apply this new knowledge to prevent and treat many environmentally-dependent livestock diseases (e.g., shipping fever) and to gain a better understanding of important livestock concerns ranging from embryo survival to selecting animals for resistance to specific diseases. The immune system is currently being exploited to develop active immunization programs for "immunocastration" in cattle and to improve fecundity in sheep. These approaches imply that the immune system affects a number of physiological systems and is important for maintaining homeostasis in livestock. The purpose of this chapter is to discuss the findings that support the concept of cross-talk between the immune and neuroendocrine systems and to highlight recent developments in this field.

II. Characteristics of the Neuroendocrine-Immune System

A substantial amount of data from a variety of disciplines supports the idea that the neuroendocrine system affects cells of the immune system, and that products from leukocytes affect the neuroendocrine system. The finding that certain monokines, such as interleukin-1 (IL-1) and tumor necrosis factor-α (TNF-α), can be found in the blood during certain autoimmune and parasitic diseases has led to the speculation that these molecules may also function as classical hormones. Similarly, the recent findings that some hormones and neuropeptides are actually synthesized by leukocytes suggest that these molecules may function in a paracrine fashion as lymphokines. The strongest supporting evidence for the existence of neuroendocrine-immune system interactions is summarized below:

1. The spleen, thymus, bone marrow, and lymph nodes are innervated with autonomic noradrenergic sympathetic neurons.
2. Lymphocytes and macrophages possess receptors for a wide variety of hormones and neuropeptides.
3. Stimulation of hormone receptors on leukocytes alters a number of functional activities of these cells.
4. Several hormones and neuropeptides are now known to be synthesized by leukocytes.
5. Changes in brain functions affect different immune responses.
6. Cytokines that are produced by leukocytes affect the neuroendocrine system and change animal behaviors such as food intake, sleep, and thermoregulation.

A. Innervation of the Immune System

Most textbooks that discuss the central and peripheral nervous systems do not mention that both primary (thymus, bone marrow) and secondary (lymph nodes, spleen, gut-associated lymphoid tissue) lymphoid tissue receive innervation from the autonomic nervous system. It has been known for years that noradrenergic neurons can be found in the spleen of almost all animal species. However, because stimulation of the splenic nerve causes the splenic capsule to contract, the belief developed that the main effect of these noradrenergic neurons was on splenic vascular smooth muscle.

Recently, David Felten and colleagues at the University of Rochester identified noradrenergic nerve profiles in the spleen as well as in the thymus and bone marrow (reviewed by Felten et al., 1987). These careful studies revealed that, in the spleen, many noradrenergic neurons are in close contact with lymphocytes and reticular cells and bear no relationship to smooth muscle. The close proximity of noradrenergic nerve terminals to lymphocytes in the spleen shares many similarities to synapses (Felten and Olschowka, 1987), thus creating the likely possibility that norepinephrine released by the nerve terminal acts at a postsynaptic receptor on lymphocytes and macrophages. Noradrenergic innervation in the parenchyma of the spleen parallels the migration of lymphocytes into the periarteriolar lymphatic sheath (Ackerman et al., 1987), and the density of these neurons declines with aging (Bellinger et al., 1987). Therefore, these workers proposed that autonomic noradrenergic innervation in the spleen is important for the development of T lymphocytes in young animals and the decline in T-dependent immune functions that occurs in old age (Kelley et al., 1987). Similar ultrastructural evidence has shown that peripheral nerves are in intimate contact with mucosal mast cells in the lamina propria (Stead et al., 1987). This structural relationship may provide a clue as to how psychologic conditions are involved in intestinal diseases, such as food sensitivity, Crohn's disease and irritable bowel disease, in which mast cells are known to accumulate.

Collectively, these data indicate that peptides and classical neurotransmitters that are released at autonomic nerve terminals in lymphoid organs are part of the microenvironment to which lymphocytes and macrophages are exposed. However, the possible existence of similar phenomena in lymphoid tissues of domestic animals has not been investigated.

B. Receptors for Hormones and Neuropeptides on Lymphoid Cells

If hormones and neuropeptides affect certain activities of leukocytes, then lymphoid and myeloid cells should possess specific receptors for these ligands. This indeed appears to be the case. Similarly, if products of leukocytes affect the central nervous system, there should be receptors for these substances in the brain. This latter issue has been explored only recently. Receptors for IL-1 have been detected in discrete areas of the brain (Farrar et al., 1987).

Leukocytes possess receptors for a wide variety of neuroendocrine peptides, including two peptides derived from the proopiomelanocortin (POMC) gene, adrenocorticotropic hormone (ACTH), and β-endorphin (Smith et al., 1987; Hazum et al., 1979; Bost et al., 1987; Clarke and Bost, 1989). Similarly, there are specific receptors for substance P (Payan and Goetzl, 1984), somatostatin (Renold et al., 1987), vasoactive intestinal peptide (Danek et al., 1983), and nerve growth factor (Thorpe et al., 1987) on leukocytes. Acetylcholine receptors are found on thymic epithelial cells (Engel et al., 1977), and specific insulin receptors can be detected on activated lymphocytes (Krug et al., 1972). Receptors for both growth hormone (Kiess and Butenandt, 1985) and the closely related hormone prolactin (Haddock Russell et al., 1985) are also found on leukocytes. Although few reports have been published in domestic animals, β-adrenergic receptors exist on porcine splenocytes (Westly and Kelley, 1987) and α-1 and α-2 adrenoceptors can be found on bovine macrophages (Ogunbiyi et al., 1988).

The presence of specific receptors on leukocytes for a variety of neuropeptides clearly establishes a biochemical means for transducing the binding of a ligand into some type of second signal that can deliver a message to the nucleus of a cell. However, for most peptides the distribution of receptors on specific subsets of cells, such as B or T lymphocytes, or on individual subsets of these cells, is totally unknown. In the limited cases in which this question has been addressed, receptors for neuropeptides appear to be present on all types of leukocytes.

C. Hormones and Neuropeptides Affect Cells of the Immune System

If receptors for neuropeptides that exist on leukocytes are physiologically important, binding of these receptors by specific ligands should alter some functional activity of leukocytes. Many studies that have been published during the past several years support this hypothesis. A complete review of all of these experiments is outside the scope of this chapter. However, a few examples of the effects of hormones and neuropeptides on lymphoid and myeloid cells will be given to demonstrate that several activities of leukocytes are affected by these substances.

1. ACTH and Glucocorticoids

Adrenocorticotropic hormone is a 39-amino-acid peptide that inhibits both T cell-dependent and -independent antibody synthesis (Johnson et al., 1982), whereas it stimulates the proliferation of B lymphocytes (Alvarez-Mon et al., 1985; Bost et al., 1987). ACTH also suppresses the synthesis of interferon-γ by T lymphocytes (Johnson et al., 1984) and inhibits the ability of IFN-γ to generate tumoricidal macrophages (Koff and Dunegan, 1985).

Although ACTH directly affects leukocytes in vitro, most of its effects in vivo are attributed to its ability to increase the synthesis of glucocorticoids from the adrenal cortex. Synthetic glucocorticoids are well known to suppress almost all cell-mediated immune events. For example, glucocorticoids inhibit synthesis of interleukin-2 (IL-2) (Gillis et al., 1979; Kelso and Munck, 1984), expression of IL-2 receptors (Reed et al., 1986), and synthesis of IFN-γ and colony stimulating factor (Kelso and Munck, 1984). Glucocorticoids also inhibit the synthesis of IL-1, TNF-α, and the expression of Class II genes of the major histocompatibility complex (Snyder and Unanue, 1982; Beutler et al., 1986; Szefler et al., 1989). These suppressive effects of glucocorticoids are mediated by inhibiting steady-state levels of messenger RNA for these cytokines (Arya et al., 1984).

Glucocorticoids are the most widely studied hormones that affect the function of leukocytes in domestic animals, and most of these results are similar to those observed in other species. For example, at physiological concentrations, glucocorticoids suppress the proliferation of concanavalin A-stimulated leukocytes *in vitro* in pigs (Westly and Kelley, 1984), chickens (Franklin et al., 1987), and cattle (Murray and Chenault, 1982). When calves are injected with ACTH, or when peripheral blood lymphocytes are cultured with cortisol *in vitro*, there is a reduction in their proliferation after stimulation with T cell lectins, and this effect is mediated by a reduction in the synthesis of IL-2 (Blecha and Baker, 1986). Glucocorticoids also inhibit a number of important activities of bovine neutrophils, as excellently summarized by Roth (1985).

Other substances produced by mammalian cells mimic these effects of glucocorticoids. We recently found that the newly discovered multipotential cytokine, transforming growth factor-$\beta 2$, is as potent as dexamethasone and 100-times more effective than cortisol in suppressing the synthesis of TNF-α by porcine alveolar macrophages (Table I).

TABLE I

TGF-$\beta 2$, Dexamethasone, and Cortisol Suppress the Production of TNF-α by Porcine Alveolar Macrophages Triggered with *Lipopolysaccharide* (LPS)[a]

Treatment	% Cytotoxicity LPS	% Change	% Cytotoxicity LPS + rPoIFN-γ	% Change
Medium	25.3 ± 6^{de}	—	49.3 ± 5^{ab}	—
TGF-$\beta 2$				
0.04 nM	37.3 ± 5^{bcd}	59	57.0 ± 5^{a}	17
0.4	21.5 ± 6^{efg}	-19	41.5 ± 5^{bc}	-18
4.0	9.2 ± 4^{fgh}	-79	28.0 ± 7^{cde}	-48
Dexamethasone				
0.4 nM	25.5 ± 4^{de}	0	44.4 ± 6^{ab}	-11
4.0	7.8 ± 2^{gh}	-86	23.5 ± 4^{def}	-58
40.0	5.5 ± 2^{h}	-98	6.5 ± 3^{gh}	-97
Cortisol				
0.4 nM	25.0 ± 3^{de}	0	50.0 ± 5^{ab}	0
4.0	25.0 ± 6^{de}	0	47.8 ± 5^{ab}	0
40.0	13.3 ± 4^{efgh}	-59	43.0 ± 6^{ab}	-14
400.0	6.8 ± 3^{gh}	-91	17.0 ± 3^{efgh}	-73

Source: From Dunham et al., 1990.
[a] Means with different superscripts are different ($p < 0.05$).

Furthermore, these suppressive effects of both TGF-$\beta 2$ and glucocorticoids can be partially reversed by preincubating the cells with porcine IFN-γ. These results are consistent with the recent results of Roth and Frank (1989), who demonstrated that the immunomodulatory effects of IFN-γ were greater in cattle that had been injected with dexamethasone.

In conclusion, glucocorticoids suppress the activities of T lymphocytes and phagocytic cells, even at physiological concentrations that are attained during acute, stressful situations. Furthermore, the administation of recombinant cytokines to domestic animals for potential prophylactic and therapeutic benefits is more likely to be successful in immunosuppressed than in normal animals.

2. Growth Hormone and Prolactin

Growth hormone is a protein synthesized by the pituitary gland. It consists of 191 amino acids and is closely related to another adenohypophyseal hormone known as prolactin. Indeed, human growth hormone is lactogenic, which is one of the classic properties of prolactin. Both of these hormones augment antibody synthesis and contact sensitivity reactions when injected into hypophysectomized rats (reviewed by Berczi and Nagy, 1990). Recently, the activity of tumoricidal macrophages has been shown to be suppressed in mice with low circulating concentrations of plasma prolactin, and this defect can be reversed with peripheral injections of prolactin (Bernton et al., 1988). The proposed mechanism for this defect is an inability of T lymphocytes from prolactin-deficient mice to synthesize and secrete IFN-γ, which therefore inhibits the generation of activated macrophages. Recently, Dardenne et al. (1989) have extended to humans the finding that prolactin, as well as human growth hormone, augments the production of thymulin by thymic epithelial cells. The immunological effects of prolactin have recently been reviewed (Bernton, 1989).

Growth hormone also affects a number of immunological events (Kelley, 1989, 1990). It is especially important to understand these effects because growth hormone is currently used in the treatment of short children with a growth hormone deficiency, and because of the potential use of growth hormone in the livestock industry. Some of the major immunological effects of growth hormone are growth of the thymus gland, an elevation in the secretion of a thymic hormone known as thymulin, increases in the synthesis of specific antibodies, stimulation of the activity of cytotoxic T lymphocytes and natural killer cells, and synergism with colony-stimulating factors to augment granulopoiesis (Table II).

TABLE II

GROWTH HORMONE AFFECTS CELLS OF THE IMMUNE SYSTEM

Growth Hormone Deficiencies and Immunoregulation
    Thymic atrophy and wasting in mice and dogs
    Reduced antibody synthesis in mice
    Delayed skin graft rejection in mice
    Normal lymphoid cell subsets and thymic histology with reduction in peripheral T and B cells
    Pituitary hypoplasia and thymic atrophy in humans
    X-linked growth hormone deficiency and complete inability to synthesize antibodies
    Reduction in activity of natural killer cells in humans
    Defective allogeneic mixed lymphocyte reaction
    Reduction in plasma thymulin in humans and mice
    Normal immunoglobulin concentrations and lymphoid cell subsets in humans
    Decreased insulin-induced growth hormone response in patients with telangiectasis and bowel disease

Growth Hormone and the Thymus Gland
    Increases thymic size and DNA synthesis in young rodents
    Improves thymic size and morphology in aged animals
    Increases plasma thymulin in humans and dogs

Growth Hormone and Lymphoid Cells
    Acts on specific receptors on lymphocytes
    Synthesized by lymphoid cells
    Augments antibody synthesis and reduces skin graft survival *in vivo*
    Increases lectin-induced T cell proliferation and IL-2 synthesis *in vivo*
    Stimulates proliferation of human lymphoblastoid cells
    Augments basal lymphocyte proliferation *in vitro*
    Increases activity of cytotoxic T lymphocytes *in vitro*
    Augments activity of natural killer cells *in vivo*

Growth Hormone and Phagocytic Cells
    Primes macrophages for superoxide anion release *in vitro* and *in vivo*
    Augments respiratory burst in neutrophils from growth hormone-deficient patients *in vivo*
    Increases basal respiratory burst of human neutrophils and inhibits activated burst *in vitro*

Growth Hormone and Hemopoiesis
    Augments neutrophil differentiation *in vitro*
    Augments erythropoiesis

Note: See Kelley (1989, 1990) for references.

We have demonstrated that growth hormone- and prolactin-secreting pituitary tumors can restore thymic size and structure, as well as defective synthesis of IL-2, when implanted into syngeneic aged rats (Kelley et al., 1986; Davila et al., 1987). Recently, we were able to show that growth hormone is also a potent primer of macrophages in both *in vitro* and *in vivo* systems as assessed by the production of superoxide anion from macrophages triggered to undergo the respiratory burst with opsonized-zymosan (Edwards et al., 1988). New results have also revealed that injections of growth hormone, as well as IFN-γ, can partially reverse the reduction in both syntheses of TNF-α and resistance to a lethal infection with *Salmonella typhimurium* that occurs in hypophysectomized rats (Edwards et al., 1989a,b).

Although the immunological effects of growth hormone have not been extensively explored in domestic livestock, preliminary results suggest that recombinant bovine growth hormone augments the number of circulating neutrophils, increases the production of reactive oxygen intermediates, and reduces clinical symptoms of acute mastitis induced experimentally with *Escherichia coli* (Burvenich et al., 1989; Heyneman et al., 1989; Vandeputte-Van Messom et al., 1988). Unpublished results from our laboratory also indicate that recombinant human growth hormone is an effective primer of both human and porcine granulocytes for the production of superoxide anion (Fu et al., 1990).

3. Thyroid Stimulating Hormone

Antibody synthesis is augmented by the anterior pituitary-derived hormone, thyroid stimulating hormone (TSH), in both *in vitro* (Blalock et al., 1985; Kruger and Blalock, 1986) and *in vivo* (Pierpaoli et al., 1969) systems. The enhancement in antibody synthesis by TSH is dependent upon the presence of T lymphocytes, but not macrophages (Kruger and Blalock, 1986). TSH is actually synthesized by activated human T lymphocytes (Smith et al., 1983) and by lymphocytes that are treated with the hypothalamic releasing hormone, thyrotropin releasing hormone (TRH) (Kruger et al., 1989). When lymphocytes are treated with TRH, the increase in antibody synthesis that occurs can be blocked with an antibody to TSH (Kruger et al., 1989). This finding suggests that the synthesis of TSH by T lymphocytes is controlled exactly as it is in the adenohypophysis, and that this molecule acts as a cytokine at antibody-producing sites to control antibody production.

The thyroid gland responds to TSH by producing the thyroid hormones, triiodothyronine (T_3) and thyroxine (T_4), and it has recently been shown that TSH interacts with IFN-γ to induce expression of Class II antigens of the major histocompatibility complex on thyroid epithelial cells (Platzer et al., (1987). This finding may be important for understanding the pathogenesis of autoimmune thyroiditis. Supplemental dietary T_3 also increases the number of splenic IgG plaque-forming cells in undernourished animals (Filteau et al., 1987). T_3, which is a more effective thyroid hormone than T_4, induces the proliferation of thymic epithelial cells (Scheiff et al., 1977). More importantly, Fabris and colleagues (Fabris and Mocchegiani, 1985; Fabris et al., 1986) have convincingly demonstrated that T_3 and T_4 augment plasma levels of a thymic hormone known as thymulin. However, excess levels of T_4 appear to suppress the activity of natural killer cells (Stein-Streilein et al., 1987), which is considered to be a thymic-independent immune event.

4. Opioids

Opioid peptides are the endogenous analogues of opiates. They are of interest in farm animals because they are elevated during acute stress and may play a role in stress-induced changes in the immune system. For example, intermittent foot shock in rats induces the release of endogenous opioid peptides and suppresses natural killer cell activity (Shavit et al., 1984). This stress effect is mediated centrally, because it can be mimicked by administering morphine directly into the brain (Shavit et al., 1986). It has recently been shown that the central effect of opiates on inhibition of natural killer cell activity is localized to the periaqueductal gray matter of the brain (Weber and Pert, 1989). Another opioid peptide, α-endorphin, suppresses the primary antibody response of human blood lymphocytes (Johnson et al., 1982) by inhibiting the production of an antigen-specific T cell helper factor (Heijnen et al., 1986). β-endorphin also indirectly inhibits the production of toxic oxygen intermediates in human mononuclear cells, presumably by inducing the release of a suppressive product from lymphocytes (Peterson et al., 1987). Unfortunately, however, very little research has been published on the role of opioids in regulating immune events in domestic animals.

The effects of opioids on leukocytes are of interest in humans because opiate addicts have an increased susceptibility to infection. Although a number of reasons could explain this observation, a substantial amount of evidence indicates that opioids directly affect functional activities of cells of the immune system (reviewed by Sibinga and Goldstein, 1988). Peptides within the opioid gene family are encoded by three genes: proopiomelanocortin, proenkephalin, and prodynorphin. The four types of opioid receptors that have been identified, mu, delta, kappa, and epsilon, have all been shown to exist on various types of leukocytes (reviewed by Carr, 1988). However, the effects of opioids on functional activities of leukocytes vary considerably. These differences in direct effects of opioids on leukocytes can be compared to indirect effects that may be mediated via the brain or other subpopulations of leukocytes, or by modulatory roles that are not mediated directly via opioid receptors (Sibinga and Goldstein, 1988).

5. Other Neuropeptides

Peptides that are synthesized and released by neurons in the central and peripheral nervous systems are now known to modulate a number of immune events. Although many of these peptides have been investigated, the most throughly characterized neuropeptides on lymphoid and myeloid tissue are substance P, somatostatin, and vasoactive intestinal peptide. For example, substance P released from afferent sensory nerve endings in diverse organ systems plays a major role in neurogenic inflammation. It has recently been shown to cause the release of IL-1, IL-6, and TNF-α from human monocytes (Lotz et al., 1988), trigger the respiratory burst in human neutrophils (Serra et al., 1988), potentiate the IL-1-induced proliferation of fibroblasts (Kimball and Fisher, 1988), and cause granulocyte infiltration through the degranulation of mast cells (Matsuda et al., 1989). These findings have initiated a search for specific substance P antagonists as a new class of antiinflammatory drugs (Payan, 1989). The major immunological effects of this and other neuropeptides have recently been summarized by Croitoru et al. (1989).

D. HORMONES ARE SYNTHESIZED BY LEUKOCYTES

Pituitary Hormones Are Synthesized by Leukocytes

Proteins that are synthesized and secreted by lymphocytes that affect the activities of other lymphocytes are known as lymphokines. It now appears that several hormones and neuropeptides can be synthesized by lymphoid cells (Table III), which creates the possibility that these molecules may be synthesized locally and act in an autocrine or paracrine fashion on leukocytes. If this were indeed the case, it would be difficult to distinguish some classic pituitary hormones from the generic list of lymphokines.

Endorphins and ACTH were the first pituitary hormones purported to be synthesized by leukocytes (Smith and Blalock, 1981). These data have been controversial because the molecules have classically been detected with the aid of either monospecific antibodies (and therefore the qualifier, immunoreactive hormone) or bioassays. However, we

TABLE III

PRODUCTION OF HORMONES AND NEUROPEPTIDES BY CELLS OF THE IMMUNE SYSTEM

Neuropeptide	Reference
ACTH, β-endorphin	Smith and Blalock (1981); Harbour-McMenamin et al. (1984); Lolait et al. (1984, 1986); Smith et al. (1986); Westly et al. (1986); Oates et al. (1988); Kavelaars et al. (1989); Buzzetti et al. (1989a)
Enkephalin	Zurawski et al. (1986)
Growth Hormone	Heistand et al. (1986); Weigent et al. (1988)
Prolactin	Heistand et al. (1986); Montgomery et al. (1987); Hartmann et al. (1989)
Vasopressin	Geenen et al. (1986); Markwick et al. (1986)
Oxytocin	Geenen et al. (1986)
Thyrotropic hormone	Smith et al. (1983); Kruger et al. (1989)
Chorionic gonadotropin	Harbour-McMenamin et al. (1986)
Vasoactive intestinal peptide	Cutz et al. (1978); O'Dorisio et al. (1980); Lygren et al. (1984)

(Westly et al., 1986) and others (Lolait et al., 1986) demonstrated that murine lymphoid cells can transcribe the appropriate gene for ACTH by Northern blot analysis with a specific cDNA probe for proopiomelanocortin. These results have recently been confirmed in humans (Kavelaars et al., 1989; Oates et al., 1988; Buzzetti et al., 1989a). However, it is important to note that neither the actual sequence of nucleotides nor the amino acid sequence of ACTH purified from lymphoid cells has yet been published. These data will provide the final proof that lymphoid cells can synthesize and secrete bona fide ACTH.

The nucleotide sequence for pre-proenkephalin derived from T helper cells is almost identical to that derived from other tissues (Zurawski et al., 1986). Leukocytes also appear to synthesize the pituitary hormones oxytocin, vasopressin, thryroid stimulating hormone, growth hormone, and prolactin (Table III), but the synthesis of these hormones has not been as thoroughly investigated as that of peptides derived from proopiomelanocortin. Although the exact subset of leukocyte that is responsible for synthesizing each of these peptides is not yet known, constitutive production of these hormones can often be detected, with even higher amounts being produced after addition of some type of inducer.

Two examples have recently been published that clearly show that leukocyte-derived hormones can function as cytokines. The TRH-induced secretion of TSH by lymphocytes enhances antibody synthesis, and addition of an antibody directed to TSH abrogates this increase in antibody synthesis (Kruger et al., 1989, vide supra). Another example has recently been published by Kavelaars et al. (1989) with leukocyte-derived β-endorphin. B lymphocytes are the primary source of β-endorphin in human leukocytes after treatment with corticotropin-releasing factor and arginine vasopressin, and this effect is dependent upon the presence of monocytes. These workers showed that corticotropin-releasing factor and arginine vasopressin induce the synthesis of IL-1 by monocytes, which in turn is responsible for causing the production of β-endorphin by B lymphocytes. These data strongly support the idea that leukocyte-derived hormones function in a paracrine fashion as cytokines during an immune response.

E. Brain Lesions Affect the Immune Response

The pituitary gland is an important organ through which the central nervous system controls a multitude of physiological processes, including the regulation of a number of immune events. Neuroendocrine peptides that are released from the hypothalamus control many functions of the adenohypophysis. It is therefore not surprising that a number of immunologic activities, such as responsiveness to antigens, natural killer cell activity, and suppressor activity of macrophages, is affected by lesions of the anterior hypothalamus (reviewed by Roszman et al., 1985). However, lesions in other areas of the brain, such as the hippocampus or amygdala, generally have less-pronounced effects.

It now appears that the brain neocortex also alters the immune response in an asymmetrical way. For example, a right cortical lesion augments the production of IL-2 by splenic lymphocytes in mice, but bilateral lesions in both the right and left cortex abrogate this response (Neveu et al., 1989). Similar results are observed with lymphoproliferation of splenocytes induced by concanavalin A. These data suggest that the left and right brain cortex are able to modulate the activities of T lymphocytes in the periphery. It is not yet known whether similar effects occur in domestic animals, or whether such lateralization of the modulation of immune events by the brain is important in the resistance of animals to infectious diseases.

F. CYTOKINES AFFECT THE CENTRAL NERVOUS SYSTEM

Fifteen years ago, Besedovsky and colleagues (1975) demonstrated that injection of an antigen increases the concentration of glucocorticoids in the blood of rodents. They later showed that this effect could be mimicked by injecting lymphokines from leukocytes stimulated with concanavalin A (Besedovsky *et al.*, 1981). They next demonstrated that the lymphokine that increased blood concentrations of glucocorticoids is IL-1 (Besedovsky *et al.*, 1986), and that IL-1 acts by stimulating the release of corticotropin-releasing factor (CRF) from the hypothalamus (Berkenbosch *et al.*, 1987). These results have been independently confirmed in a number of other laboratories, and all of these findings have been recently reviewed by Buzzetti *et al.* (1989b). Tumor necrosis factor-α probably shares the CRF-releasing property of IL-1.

Del Rey and Besedovsky (1989) have most recently demonstrated that IL-1 is a potent antidiabetic agent because it reduces blood glucose levels, even in genetically diabetic, insulin-resistant mice. It has also been recently shown that specific receptors for IL-1 exist in the brain (Farrar *et al.*, 1987) and that there are IL-1-containing neurons in the brain (Breder *et al.*, 1988). These data show that a protein released by activated macrophages affects the central nervous system, and they also suggest that IL-1 is involved in a regulatory feedback loop with the pituitary gland that controls its own production. IL-1 secretion by activated macrophages augments the synthesis of ACTH. Elevated plasma concentrations of glucocorticoids negatively feedback to suppress the synthesis of IL-1. This may help control hyperthermia and acute-phase reactions that are induced by IL-1.

Interleukin-6 (IL-6) has recently been identified as a T cell-derived lymphokine that causes dividing B lymphocytes to develop into immunoglobulin-secreting cells. However, it is now known to possess other biological properties as well, such as the stimulation of hepatocytes and the production of acute-phase proteins. Indeed, this molecule is identical to hybridoma growth factor, hepatocyte-stimulating factor, interferon-β2, and the human 26-kDa protein. Frei *et al.* (1989) recently demonstrated that IL-6 is synthesized by virus-infected microglial cells and astrocytes. Interleukin-6 acts in an autocrine fashion to increase the production of nerve growth factor by astrocytes, which again supports the idea that many cytokines have major pleiotropic effects. The important concepts of pleiotropy and redundancy have recently been discussed by Paul (1989).

The immunological properties of most of the newly discovered inter-

TABLE IV

COMPARISON OF THE EFFECTS OF CENTRAL OR
PERIPHERAL ADMINISTRATION OF CYTOKINES
WITH NONSPECIFIC SYMPTOMS OF SICKNESS

CNS effects of cytokines	Nonspecific symptoms of sickness
General malaise	Feeling sick
Decreased activity	Loss of energy or fatigue
Decreased social investigation	Loss of interest in usual activities
Decreased food and water intake, weight loss	Poor appetite and significant weight loss
Sleep changes	Sleep changes
Fever	Fever

Note: See Dantzer and Kelley (1989) for references.

leukins have been the most thoroughly investigated, but it is now becoming clear that these molecules probably serve other roles that help the body to maintain homeostasis during an infectious disease. For example, many diseases are associated with a number of nonspecific symptoms of illness, such as anorexia, sleepiness, apathy, irritability, fatigue, and fever. Many of the recombinant interferons and interleukins that have been tested in humans and animals, particularly IL-1 and TNF-α, cause similar kinds of side effects (Table IV). These data suggest that another important function of cytokines that are released from leukocytes during acute infections is to inform the brain that a pathogenic insult has occurred in peripheral tissues. The brain then integrates this information and initiates appropriate physiological and behavioral responses to aid in the maintenance of homeostasis.

III. Conclusions

An important practical application of these new findings in immunophysiology is increased understanding of the effects of stress on the immune system of farm animals (Fig. 1). Stimuli that are not sensed by classical sensory organs, such as pathogenic microbes, can now be included in the list of stimuli that induce the release of ACTH from the

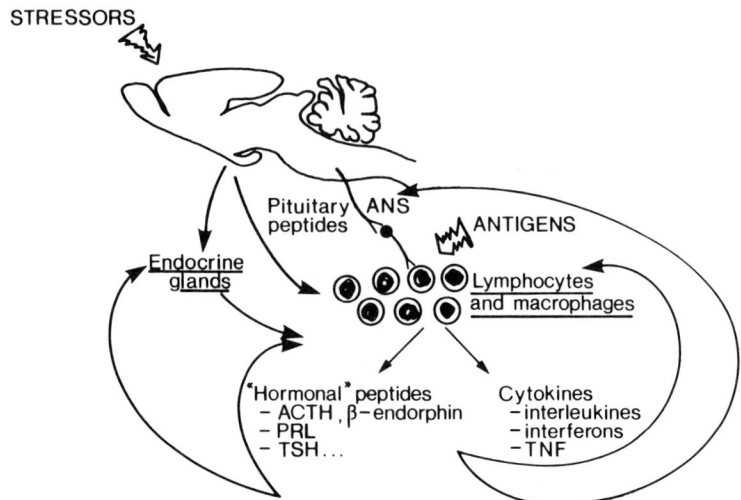

FIG. 1. Hormones from the pituitary gland affect lymphocytes and macrophages, and cytokines released by leukocytes affect the pituitary gland. The existence of bidirectional pathways between the brain and the immune system enables the coupling of functions between these two essential organ systems during the course of infection and inflammation. Messengers involved in this communication are cytokines and hormonal peptides that are elaborated by the immune system, and hormones and neuropeptides that originate from the neuroendocrine and autonomic nervous systems (ANS). Note that because of the commonality of signals, hormones and peptides released during exposure to stressors can influence the functions of lymphocytes and macrophages (modified from Dantzer and Kelley, 1989).

adenohypophysis. The mechanism by which these stimuli (e.g., endotoxin from Gram-negative bacteria) increase plasma levels of glucocorticoids is induction of the release of IL-1 from cells such as macrophages. IL-1 increases the release of ACTH from the pituitary gland, which stimulates the synthesis and release of glucocorticoids from the adrenal cortex. Glucocorticoids are potent immunosuppressive agents. Other pituitary hormones (e.g., growth hormone and prolactin) or T cell-derived lymphokines (e.g., interferon-γ) may counteract the immunosuppressive effects of glucocorticoids (Kelley and Dantzer, 1990). It is now clear that bidirectional communication exists between the brain and the immune systems. Cytokines serve as hormones to relay information to the brain, and classical pituitary hormones and neuropeptides modulate a number of immune functions. In addition, neuropeptides are actually synthesized by leukocytes and may function as cytokines in the microenvironment of lymph nodes. The expanding area of immunophysiology will continue to be important in understanding how cells of the immune system interact with other physiological systems to preserve homeostasis during pathological disorders.

Note added in proof: The amino acid and nucleotide sequence of lymphocyte-derived ACTH has been determined and shown to be identical to pituitary ACTH (1–25) (Smith, 1990).

ACKNOWLEDGMENTS

Supported by NIH Grant AG 06246, Office of Naval Research Grant N00014-89-J-1956, U.S. Department of Agriculture Grant 89-37265-4536, and the Moorman Mfg. Co.

REFERENCES

Ackerman, K. D., Felten, S. Y., Bellinger, D. L., and Felten, D. L. (1987). Noradrenergic sympathetic innervation of the spleen. III. Development of innervation in the rat spleen. *J. Neurosci. Res.* **18**, 49–54.

Alvarez-Mon, A., Kehrl, J. H., and Fauci, A. S. (1985). A potential role for adrenocorticotropin in regulating human B lymphocyte functions. *J. Immunol.* **135**, 3823–3826.

Arya, S. K., Wong-Staal, F., and Gallo, R. C. (1984). Dexamethasone-mediated inhibition of human T cell growth factor and γ-interferon messenger RNA. *J. Immunol.* **133**, 273–276.

Bellinger, D. L., Felten, S. Y., Collier, T. J., and Felten, D. L. (1987). Noradrenergic sympathetic innervation of the spleen. IV. Morphometric analysis in adult and aged F344 rats. *J. Neurosci. Res.* **18**, 55–63.

Berczi I., and Nagy E. (1990). Effects of hypophysectomy on immune function. In "Psychoneuroimmunology II" (R. Ader, N. Cohen, and D. Felton, eds.), 2nd ed. Academic Press, San Diego, California. In press.

Berkenbosch, F., Van Oers, J., Del Rey, A., Tilders, F., and Besedovsky, H. (1987). Corticotropin-releasing factor-producing neurons in the rat activated by interleukin-1. *Science* **238**, 524–526.

Bernton, E. W. (1989). Prolactin and immune host defenses. *Prog. NeuroEndocrin Immunol.* **2**, 21–29.

Bernton, E. W., Meltzer, M. S., and Holaday, J. W. (1988). Suppression of macrophage activation and T-lymphocyte function in hypoprolactinemic mice. *Science* **239**, 401–404.

Besedovsky, H. O., Sorkin, E., Keller, M., and Muller, J. (1975). Changes in blood hormone levels during the immune response. *Proc. Soc. Exp. Biol. Med.* **150**, 466–470.

Besedovsky, H. O., Del Rey, A., and Sorkin, E. (1981). Lymphokine containing supernatants from ConA stimulated cells increase corticosterone blood levels. *J. Immunol.* **126**, 385–387.

Besedovsky, H. O., Del Rey, A., Sorkin, E., and Dinarello, C. (1986). Immunoregulatory feedback between interleukin-1 and glucocorticoid hormones. *Science* **233**, 652–654.

Beutler, B., Krochin, N., Milsark, I. W., Luedke, C., and Cerami, A. (1986). Control of cachectin (tumor necrosis factor) synthesis: Mechanisms of endotoxin resistance. *Science* **232**, 977–980.

Blalock, J. E. (1989). A molecular basis for bidirectional communication between the immune and neuroendocrine systems. *Physiol. Rev.* **69**, 1–32.

Blalock J. E., Johnson, H. M., Smith, E. M., and Torres, B. A. (1985). Enhancement of the in vitro antibody response by thyrotropin. *Biochem. Biophys. Res. Commun.* **125**, 30–34.
Blecha, F., and Baker, P. E. (1986). Effect of cortisol in vitro and in vivo on production of bovine interleukin 2. *Am. J. Vet. Res.* **47**, 841–845.
Bost, K. L., Smith, E. M., Wear, L. B., and Blalock, J. E. (1987). Presence of ACTH and its receptor on a B lymphocytic cell line: A possible autocrine function for a neurendocrine hormone. *J. Biol. Regul. Homeostatic Agents* **1**, 23–27.
Breder, C. D., Dinarello, C. A., and Saper, C. B. (1988). Interleukin-1 immunoreactive innervation of the human hypothalamus. *Science* **240**, 321–324.
Burvenich, C., Heyneman R., Vandeputte-Van Messom, G., and Roets, E. (1989). Role of neutrophil activity in the outcome of hyperacute experimentally-induced *Escherichia coli* mastitis in cattle immediately post-partum and effect of rBST. *Am. Dairy Sci. Am. Soc. Anim. Sci. Meet.*, Abstr. 25, p. 11.
Buzzetti, R., McLoughlin, L., Lavender, P. M., Clark, A. J. L., and Rees, L. H. (1989a). Expression of pro-opiomelanocortin gene and quantification of adrenocorticotropic hormone-like immunoreactivity in human normal peripheral mononuclear cells and lymphoid and myeloid malignancies. *J. Clin. Invest.* **83**, 733–737.
Buzzetti, R., McLoughlin, L., Scavo, D., and Rees, L. H. (1989b). A critical assessment of the interactions between the immune system and the hypothalamo-pituitary-adrenal axis. *J. Endocrinol.* **120**, 183–187.
Carr, D. J. J. (1988). Opioid receptors on cells of the immune system. *Prog. NeuroEndocrinImmunol.* **1**, 8–14.
Clarke, B. L., and Bost, K. L. (1989). Differential expression of functional adrenocorticotropic hormone receptors by subpopulations of lymphocytes. *J. Immunol.* **143**, 464–469.
Croitoru, K., Stead, R. H., Bienenstock, J., and Stanisz, A. M. (1989). The role of neuropeptides in modulating the intestinal immune response. *In* "Interactions Among Central Nervous System, Neuroendocrine and Immune Systems" (J. W. Hadden, K. Masek, and G. Nistico, eds.), pp. 437–458. Pythagora Press, Rome-Milan.
Cutz, E., Chan, W., Track, N., Goth, A., and Said, S. (1978). Release of vasoactive intestinal peptide in mast cells by histamine liberators. *Nature (London)* **275**, 661–662.
Danek, A., O'Dorisio, M. S., O'Dorisio, T. M., and George, J. M. (1983). Specific binding sites for vasoactive intestinal polypeptide on nonadherent peripheral blood lymphocytes. *J. Immunol.* **131**, 1173–1177.
Dantzer, R., and Kelley, K. W. (1989). Stress and immunity: An integrated view of relationships between the brain and the immune system. *Life Sci.* **44**, 1995–2008.
Dardenne, M., Savino, W., Gagnerault, M. C., Itoh, T., and Bach, J. F. (1989). Neuroendocrine control of thymic hormonal production. I. Prolactin stimulates in vivo and in vitro the production of thymulin by human and murine thymic epithelial cells. *Endocrinology (Baltimore)* **125**, 3–12.
Davila, D. R., Brief, S., Simon, J., Hammer, R. E., Brinster, R. L., and Kelley, K. W. (1987). Role of growth hormone in regulating T-dependent immune events in aged, nude, and transgenic rodents. *J. Neurosci. Res.* **18**, 108–116.
Del Rey, A., and Besedovsky, H. (1989). Antidiabetic effects of interleukin 1. *Proc. Natl. Acad. Sci. U.S.A.* **86**, 5943–5947.
Dunham, D., Arkins, S., Edwards, C. K., Dantzer, R., and Kelley, K. W. (1990). Role of interferon-γ in counteracting the suppressive effects of transforming growth factor-β2 and glucocorticoids on the production of tumor necrosis factor-γ. *J. Leuk. Biol.* **48**, In press.

Edwards, C. K., III, Ghiasuddin, S. M., Schepper, J. M., Yunger, L. M., and Kelley, K. W. (1988). A newly defined property of somatotropin: Priming of macrophages for production of superoxide anion. *Science* **239**, 769–771.

Edwards, C. K., III, Lorence, R. M., Dunham, D. M., Yunger, L. M., and Kelley, K. W. (1989a). Peritoneal macrophages from hypophysectomized rats treated *in vivo* with interferon-γ or growth hormone are primed to release tumor necrosis factor-α. *Proc. Int. Congr. Immunol., 7th, 1989,* Abstr. 93–20, p. 618.

Edwards, C. K., III, Lorence, R. M., Yunger, L. M., and Kelley, K. W. (1989b). Rats treated with interferon-γ or growth hormone have enhanced host protection to *Salmonella typhimurium*. *J. Leuk. Biol.* **46**, 293 (Abstr. 10).

Engel, W. K., Trotter, J. L., McFarlin, D. E., and McIntosh, C. L. (1977). Thymic epithelial cell contains acetylcholine receptor. *Lancet* **1**, 1310–1311.

Fabris, N., and Mocchegiani, E. (1985). Endocrine control of thymic serum factor production in young-adult and old mice. *Cell. Immunol.* **91**, 325–335.

Fabris, N., Mocchegiani, E., Mariotti, S., Pacini, F., and Pinchera, A. (1986). Thyroid function modulates thymic endocrine activity. *J. Clin. Endocrinol. Metab.* **62**, 474–478.

Farrar, W. L., Kilian, P. L., Ruff, M. R., Hill, J. M., and Pert, C. B. (1987). Visualization and characterization of interleukin 1 receptors in brain. *J. Immunol.* **139**, 459–463.

Felten, D. L., Felten, S. Y., Bellinger, D. L., Carlson, S. L., Ackerman, K. D., Madden, K. S., Olschowki, J. A., and Livnat, S. (1987). Noradrenergic sympathetic neural interactions with the immune system: Structure and function. *Immunol. Rev.* **100**, 225–260.

Felten, S. Y., and Olschowka, J. (1987). Noradrenergic sympathetic innervation of the spleen. II. Tyrosine hydroxylase (TH)-positive nerve terminals form synapticlike contacts on lymphocytes in the splenic white pulp. *J. Neurosci. Res.* **18**, 37–48.

Filteau, S. M., Perry, K. J., and Woodward, B. (1987). Triiodothyronine improves the primary antibody response to sheep red blood cells in severely undernourished weanling mice. *Proc. Soc. Exp. Biol. Med.* **185**, 427–433.

Franklin, R. A., Davila, D. R., and Kelley, K. W. (1987). Chicken serum inhibits lectin-induced proliferation of autologous splenic mononuclear cells. *Proc. Soc. Exp. Biol. Med.* **184**, 225–233.

Frei, K., Malipiero, U. V., Leist, T. P., Zinkernagel, R. M., Schwab, M. E., and Fontana, A. (1989). On the cellular source and function of interleukin 6 produced in the central nervous system in viral diseases. *Eur. J. Immunol.* **19**, 689–694.

Fu, Y.-K., Arkins, S., and Kelley, K. W. (1990). Growth hormone (GH) and insulin-like growth factor-I (IGF-I) prime granulocytes for superoxide anion secretion. *FASEB J.* **4**, p. A 1908 (Abstr. 1248).

Geenen, V., Legros, J. J., Franchimont, P., Baudrihaye, M., Defresne, M. P., and Boniver, J. (1986). The neuroendocrine thymus: Coexistence of oxytocin and neurophysin in the human thymus. *Science* **232**, 508–511.

Gillis, S., Crabtree, G. R., and Smith, K. A. (1979). Glucocorticoid-induced inhibition of T cell growth factor production. I. The effect on mitogen-induced lymphocyte proliferation. *J. Immunol.* **123**, 1624–1631.

Haddock Russell, D. H., Kibler, R., Matrisian, L., Larson, D. F., Poulos, B., and Magun, B. E. (1985). Prolactin receptors on human T and B lymphocytes: Antagonism of prolactin binding by cyclosporine. *J. Immunol.* **134**, 3027–3031.

Harbour-McMenamin, D. V., Smith, E. M., and Blalock, J. E. (1984). Endotoxin induction of leukocyte-derived proopiomelanocortin related peptides. *Infect. Immun.* **48**, 813–819.

Harbour-McMenamin, D. V., Smith, E. M., and Blalock, J. E. (1986). Production of immunoreactive chorionic gonadotropin during mixed lymphocyte reactions: A possible selective mechanism for genetic diversity. *Proc. Natl. Acad. Sci. U.S.A.* **83**, 6834–6838.

Hartmann, D. P., Holaday, J. W., and Bernton, E. W. (1989). Inhibition of lymphocyte proliferation by antibodies to prolactin. *FASEB J.* **3**, 2194–2202.

Hazum, E. K., Chang, K., and Cuatrecasas, P. (1979). Specific non opiate receptors for β-endorphin. *Science* **205**, 1033–1035.

Heijnen, C. J., Bevers, C., Kavelaars, A., and Ballieux, R. E. (1986). Effect of α-endorphin on the antigen-induced primary antibody response of human blood B cells *in vitro*. *J. Immunol.* **136**, 213–216.

Heistand, P. C., Mekler, P., Nordmann, R., Grieder, A., and Perminongkol, C. (1986). Prolactin as a modulator of lymphocyte responsiveness provides a possible mechanism of action for cyclosporine. *Proc. Natl. Acad. Sci. U.S.A.* **83**, 2599–2603.

Heyneman, R., Burvenich, C., Van Hoegaerden, M., and Peeters, G. (1989). Influence of recombinant methionyl bovine somatotropin (rBST) on blood neutrophil respiratory burst activity in healthy cows. *Am. Dairy Sci. Am. Soc. Anim. Sci. Meet.*, Abstr. 848, p. 349.

Johnson, H. M., Smith, E. M., Torres, B. A., and Blalock, J. E. (1982). Regulation of the *in vitro* antibody response by neuroendocrine hormones. *Proc. Natl. Acad. Sci. U.S.A.* **79**, 4171–4174.

Johnson, H. M., Torres, B. A., Smith, E. M., Dion, L. D., and Blalock, J. E. (1984). Regulation of lymphokine (γ-interferon) production by corticotropin. *J. Immunol.* **132**, 246–250.

Kavelaars, A., Ballieux, R. E., and Heijnen, C. J. (1989). The role of IL-1 in the corticotropin-releasing factor and arginine-vasopressin-induced secretion of immunoreactive β-endorphin by human peripheral blood mononuclear cells. *J. Immunol.* **142**, 2338–2342.

Kelley, K. W. (1988). Cross-talk between the immune and endocrine systems. *J. Anim. Sci.* **66**, 2095–2108.

Kelley, K. W. (1989a). Growth hormone, lymphocytes and macrophages. *Biochem. Pharmacol.* **38**, 705–713.

Kelley, K. W. (1990). Growth hormone in immunobiology. *In* "Psychoneuroimmunology II" (R. Ader, N. Cohen, and D. Felton, eds), 2nd ed. Academic Press, San Diego, California. pp. 377–402.

Kelley, K. W., and Dantzer, R. (1990). Growth hormone and prolactin as natural antagonists of glucocorticoids in immunoregulation. *In* "Stress and Immunity" (N. Plotnikoff, R. Faith, J. Wybran, and A. J. Murgo, eds.). Telford Press, Caldwell, New Jersey (accepted for publication).

Kelley, K. W., Brief, S., Westly, H. J., Novakofski, J., Bechtel, P. J., Simon, J., and Walker, E. B. (1986). GH_3 pituitary adenoma cells can reverse thymic aging in rats. *Proc. Natl. Acad. Sci. U.S.A.* **83**, 5663–5667.

Kelley, K. W., Brief, S., Westly, H. J., Novakofski, J., Bechtel, P. J., Simon, J., and Walker, E. B. (1987). Hormonal regulation of the age-associated decline in immune function. *Ann. N. Y. Acad. Sci.* **496**, 91–97.

Kelso, A., and Munck, A. (1984). Glucocorticoid inhibition of lymphokine secretion by alloreactive T lymphocyte clones. *J. Immunol.* **133**, 784–791.

Kiess, W., and Butenandt, O. (1985). Specific growth hormone receptors on human peripheral mononuclear cells: Reexpression, indentification, and characterization. *J. Clin. Endocrinol. Metab.* **60**, 740–746.

Kimball, E. S., and Fisher, M. C. (1988). Potentiation of IL-1 induced BALB/3T3 fibroblast proliferation by neuropeptides. *J. Immunol.* **141**, 4203–4208.
Koff, W. C., and Dunegan, M. A. (1985). Modulation of macrophage-mediated tumoricidal activity by neuropeptides and neurohormones. *J. Immunol.* **135**, 350–354.
Krug, U., Krug, F., and Cuatrecasas, P. (1972). Emergence of insulin receptors on human lymphocytes during *in vitro* transformation. *Proc. Natl. Acad. Sci. U.S.A.* **69**, 2604–2607.
Kruger, T. E., and Blalock, J. E. (1986). Cellular requirements for thyrotropin enhancement of *in vitro* antibody production. *J. Immunol.* **137**, 197–200.
Kruger, T. E., Smith, L. R., Harbour, D. V., and Blalock, J. E. (1989). Thyrotropin: An endogenous regulator of the *in vitro* immune response. *J. Immunol.* **142**, 744–747.
Lolait, S. J., Lim, A. T. W., Toh, B. W., and Funder, J. W. (1984). Immunoreactive β-endorphin in a subpopulation of mouse spleen macrophages. *J. Clin. Invest.* **75**, 277–280.
Lolait, S. J., Clements, J. A., Markwick, A. J., Cheng, C., McNally, M., Smith, A. I., and Funder, J. W. (1986). Pro-opiomelanocortin messenger RNA and post-translational processing of beta-endorphin in spleen macrophages. *J. Clin. Invest.* **77**, 1776–1779.
Lotz, M., Vaughan, J. H., and Carson, D. A. (1988). Effect of neuropeptides on production of inflammatory cytokines by human monocytes. *Science* **241**, 1218–1221.
Lygren, I., Revhaug, P., Barhol, P. G., Giercksky, K. E., and Jenssen, T. G. (1984). Vasoactive intestinal peptide and somatostatin in leukocytes. *Scand. J. Clin. Lab. Invest.* **44**, 347–351.
Markwick, A. J., Lolait, S. J., and Funder, J. W. (1986). Immunoreactive arginine vasopressin in the rat thymus. *Endocrinology (Baltimore)* **119**, 1690–1696.
Matsuda, H., Kawakita, K., Kiso, Y., Nakano, T., and Kitamura, Y. (1989). Substance P induces granulocyte infiltration through degranulation of mast cells. *J. Immunol.* **142**, 927–931.
Möller, G., ed. (1987). Neuroimmunology. *Immunol. Rev.* **100**, 1–378.
Montgomery, D. W., Zukoski, C. F., Shah, N. G., Buckley, A. R., Pacholczyk, T., and Russell, D. H. (1987). Concanavalin A-stimulated murine splenocytes produce a factor with prolactin-like bioactivity and immunoreactivity. *Biochem. Biophys. Res. Commun.* **145**, 692–698.
Murray, F. A., and Chenault, J. R. (1982). Effects of steroids on bovine T-lymphocyte blastogenesis *in vitro*. *J. Anim. Sci.* **55**, 1132–1138.
Neveu, P. J., Barnéoud, P., Vitiello, S., Kelley, K. W., and Le Moal, M. A. (1989). Brain neocortex modulation of mitogen-induced interleukin 2, but not interleukin 1, production. *Immunol. Lett.* **21**, 307–310.
Oates, E. L., Allaway, G. P., Armstrong, G. R., Boyajian, R. A., Kehrl, H. H., and Prabhakar, B. S. (1988). Human lymphocytes produce pro-opiomelanocortin gene-related transcripts. *J. Biol. Chem.* **263**, 10041–10044.
O'Dorisio, M. S., O'Dorisio, T. M., Cataland, S., and Balcerzak, S. P. (1980). Vasoactive intestinal peptide as a biochemical marker for polymorphonuclear leukocytes. *J. Lab. Clin. Med.* **96**, 666–670.
Ogunbiyi, P. O., Conlon, P. D., Black, W. D., and Eyre, P. (1988). Levamisole-induced attenuation of alveolar macrophage dysfunction in respiratory virus-infected calves. *Int. J. Immunopharmacol.* **10**, 377–385.
Paul, W. E. (1989). Pleiotropy and redundancy: T cell-derived lymphokines in the immune response. *Cell (Cambridge, Mass.)* **87**, 521–524.
Payan, D. G. (1989). Neuropeptides and inflammation: The role of substance P. *Annu. Rev. Med.* **40**, 341–352.

Payan, D. G., and Goetzl, E. J. (1984). Stereospecific receptors for substance P on cultured human IM-9 lymphoblasts. *J. Immunol.* **133**, 3260–3265.

Peterson, P. K., Sharp, B., Gekker, G., Brummitt, C., and Keane, W. F. (1987). Opioid-mediated suppression of cultured peripheral blood mononuclear cell respiratory burst activity. *J. Immunol.* **138**, 3907–3912.

Pierpaoli, W., Baroni, C., Fabris, N., and Sorkin, E. (1969). Hormones and immunological capacity. II. Reconstitution of antibody production in hormonally deficient mice by somatotropic hormone, thyrotropic hormone and thyroxin. *Immunology* **16**, 217–230.

Platzer, M., Neufeld, D. S., Piccinini, A., and Davies, T. F. (1987). Induction of rat thyroid cell MHC class II antigen by thyrotropin and γ-interferon. *Endocrinology (Baltimore)* **121**, 2087–2092.

Reed, J. C., Abidi, A. H., Alpers, J. D., Hoover, R. G., Robb, R. J., and Nowell, P. C. (1986). Effect of cyclosporin A and dexamethasone on interleukin 2 receptor gene expression. *J. Immunol.* **137**, 150–154.

Renold F. K., Dazin, P., Goetzl, E. J., and Payan, D. G. (1987). Interleukin-3 modulation of mouse bone marrow derived mast cell receptors for somatostatin. *J. Neurosci. Res.* **18**, 195–202.

Roszman, T. L., Jackson, J. C., Cross, R. J., Titus, M. J., Markesbery, W. R., and Brooks, W. H. (1985). Neuroanatomic and neurotransmitter influences on immune function. *J. Immunol.* **135**, 769s–772s.

Roth, J. A. (1985). Cortisol as mediator of stress-associated immunosuppression in cattle. In "Animal Stress" (G. Moberg, ed.), pp. 225–243. Am. Physiol. Soc., Bethesda, Maryland.

Roth, J. A., and Frank, D. E. (1989). Recombinant bovine interferon-γ as an immunomodulator in dexamethasone-treated and nontreated cattle. *J. Interferon Res.* **9**, 143–151.

Scheiff, J. M., Cordier, A. C., and Haumont, S. (1977). Epithelial cell proliferation in thymic hyperplasia induced by triiodothyronine. *Clin. Exp. Immunol.* **27**, 516–521.

Serra, M. C., Bazzoni, F., Bianca, V. D., Greskowiak, M., and Rossi, F. (1988). Activation of human neutrophils by substance P: Effect on oxidative metabolism, exocytosis, cytosolic Ca^{2+} concentration and inositol phosphate formation. *J. Immunol.* **141**, 2118–2124.

Shavit, Y., Lewis, J. W., Terman, G. W., Gale, R. P., and Liebeskind, J. C. (1984). Opioid peptides mediate the suppressive effect of stress on natural killer cell cytotoxicity. *Science* **223**, 188–190.

Shavit, Y., Depaulis, A., Martin, F. C., Terman, G. W., Pechnick, R. N., Zane, C. J., Gale, R. P., and Liebeskind, J. C. (1986). Involvement of brain opiate receptors in the immune-suppressive effect of morphine. *Proc. Natl. Acad. Sci. U.S.A.* **83**, 7114–7117.

Sibinga, N. E. S., and Goldstein, A. (1988). Opioid peptides and opioid receptors in cells of the immune system. *Annu. Rev. Immunol.* **6**, 219–249.

Smith, E. M., and Blalock, J. E. (1981). Human lymphocyte production of corticotropin and endorphin like substances: Association with leukocyte interferon. *Proc. Natl. Acad. Sci. U.S.A.* **75**, 7530–7534.

Smith, E. M., Phan, M., Kruger, T. E., Coppenhaver, D., and Blalock, J. E. (1983). Human lymphocyte production of immunoreactive thyrotropin. *Proc. Natl. Acad. Sci. U.S.A.* **80**, 6010–6013.

Smith, E. M., Morrill, A. C., Meyer, W. J., III, and Blalock, J. E. (1986). Corticotropin releasing factor induction of leukocyte-derived immunoreactive ACTH and endorphins. *Nature (London)* **321**, 881–882.

Smith, E. M., Brosnan, P., Meyer, W. J., and Blalock, J. E. (1987). A corticotropin receptor on human mononuclear lymphocytes: Correlation with adrenal ACTH receptor activity. *N. Engl. J. Med.* **317**, 1266–1269.

Smith, E. M., Galin, F. S., LeBoeuf, R. D., Coppenhaver, D. H., Harbour, D. V., and Blalock, J. E. (1990). Nucleotide and amino acid sequence of lymphocyte-derived corticotropin: Endotoxin induction of a truncated peptide. *Proc. Natl. Acad. Sci. U.S.A.* **87**, 1057–1060.

Snyder, D. S., and Unanue, E. R. (1982). Corticosteroids inhibit murine macrophage I_a expression and interleukin 1 production. *J. Immunol.* **129**, 1803–1805.

Stead, R. H., Tomioka, M., Quinonez, G., Simon, G. T., Felten, S. Y., and Bienenstock, J. (1987). Intestinal mucosal mast cells in normal and nematode-infected rat intestines are in intimate contact with peptidergic nerves. *Proc. Natl. Acad. Sci. U.S.A.* **84**, 2975–2979.

Stein-Streilein, J., Zakarija, M., Papic, M., and McKenzie, J. M. (1987). Hyperthyroxinemic mice have reduced natural killer cell activity. Evidence for a defective trigger mechanism. *J. Immunol.* **139**, 2502–2507.

Szefler, S. J., Norton, C. E., Ball, B., Gross, J. M., Aida, Y., and Pabst, M. J. (1989). IFN-γ and LPS overcome glucocorticoid inhibition of priming for superoxide release in human monocytes: Evidence that secretion of IL-1 and tumor necrosis factor-α is not essential for monocyte priming. *J. Immunol.* **142**, 3985–3992.

Thorpe, L. W., Stach, R. W., Hashim, G. A., Marchetti, D., and Perez-Polo, J. R. (1987). Receptors for nerve growth factor on rat splenic mononuclear cells. *J. Neurosci. Res.* **17**, 128–134.

Vandeputte-Van Messom, G., Burvenich, C., Roets, E., and Devriese, L. A. (1988). Effect of bovine somatotropin on milk yield and composition during *Escherichia coli* induced mastitis in lactating cows: Some preliminary results. *Vlaams Diergeneeskd. Tijdschr.* **57**, 53–61.

Weber, R. J., and Pert, A. (1989). The periaqueductal gray matter mediates opiate-induced immunosuppression. *Science* **245**, 188–190.

Weigent, D. A., Baxter, J. B., Wear, W. E., Smith, L. R., Bost, K. L., and Blalock, J. E. (1988). Production of immunoreactive growth hormone by mononuclear leukocytes. *FASEB J.* **2**, 2812–2818.

Westly, H. J., and Kelley, K. W. (1984). Physiologic concentrations of cortisol suppress cell-mediated immune events in the domestic pig. *Proc. Soc. Exp. Biol. Med.* **177**, 156–164.

Westly, H. J., and Kelley, K. W. (1987). Down-regulation of glucocorticoid and β-adrenergic receptors on lectin-stimulated splenocytes. *Proc. Soc. Exp. Biol. Med.* **185**, 211–218.

Westly, H. J., Kleiss, A. J., Kelley, K. W., and Wong P. H. (1986). Newcastle disease virus-infected splenocytes express the pro-opiomelanocortin gene. *J. Exp. Med.* **163**, 1589–1594.

Zurawski, G., Benedik, M., Kamp, B. J., Abrams, J. S., Zurawski, S. M., and Lee, F. D. (1986). Activation of mouse T-helper cells induces abundant preproenkephalin mRNA synthesis. *Science* **232**, 772–775.

Potential for Improving Animal Health by Modulation of Behavior and Immune Function

JOHN J. McGLONE

Department of Animal Science, Texas Tech University, Lubbock, Texas 79409

I. Introduction
II. Behavior of Farm Animals
III. Social Behavior and Immune Function
   A. The Subordinate Syndrome
   B. The Dominant Syndrome
   C. Penmates as an Aid to Coping with Stress
IV. Nonsocial Behaviors and Immune Function
V. Brain-Immune Interactions
   A. Direct Brain-Immune Interactions
   B. Brain and Gut Immunity
   C. Teaching the Immune System
VI. Concluding Remarks
   References

I. Introduction

Many scientists seek to better understand and improve animal health. Some study how animals deal with infectious agents. In outbreaks of infectious disease, a common observation is that animals die at a certain rate. A typical report of a disease outbreak might be that when nursing pigs and their lactating mothers were exposed to the transmissible gastroenteritis virus, it would be said that 50% (or some percentage) of the piglets died. The truly impressive fact is actually that 50% of the exposed piglets *lived*. Why is it that some animals live and others die when exposed to pathogens? Why do some animals get sick and others do not? Clearly, there are interacting variables that have major effects on animal health that have not been discovered by use of conventional scientific techniques in traditional scientific disciplines.

The literature on stress effects on immune function is riddled with inconsistencies (Kelley, 1980, 1985). Reasons are many, but without question, little attention has been paid to potential interacting variables that probably have large effects on animal stress responses.

I believe that the two most likely interacting variables that influence animal susceptibility to disease are genotype and brain–behavior interactions. Many traditional animal and veterinary scientists will be more comfortable with the possibility of genotype influencing animal health rather than the brain (for a recent review of genotype variation in immunity, see Templeton et al., 1988). This chapter should at least spark some degree of interest in the possibility that the brain is an important organ that modulates immune function. And, I hope to convince readers that manipulation of the brain and(or) behavior can result in suppression or enhancement of immune function. I am not alone in my view of the brain–immune network. Just three years ago, Solomon (1987) gave 35 examples of brain and immune function interactions.

In this chapter, I will first discuss how behavior and immune function are known to interact. Then, I will provide a sampling of the literature on how the brain can be manipulated directly in order to impact immune function.

II. Behavior of Farm Animals

From the perspective of an ethologist, the farm animal pen is a lively setting. Farm animals are not inanimate objects—they interact with each other and sense each other's presence continuously.

All farm animals, with the possible exception of the adult boar, are highly social animals. When first introduced, farm animals fight with the apparent objective of establishing a social dominance order (Craig, 1986; McGlone, 1986). Then, once social order is established, animals socially interact on a daily basis. The dominant animals would be said to have preferred access to limited resources. The subordinate animal would be worst off in a social group when it came to obtaining resources.

If all pens of animals have a social dominance order, what influence do the various social relationships have on animal health? A similar question has been asked in human health. House et al. (1988) concluded that certain human social relationships are more important than cigarette smoking in increasing risks of reduced health. Of greatest concern for human health are the socially isolated people—they have a higher incidence of mental and infectious diseases than people more integrated into society.

I believe humans provide a good model for domestic animals (people usually argue the reverse). And thus, social relationships probably play an important role in animal health. A better understanding of how social behavior influences animal health may eventually lead to improvements in animal health by appropriate immunomodulation.

III. Social Behavior and Immune Function

We know little about how farm animals perceive their environment, but two things are certain. First, social status has a powerful effect on how animals perceive their environment. Second, social stress has long been known to influence immune function (reviewed by Kelley, 1980).

I can imagine a future management scheme identifying animals of particular social types (for example, subordinates) and applying immunostimulants to those animals only (of course, if therapy is inexpensive, all animals could be stimulated). But at this time, we would have trouble at both ends; we have difficulty identifying social types and we do not know in what ways these animals require immunostimulation.

A. The Subordinate Syndrome

Data from humans suggests that being a social outcast is detrimental to health. The animal that most resembles the human with problems in social relationships is the subordinate animal.

Subordinate animals may experience a stress response most of the time (Arnone and Dantzer, 1980). Socially subordinate animals are also likely to be immunosuppressed because they have elevated blood glucocorticoids, which are known to be immunosuppressive (Roth, 1985). Conventional wisdom would hold that social subordinates have more health problems than other social types.

B. The Dominant Syndrome

With power comes stress, at least in humans. The dominant animal must expend some energy to maintain its social status, but at what cost?

We recently completed a study in which we examined relationships between social status and immune function in young pigs. Pigs were placed together and their behavior was video taped. From video records we could establish which pigs were socially dominant, intermediate, and subordinate. At the same time, we measured immune function before and after establishment of the new social groups.

Presented in Fig. 1 is the lymphocyte blastogenic response to pokeweed mitogen. What is clear is that the socially intermediate pigs had enhanced blastogenic response compared with social dominants and subordinates. A complete understanding of the immune mechanisms causing this effect remain to be identified.

The response among social subordinates was expected, but suppressed blastogenic response was not expected among dominant pigs. Clearly, the cost to maintain dominance is great.

The other striking aspect of this study is the variation that social behavior adds to immune data. If we examine any particular treatment

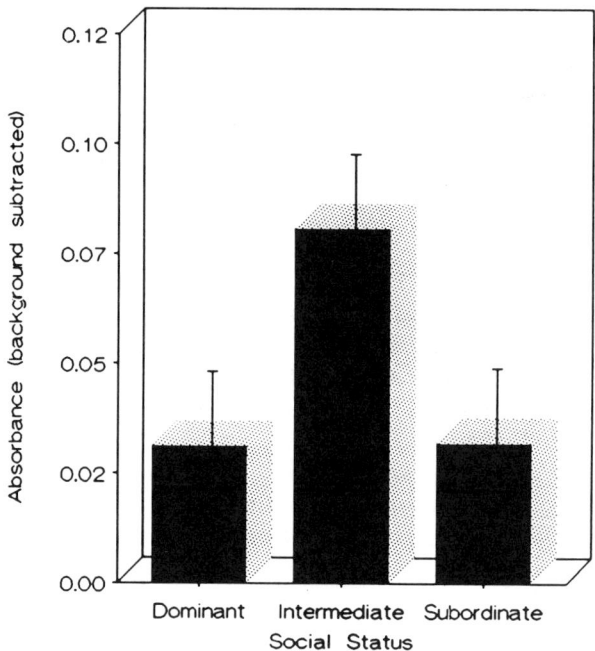

FIG. 1. Lymphocyte blastogenic response to pokeweed mitogen for pigs of three social types: dominant, intermediate, and subordinate. Y-axis is absorbance minus background while peripheral mononuclear cells were incubated with mitogen (MTT added the last 4 hours of a 72-hour culture). Socially intermediate pigs had a higher blastogenic response to mitogen than socially dominant or subordinate pigs. Data have since been replicated using more sensitive isotope assays.

for its effect on blastogenic response, we might easily come to the wrong conclusion. Assuming the social intermediates have "normal" lymphocyte function and other social types are suppressed, we would expect immunostimulants to be effective only among dominant and subordinate pigs. Thus, social status may mask beneficial effects of immunomodulators. We now know a proper evaluation of immunomodulators should include knowledge of each animal's social status.

C. Penmates as an Aid to Coping with Stress

It seems that misery loves company, even in the animal kingdom. House *et al.* (1988) reviewed several studies that show quite clearly the buffering effect of conspecifics on stress responses. Having members of the same species reduces stress-induced ulcers, hypertension neurosis, and adrenal-pituitary activation. One would predict penmates would have a beneficial effect on stress-induced immunosuppression.

Besides penmates, other physical manipulations may reduce stress effects on the pituitary-adrenal axis. Pigs that were able to develop stereotyped chain chewing had a reduced cortisol response to hunger stress (Dantzer and Mormede, 1981). There is little doubt that food animals are able to adapt to a variety of stressors. Helping them cope fully should be the subject of extensive research efforts.

IV. Nonsocial Behaviors and Immune Function

Animals express a wide array of behaviors, many of which may impact animal health directly or indirectly. One can imagine how feeding, drinking, thermoregulatory, and play behaviors can influence health. Receiving insufficient nutrients or inability to behaviorally thermoregulate would have major effects on health and well-being. But, more subtle behavioral effects are also likely, such as providing play objects that may reduce boredom and enhance animal health (these are only now being studied).

In the early 1980s a classic example showed how looking towards behavioral biology may answer a practical immunobiology question. Baby pigs exposed to cold stress have suppressed acquisition of immunoglobulins from colostrum (Blecha and Kelley, 1981). There are many possible immunological causes of this effect such as decreased absorption of macromolecules in colostrum or increased catabolism of immunoglobulins. As it turns out, cold-stressed pigs consume considerably less colostrum and therefore have less immunoglobulins absorbed (Le

Dividich and Noblet, 1981). This is now a classic example of how behavior impacts immunity. The way to manage cold-stressed piglets is, at least, to stimulate nursing behavior.

V. Brain-Immune Interactions

Many possibilities exist for brain-immune interactions, but only a few will be touched upon here. The neuroendocrine-immune interactions are discussed in recent reviews (Kelley and Dantzer, Ch. 11, this volume; Weigent and Blalock, 1989), so this important brain-immune network will not be repeated here. Suffice it to say neuroendocrine-immune manipulations will probably lead to significant animal health improvements in the future.

A. Direct Brain-Immune Interactions

A developing literature on brain region effects on immune function leads to the hope of great advances in manipulating the brain in order to enhance immune function. Lesions in the left neocortex depressed T lymphocyte responses, while not influencing B-lymphocyte function (Renoux et al., 1980, 1987). In contrast, right hemisphere lesions enhance T-lymphocyte function. Bilateral lesions in the neocortex reduce thymus and spleen weights and these immune organ weights are restored by use of the T-lymphocyte stimulant imuthiol.

Immunosuppression and immunoenhancement of peripheral natural killer cell activity seems to be modulated by the brain, especially via opiate systems. Microinjections of morphine in the periaqueductal gray area (and not other brain regions) had a large suppressive effect on natural killer cell activity in peripheral blood (Weber and Pert, 1989).

At least two general ideas predominate conventional wisdom on how the brain may influence immune function. First, any brain manipulation that influences the pituitary-adrenal axis is likely to have an effect in immune function. Second, immune organs are thought to have neural inputs that may modulate cellular maturation or function. The extent that each general mechanism may explain brain-immune effects remains to be determined.

B. Brain and Gut Immunity

The brain has many known effects on gut physiology, including gut immunity. Diarrhea is a symptom of stress in farm animals, but as with other aspects of immunity, not all animals become sick with exposure to the same pathogen or stressor. Brain peptides have significant effects on gut peptides and gut immunity (see Bienenstock et al., 1989, for a recent review). Generally, substance P stimulated gut immunity (lymphocyte numbers and function) while somatostatin and vasoactive intestinal peptide were generally inhibitory towards gut immunity (but see Pawlikowski et al., 1989, on stimulation of peripheral NK activity by somatostatin). There is every reason to believe that similar brain–respiratory tract and brain–reproductive tract immune relationships also exist.

Recent evidence suggests a peptide, found in the pituitary and in milk, prevents piglet diarrhea (Lonnroth and Lange, 1988; Lonnroth et al., 1988). Stressed animals have low levels of this peptide in their pituitary and they show clinical diarrhea. When stressed animals (rats and pigs) were given a neuroleptic (Amperozide) known to bind brain catecholamine receptors, the diarrhea was halted and pituitary levels of antisecretory factor was normal (i.e., not suppressed). Similar results were found in a rat-stress and a pig-stress model (Lonnroth et al., 1988; Kyriakis, 1989). This is clear evidence of a brain effect on animal health and of a brain-active drug improving animal health. We await more detailed mechanisms to explain this phenomenon, but early results are promising.

C. Teaching the Immune System

Many physiological systems can be conditioned or taught to respond to stimuli. Interested readers are directed towards the work of Ader and others who have studied and reviewed conditioning of the immune system for over a decade (Ader, 1981). While most studies have documented conditioned suppression of immune function, the potential exists for conditioned enhancement of immunity also (Ghanta et al., 1987). This type of research has largely not been investigated in food animals, except for one failed attempt to condition enhanced antibody titers (McGlone and Blecha, 1985). Without question, conditioned enhancement of immune function would be advantageous, but effective procedures remain to be described.

VI. Concluding Remarks

Animal health can certainly be improved by traditional methods of antibiotic therapy and vaccines. However, in many studies the background variation in immune measures remains high (and certainly greater than for most biological processes, for example, body growth).

The reason livestock and poultry weight gains are fairly uniform is that our present population has been selected for uniformity (presumably uniformly high) and because the major factors influencing growth are known and controlled (diet, temperature, social status, etc.).

I feel confident that the major factors controlling animal health have not yet been identified (except for the identification of pathogenic organisms). The most likely avenues of animal health improvement, in my opinion, are genetic manipulation (by selection *in vivo* or *in vitro*) and brain-behavior interactions with immune function.

To begin research in this area requires a break in tradition and special training. Most immunologists have little training in neuroscience and most neuroscientists have little training in immunology. This will change over time. In the mean time, some communication between scientists in the two disciplines will, at least, be a broadening experience for all and, at best, will greatly benefit animal health.

REFERENCES

Ader, R., ed. (1981). "Psychoneuroimmunology." Academic Press. New York.

Arnone, M., and Dantzer, R. (1980). Does frustration induce aggression in pigs? *Appl. Anim. Ethol.* **6,** 351–362.

Bienenstock, J., Croitoru, K., Ernst, P. B., Stead, R. H., and Stanisz, A. (1989). Neuroendocrine regulation of mucosal immunity. *Immunol. Invest.* **18,** 69–76.

Blecha, F., and Kelley, K. W. (1981). Cold stress reduces acquisition of colostral immunoglobulins in piglets. *J. Anim. Sci.* **52,** 594–600.

Craig, J. V. (1986). Measuring social behavior: Social dominance. *J. Anim. Sci.* **62,** 1120–1129.

Dantzer, R., and Mormede, P. (1981). Pituitary-adrenal consequences of adjunctive activities in pigs. *Horm. Behav.* **15,** 386–395.

Ghanta, V. K., Hiramoto, N. S., Solvason, H. B., Tyring, S. K., Spector, N. H., and Hiramoto, R. N. (1987). Conditioned enhancement of natural killer cell activity, but not interferon, with camphor or saccharin-LiCl conditioned stimulus. *J. Neurosci. Res.* **18,** 10–15.

House, J. S., Landis, K. L., and, Umberson, D. (1988). Social relationships and health. *Science* **241,** 540–545.

Kelley, K. W. (1980). Stress in farm animals: A bibliographic review. *Ann. Rech. Vet.* **11,** 445–478.

Kelley, K. W. (1985). Immunological consequences of changing environmental stimuli. *In* "Animal Stress" (G. P. Moberg, ed.), Am. Physiol. Soc., pp. 193–224. Bethesda, Maryland.

Kyriakis, S. C. (1989). New aspects of the prevention and/or treatment of the major stress induced diseases of the early weaned piglet. *Pig News Inf.* **10,** 177–181.

Le Dividich, J., and Noblet, J. (1981). Colostrum intake and thermoregulation in the neonatal pig in relation to environmental temperature. *Biol. Neonate* **40,** 167–174.

Lonnroth, I., and Lange, S. (1988). Antisecretory factors from the pituitary gland regulates intestinal fluid transport and reverse diarrhoea in piglets. *Proc. Symp. Social Stress Pigs, 1988.* pp. 90–91.

Lonnroth, I., Martinsson, K., and Lange, S. (1988). Evidence of protection against diarrhea in suckling piglets by a hormone-like protein in sow's milk. *J. Vet. Med.* **35,** 628–635.

McGlone, J. J. (1986). Agonistic behavior in food animals: Review of research and techniques. *J. Anim. Sci.* **62,** 1130–1139.

McGlone, J. J., and Blecha, F. (1985). Attempt to condition antibody production in young pigs. *Tex. Tech Univ. Swine Res. Rep.,* p. 19.

Pawlikowski, M., Zelazowski, P., and Stepien, H. (1989). Enhancement of human lymphocyte natural killer cell activity by somatostatin. *Neuropeptides (Edinburgh)* **13,** 75–77.

Renoux, G., Bizière, K., Renoux, M., and Guillaumin, J. M. (1980). Le cortex cérébral regle les responses immunes des souris. *C. R. Hebd. Seances Acad. Sci., Ser. D* **290,** 719–722.

Renoux, G., Bizière, K., Ronoux, M., Bardos, P., and Degenne, D. (1987). Consequences of bilateral brain neocortical ablation on imuthiol-induced immunostimulation in mice. *Ann. N. Y. Acad. Sci.* **496,** 346–253.

Roth, J. A. (1985). Cortisol as a mediator of stress-associated immunosuppression in cattle. *In* "Animal Stress" (G. P. Moberg, ed.), Am. Physiol. Soc., pp. 225–244. Bethesda, Maryland.

Solomon, G. F. (1987). Psychoneuroimmunology: Interactions between central nervous system and immune system. *J. Neurosci. Res.* **18,** 1–9.

Templeton, J. W., Smith, R., and Adams, G. (1988). Natural disease resistance in domestic animals. *J. Am. Vet. Med. Assoc.* **192,** 1306–1315.

Weber, R. J., and Pert, A. (1989). The periaqueductal gray matter mediates opiate-induced immunosuppression. *Science* **245,** 188–190.

Weigent, D. A., and Blalock, J. E. (1989). Structural and functional relationships between the immune and neuroendocrine systems. *Bull. Inst. Pasteur (Paris)* **87,** 61–92.

Index

A

Acquired immune deficiency syndrome, immunomodulators and, 109, 112, 115
ACTH
 interleukins and, 236
 neuroendocrine-immune interactions and, 286–288, 293, 294, 296–298
Actinobacillus pleuropneumoniae, interleukins and, 237, 238, 240, 241
Activation
 cytokines and, 183, 185, 187, 207
 immunomodulators and, 14
  chemical induction, 106, 109, 111
  mechanisms of action, 43, 48–50, 81
 interleukins and, 234, 235
 neuroendocrine-immune interactions and, 286, 289, 291
 nutrition and, 263
 thymosin-tuftsin conjugate and, 163–168, 172
Adjuvants, 121, 122, 145–147
 aluminum salts, 122–124
 cytokines and, 184, 185
 immunomodulators and, 6, 104, 115
 interferon immunomodulators and, 216, 221
 interleukins and, 244, 246
 ISCOMS, 138–141
 muramyldipeptides, 141, 142
 nutrition and, 265
 oil emulsions, 124–128
 polymeric, 142–145
 surface active agents
  lipophilic amines, 128–130
  nonionic block polymers, 130, 131
  saponins, 132–138
  supholipopolysaccharides, 131, 132
Aluminum salts, adjuvants and, 122–124
Alveolar macrophages
 cytokines and, 190, 204

 immunomodulators and, 7, 9, 14, 77, 82
 neuroendocrine-immune interactions and, 288, 289
Amino acids
 adjuvants and, 142, 147
 cytokines and, 204–206
  biology, 184, 186, 187
  recombinant bovine, 191, 193, 197, 198, 202
 immunomodulators and, 114
 neuroendocrine-immune interactions and, 287, 289, 294
 thymosin-tuftsin conjugate and, 164, 166
τ-Aminobutyric acid, immunomodulators and, 114
Antibiotics, immunomodulators and, 5
 chemical induction, 106
 mechanism of action, 54, 86, 87
Antibodies
 adjuvants and, 145, 147
  ISCOMS, 139, 140
  muramyldipeptides, 142
  polymeric adjuvants, 143, 144
  surface active agents, 128–130, 135, 137, 138
 cytokines and, 187, 205
 immunomodulators and, 9, 10
  chemical induction, 106–109, 111, 113–115
  immune system, 46–48, 53
  mechanism of action, 44, 83, 85
  model systems, 26
  physiology, 60, 61, 63, 67, 70
  synthetic compounds, 74, 75, 79
 interferon immunomodulators and, 220, 221, 224, 225
 interleukins and, 231, 239, 240, 245
 modulation of behavior and, 313
 neuroendocrine-immune interactions and, 283, 287, 289, 291–295
 nutrition and, 258, 259, 261

317

minerals, 269, 270
vitamins, 263–265, 267, 268
thymosin-tuftsin conjugate and, 165, 167, 168
Antibody-dependent cell-mediated cytotoxicity
cytokines and, 186, 188
immunomodulators and, 46, 71
interleukins and, 240
nutrition and, 268
Antigens
adjuvants and, 121, 122, 146, 147
aluminum salts, 122–124
ISCOMS, 138–141
muramyldipeptides, 142
oil emulsions, 124–128
polymeric adjuvants, 142–145
surface active agents, 128–135, 137
cytokines and, 188, 205
immunomodulators and, 5–7
chemical induction, 104, 106, 107, 109, 111, 113, 114
mechanism of action, 44, 46–49, 53, 55, 85
model systems, 25, 26
physiology, 59, 61, 64–67, 70, 71
synthetic compounds, 73, 77–79
interferon immunomodulators and, 218, 220, 221
neuroendocrine-immune interactions and, 292, 295, 296
nutrition and, 257, 261, 262, 267
thymosin-tuftsin conjugate and, 165, 167
Antimicrobial mechanisms in gut, interferon and, 221, 222
Ascorbic acid, *see* Vitamin C
Aujeszky's disease, adjuvants and, 126, 140, 141
Autonomic nervous system, neuroendocrine-immune interactions and, 285, 286
Avridine
adjuvants and, 128–130, 146
immunomodulators and
chemical induction, 108, 109
model systems, 29, 30

B

B cells
adjuvants and, 132, 137, 144, 147

cytokines and, 184, 185, 187, 188
immunomodulators and, 8
mechanism of action, 44, 46–49, 77, 83
physiology, 64, 65, 67, 70
interferon immunomodulators and, 220, 221
interleukins and, 232, 233, 235
nutrition and, 263, 266
thymosin-tuftsin conjugate and, 166, 172
B-complex vitamins, nutrition and, 259, 266, 267
B lymphocytes, immunomodulators and
chemical induction, 109, 111
mechanism of action, 46, 47, 55, 64
Bacteria
adjuvants and, 122, 147
oil emulsions, 127
surface active agents, 129, 130, 132, 135
cytokines and, 187, 190, 193, 202, 207
immunomodulators and, 4–6, 8, 9, 12
chemical induction, 108, 110, 111, 113
mechanism of action, 46, 47, 53, 54, 57
microbial products, 81–84
model systems, 27, 29, 30, 32–36
synthetic compounds, 77, 80
interferon immunomodulators and, 216, 218, 219, 221, 222, 224, 225
interleukins and, 237, 238, 245
nutrition and, 265, 266, 270, 271
thymosin-tuftsin conjugate and, 161, 165, 170, 171
Behavior, modulation of, 307–309, 313, 314
brain-immune interactions, 312, 313
immune function, 309–312
Biological response modifiers, thymosin-tuftsin conjugate and, 163
Biology
adjuvants and, 121, 146
of cytokines, 181–189, 205, 207
immunomodulators and
chemical induction, 105
mechanism of action, 57, 63, 64, 73, 85, 88
model systems, 23, 28–30
interferon immunomodulators and, 215

interleukins and, 231, 240
modulation of behavior and, 311, 313
thymosin-tuftsin conjugate and,
163–167, 169–173
Biostim, immunomodulators and, 111,
112
Blast transformation assay,
thymosin-tuftsin conjugate and, 172
Blastogenesis
cytokines and, 193
immunomodulators and
chemical induction, 106–108, 110,
113
mechanism of action, 70, 73
model systems, 25, 34–36
interleukins and, 239, 240
modulation of behavior and, 310, 311
nutrition and, 261, 262
Bone marrow
cytokines and, 184, 188, 189, 201, 202
immunomodulators and
chemical induction, 114
mechanism of action, 44–46, 48, 49
microbial products, 82
physiology, 62, 70
thymosin-tuftsin conjugate and, 166,
167
Bovine herpesvirus-1
adjuvants and, 139
immunomodulators and, 12, 13
chemical induction, 109, 110
mechanism of action, 68, 77
model systems, 33, 34
interferon immunomodulators and,
216, 218–220
interleukins and, 241–245
nutrition and, 260, 264, 265, 271–273
Bovine leukemia virus,
immunomodulators and, 33, 74, 107
Bovine respiratory disease
immunomodulators and, 4, 5
chemical induction, 105
model systems, 33–35
interferon immunomodulators and,
216, 221
interleukins and, 235, 241
thymosin-tuftsin conjugate and, 162
Bovine respiratory synctial virus,
immunomodulators and, 33, 34
Bovine rhinotracheitis virus,
immunomodulators and, 73, 74

Bovine serum albumin, adjuvants and,
130, 131, 133, 136, 143
Bovine viral diarrhea
adjuvants and, 144
immunomodulators and
chemical induction, 107
mechanism of action, 73
model systems, 33–35
Brain
modulation of behavior and, 308,
312–314
neuroendocrine-immune interactions
and, 286, 292, 293, 295, 297, 298
Brucella, immunomodulators and, 72,
73, 82
Bryostatins, immunomodulators and, 113

C

Calcium
adjuvants and, 144
cytokines and, 183, 185–188
nutrition and, 271
thymosin-tuftsin conjugate and, 166
Calves
adjuvants and, 127, 130, 143
immunomodulators and
chemical induction, 107, 110, 112
mechanism of action, 68, 74, 77,
82, 83
model systems, 23, 25, 30, 31, 33–35
interferon immunomodulators and,
216–219, 221, 222
interleukins and, 235, 241–246
nutrition and, 256–259, 261
minerals, 270, 271, 274
vitamins, 262, 264–268
thymosin-tuftsin conjugate and, 161,
171
Cancer, immunomodulators and, 112, 115
β-Carotene, nutrition and, 262, 263
Cattle
adjuvants and, 126, 127, 129, 133–135
cytokines and, 181, 184, 188, 190, 207
immunomodulators and, 4–6, 12
chemical induction, 105–109, 111,
112
mechanism of action, 71, 73, 74, 86
model systems, 25–29, 34, 35
interferon immunomodulators and,
219–221, 224, 225

interleukins and, 236, 237, 239, 240, 244, 246
  neuroendocrine-immune interactions and, 284, 288, 289
  nutrition and, 258–260, 264, 272, 274
cDNA
  cytokines and, 204, 207
    biology, 186, 187
    recombinant bovine, 190, 191, 193, 197, 198, 202
  neuroendocrine-immune interactions and, 294
Cell-mediated immunity
  adjuvants and, 123, 129, 136, 141, 142
  immunomodulators and
    chemical induction, 113, 115
    mechanism of action, 44, 49, 50, 53, 56, 84, 89
  nutrition and, 256–259, 261, 265, 268
  thymosin-tuftsin conjugate and, 167, 172
Cellular immune response
  adjuvants and, 128, 131
  interferon immunomodulators and, 218–221
  interleukins and, 231, 240
Central nervous system
  immunomodulators and, 58–62, 65
  neuroendocrine-immune interactions and, 286, 295–297
Chemical induction, immunomodulators and, *see* Immunomodulators, chemical induction and
Chemotaxis, thymosin-tuftsin conjugate and, 170, 171
Chemotherapy, immunomodulators and, 53–55, 86
Chicken
  adjuvants and, 129
  immunomodulators and, 12
    chemical induction, 105, 106
    mechanism of action, 63, 74, 77
    model systems, 26, 33
  neuroendocrine-immune interactions and, 288
  nutrition and, 259, 260, 264, 267, 268, 270
Cholesterol, adjuvants and, 137
Chromatography, thymosin-tuftsin conjugate and, 169

Ciprofloxacin, immunomodulators and, 114
Clones
  cytokines and, 204, 207
    biology, 184, 186–188
    recombinant bovine, 190, 193, 197, 198
  interferon immunomodulators and, 216
  interleukins and, 232
Cobalt, nutrition and, 260, 273, 274
Colony-stimulating factors, biology of, 182, 184, 189
Colostrum
  adjuvants and, 135
  immunomodulators and, 46, 47
  modulation of behavior and, 311
  nutrition and, 262, 268
Complement 3, immunomodulators and, 7, 9
Concanavalin A, nutrition and, 266, 271
Copper, nutrition and, 260, 272, 273
Corticotropin-releasing factor, neuroendocrine-immune interactions and, 295, 296
Cortisol
  immunomodulators and
    mechanism of action, 69, 71
    model systems, 26, 27, 31
  interleukins and, 236
  modulation of behavior and, 311
  neuroendocrine-immune interactions and, 288
COS cells, cytokines and, 201, 204
Cyclic AMP
  cytokines and, 187
  immunomodulators and, 57, 66, 78, 88
  thymosin-tuftsin conjugate and, 166, 167
Cyclic GMP
  cytokines and, 187
  immunomodulators and, 57, 62, 75, 77, 78, 88
  thymosin-tuftsin conjugate and, 166
Cytokines
  adjuvants and, 134
  biology, 181–183, 205, 207
    characteristics, 183–188
    regulation, 188, 189
  immunomodulators and, 12

mechanism of action, 55, 60, 61,
63–68, 88
model systems, 22, 29
interferon immunomodulators and,
223–225
interleukins and, 244, 246
neuroendocrine-immune interactions
and, 287–289, 295–297
nutrition and, 256
recombinant bovine, 189, 190
GM-CSF, 198–202
interferon-τ, 202, 203
interleukin-1, 190–196
interleukin-2, 193, 196–198
recombinant porcine interleukin-1,
190, 204
structure, 204–206
thymosin-tuftsin conjugate and, 169,
171, 172
Cytoplasm
cytokines and, 205
immunomodulators and, 7
Cytotoxicity
cytokines and, 186–188
immunomodulators and, 48, 84, 107
interferon immunomodulators and,
217–219
interleukins and, 236, 239–242, 245
neuroendocrine-immune interactions
and, 288–290
thymosin-tuftsin conjugate and, 165,
166, 169, 172

D

Defenses
cytokines and, 189
immunomodulators and
chemical induction, 103, 107
mechanism of action, 44, 49, 54, 78
model systems, 23, 27, 34, 35
nutrition and, 256
thymosin-tuftsin conjugate and, 162
Delayed-type hypersensitivity
adjuvants and, 128, 136
immunomodulators and, 110, 112
nutrition and, 261, 271
Dexamethasone
immunomodulators and
chemical induction, 107, 108, 111

model systems, 26–30, 32
interleukins and, 236, 239, 240, 245,
246
neuroendocrine-immune interactions
and, 288, 289
nutrition and, 268
thymosin-tuftsin conjugate and, 171,
173
Dextran sulfate, adjuvants and, 143–146
Diarrhea
adjuvants and, 125
bovine viral, *see* Bovine viral diarrhea
interferon immunomodulators and,
221, 222
interleukins and, 240, 241
modulation of behavior and, 312, 313
nutrition and, 262, 270
Diethylaminoethyl-dextran, adjuvants
and, 143, 144
Differentiation
cytokines and, 185, 187, 188
immunomodulators and
chemical induction, 109, 113
mechanism of action, 43, 46–48, 77
physiology, 67, 70, 71
interferon immunomodulators and, 221
nutrition and, 262
thymosin-tuftsin conjugate and, 166
Dihydroheptaprenol, immunomodulators
and, 112
Dimethyldioctadecylammonium bromide,
adjuvants and, 128–130, 143
Dinitrophenyl, adjuvants and, 130, 131,
137, 143
Disease-free interval, thymosin–tuftsin
conjugate and, 167
DNA
adjuvants and, 122, 143
cytokines and, 191, 193, 197, 204, 206
immunomodulators and
chemical induction, 113
mechanism of action, 48, 63, 72,
76, 78
interferon immunomodulators and,
216
neuroendocrine-immune interactions
and, 290
thymosin-tuftsin conjugate and, 166
Dominance, modulation of behavior and,
308–311

E

Economics, immunomodulators and, 3–5, 7, 14
  model systems, 24, 25, 36
Electrophoresis
  cytokines and, 193
  thymosin-tuftsin conjugate and, 169
Endorphins
  immunomodulators and, 58–60, 65
  neuroendocrine-immune interactions and, 286, 292–295
Energy, nutrition and, 257, 258, 261, 262
Enkephalins, immunomodulators and, 58, 60, 65
Environment, immunomodulators and, 44, 53, 54, 61, 87, 89
Enzymes
  adjuvants and, 145
  cytokines and, 183, 184, 188, 207
  immunomodulators and, 7
    mechanism of action, 49, 67, 77, 78, 81, 83
  interferon immunomodulators and, 217
  nutrition and, 262, 264, 269, 272
  thymosin-tuftsin conjugate and, 163, 164
Eosinophils
  cytokines and, 186, 187, 189
  immunomodulators and, 70, 72, 78
  interferon immunomodulators and, 217
Epidermal growth factor, cytokines and, 182, 183, 185, 186
Epstein-Barr virus, adjuvants and, 139
Escherichia coli
  adjuvants and, 135
  cytokines and, 191, 194–198, 202
  immunomodulators and, 109, 112
  interferon immunomodulators and, 216
  interleukins and, 239, 240
  neuroendocrine-immune interactions and, 291
  nutrition and, 260, 265, 270
Experimental autoimmune thyroiditis, adjuvants and, 137

F

Feedback, immunomodulators and, 59, 69
Feline leukemia virus, adjuvants and, 140
Foot-and-mouth disease, adjuvants and, 126, 127, 132–134, 143
Free fatty acids, nutrition and, 264
Free radicals
  immunomodulators and, 113, 114
  nutrition and, 264
Freund's complete adjuvant, 121, 122, 141
Freund's incomplete adjuvant, 124, 126, 135, 136
Fungi, immunomodulators and, 81, 83
Fusion protein, cytokines and, 198

G

Genetics
  cytokines and, 204, 205
  immunomodulators and, 24, 58, 66
  interferon immunomodulators and, 223, 224
  modulation of behavior and, 314
Glucocorticoids
  immunomodulators and, 12
    mechanism of action, 57, 61, 68–72
    model systems, 23, 26–32
  interleukins and, 236, 240
  modulation of behavior and, 309
  neuroendocrine-immune interactions and, 287–289, 296, 298
Glutathione peroxidase, nutrition and, 269
Glycoprotein
  adjuvants and, 140
  cytokines and, 182, 186
  interferon immunomodulators and, 215
Granulocyte/macrophage-CSF
  biology of, 182, 183, 186, 187, 189
  recombinant bovine cytokines and, 190, 191
  structure of, 204, 205
Granulocytes
  immunomodulators and, 55, 64
  thymosin-tuftsin conjugate and, 162, 164
Growth hormone,
  neuroendocrine-immune interactions and, 286, 289–291, 294
Guinea pig
  adjuvants and, 134, 139
  immunomodulators and, 63, 82, 105

Gut
  interferon immunomodulators and, 221, 222
  modulation of behavior and, 312, 313

H

Haemophilus pleuropneumoniae, interleukins and, 237, 238, 240, 241
Haemophilus somnus, immunomodulators and, 30, 31, 33, 34
Hematopoietic cells, cytokines and, 188, 189
Herpes simplex virus, adjuvants and, 140, 145
High-performance liquid chromatography
  adjuvants and, 133
  cytokines and, 198
  thymosin-tuftsin conjugate and, 169
Homology
  cytokines and, 184, 186, 191
  interferon immunomodulators and, 215, 223
Hormones
  cytokines and, 182, 183, 186, 207
  immunomodulators and, 46, 58–64, 69, 76, 87
  neuroendocrine-immune interactions and, 283–288, 293–295, 298
  thymosin-tuftsin conjugate and, 165, 168
Human immunodeficiency virus, adjuvants and, 140, 145
Humoral immunity
  adjuvants and, 128, 131, 136, 143, 146
  immunomodulators and
    chemical induction, 106, 113
    mechanism of action, 44, 50, 53, 56, 89
    microbial products, 84
    physiology, 62, 67
  nutrition and, 256–259, 261, 264, 268, 269
Hybrids, cytokines and, 190, 191, 193, 198, 204, 207

I

Immune function, behavior and, 307–314
Immunity
  neuroendocrine-immune interactions and, *see* Neuroendocrine-immune interactions
  nutritional modulation of, *see* Nutritional modulation of immunity
Immunoglobulin
  adjuvants and, 123, 129, 135, 137, 139
  immunomodulators and, 7
    chemical induction, 106, 107
    mechanism of action, 46–48
    physiology, 62, 64, 65, 67, 70
  interferon immunomodulators and, 221
  modulation of behavior and, 311
  neuroendocrine-immune interactions and, 290, 292, 296
  nutrition and, 256, 257, 261, 263
  in vivo use of, 231, 234
Immunoglobulin G
  cytokines and, 188
  thymosin-tuftsin conjugate and, 163, 165, 171
Immunomodulators, 3–6, 14
  adjuvants and, 124, 142
  behavior and, 309, 311
  chemical induction and, 103–105, 112–115
    ascorbic acid derivatives, 111
    avridine, 108, 109
    biostim, 111, 112
    dihydroheptaprenol, 112
    glucan, 110
    imuthiol, 108
    indomethacin, 110, 111
    isoprinosine, 109, 110
    levamisole, 105–108
    thiabendazole, 108
  cytokines and, 182, 184, 204
  interferon, 215, 216, 224, 225
    antimicrobial defense mechanisms, 216–218
    cellular immune response, 218–221
    in gut, 221, 222
    noninfectious diseases, 222–224
  interleukins and, 235, 242
  mechanism of action of, 43–46, 86–89
    B lymphocytes, 46, 47
    cytokines, 63–68
    glucocorticoids, 68–72
    history, 54, 55
    immunomodulation, 53, 54, 57, 58
    isoprinosine, 75–78
    lentinan, 83–85
    levamisole, 72–75

liposomes, 85, 86
macrophages, 49, 50
microbial products, 80, 81
neuroendocrine hormones, 58–61
objectives, 55, 56
polynucleotides, 78–80
Proprionibacterium acnes, 81–83
T lymphocytes, 47–49
thymic hormones, 61–63
model systems, 21–23, 36
glucocorticoid immunosuppression, 26–32
infectious disease, 32–36
stress, 23–25
neonatal period, 6–9
pathogens, 12–14
stress, 9–12
Immunopotentiators, *see* Immunomodulators
Immunoregulation, interleukins and, 235–237
Immunostimulating complexes, adjuvants and, 138–141, 147
Immunostimulation
adjuvants and, 132, 134, 142, 146
immunomodulators and
chemical induction, 107
mechanism of action, 55–57, 76, 81, 83–85
Immunosuppression
behavior and, 311, 312
immunomodulators and, 12–14
chemical induction, 104–106, 108, 109, 111, 112, 114, 115
mechanism of action, 55–57, 86, 89
microbial products, 83
model systems, 21–24, 26–36
physiology, 60, 67, 68
synthetic compounds, 73, 76–78
interferon immunomodulators and, 219
interleukins and, 235–237, 239, 240
neuroendocrine-immune interactions and, 289, 298
nutrition and, 264, 267, 268
thymosin–tuftsin conjugate and, 162, 167, 173
IMP-1, 168–174
Imuthiol, immunomodulators and, 108
Indomethacin, immunomodulators and, 110

Inflammation
adjuvants and, 129, 137, 141, 142
cytokines and, 184
immunomodulators and
chemical induction, 108
mechanism of action, 44, 49, 87
microbial products, 85
physiology, 63, 64, 66, 68–70
interferon immunomodulators and, 220
neuroendocrine-immune interactions and, 293
Inhibition
adjuvants and, 137, 139
cytokines and, 186, 188
immunomodulators and
chemical induction, 110, 114, 115
mechanism of action, 57
model systems, 26, 35
physiology, 61, 65–67, 69, 71
synthetic compounds, 76
interferon immunomodulators and, 219, 221, 223
interleukins and, 240
modulation of behavior and, 313
neuroendocrine-immune interactions and, 287, 290, 292
nutrition and, 257, 262, 263, 267, 269, 272
thymosin-tuftsin conjugate and, 163, 164
Inoculation
adjuvants and, 140
immunomodulators and, 25, 32, 33
Insulin
cytokines and, 182, 183, 186, 207
neuroendocrine-immune interactions and, 286, 290, 296
Interferon
adjuvants and, 130, 134
immunomodulators and, 6, 8, 215, 216, 224, 225
antimicrobial defense mechanisms, 216–218
cellular immune response, 218–221
chemical induction, 106, 108, 111, 114, 115
gut, 221, 222
mechanism of action, 56
microbial products, 84
model systems, 29

noninfectious diseases, 222–224
physiology, 64–68, 71
synthetic compounds, 77–80
neuroendocrine–immune interactions and, 297
nutrition and, 267
Interferon-α
  immunomodulators and, 34, 216
    mechanism of action, 59, 60, 64, 66–68
  thymosin-tuftsin conjugate and, 167
Interferon-β2, neuroendocrine-immune interactions and, 296
Interferon-τ
  biology, 182, 183, 187, 188
  immunomodulators and, 218–220, 222
    chemical induction, 113
    liposomes, 85, 86
    mechanism of action, 48–50
    model systems, 29–32
    physiology, 60, 64–68
    synthetic compounds, 76, 78
  neuroendocrine-immune interactions and, 287, 289, 291, 298
  recombinant bovine, 189–196
  structure, 204, 205
  thymosin-tuftsin conjugate and, 163, 170, 172, 173
Interleukin
  neuroendocrine-immune interactions and, 296, 297
  in vivo use of, 231–235, 245, 246
    immunoregulation defects, 235–237
    recombinant bovine IL-1β, 244, 245
    recombinant bovine IL-2, 241–244
    recombinant human IL-2, 237–240
Interleukin-1
  adjuvants and, 123
  biology, 182–185, 189
  immunomodulators and
    chemical induction, 115
    mechanism of action, 46–48, 57
    microbial products, 84
    physiology, 64, 65
    synthetic compounds, 76, 77, 79
  interferon immunomodulators and, 218
  neuroendocrine-immune interactions and, 284, 286, 287, 293, 295–298
  recombinant bovine, 189–196
  structure, 204–206

thymosin-tuftsin conjugate and, 170–172
in vivo use of, 232, 234, 236, 237, 244–246
Interleukin-2
  adjuvants and, 144
  biology, 182–186
  immunomodulators and, 6, 84
    chemical induction, 108, 109, 111, 113, 114
    mechanism of action, 48
    model systems, 26, 29, 34
    physiology, 64, 65, 68, 71
    synthetic compounds, 76, 77, 80
  interferon immunomodulators and, 219
  neuroendocrine-immune interactions and, 287, 288, 295
  nutrition and, 257, 258, 263
  recombinant bovine, 190, 191, 193, 196–198
  structure, 204, 205
  thymosin-tuftsin conjugate and, 162, 167, 170–173
  in vivo use of, 232, 234–246
Interleukin-3, 48, 65, 189, 233
Interleukin-4, 48, 64, 113, 233
Interleukin-5, 48, 233
Interleukin-6, 48, 233, 296
Interleukin-7, 48, 233
Interleukin-8, 233
Intestinal infections, immunomodulators and, 7, 9
Iron, nutrition and, 260, 270, 271, 273
Isoprinosine, immunomodulators and, 8
  chemical induction, 109, 110, 114
  mechanism of action, 75–78
  model systems, 24, 34

L

Lactic dehydrogenase, nutrition and, 264
Lentinan, immunomodulators and, 83–85
Lesions
  immunomodulators and, 14, 50
  modulation of behavior and, 312
  neuroendocrine-immune interactions and, 295
  thymosin-tuftsin conjugate and, 162

Leukocytes
  immunomodulators and, 8, 112
  interferon immunomodulators and, 222
  interleukins and, 232, 240
  neuroendocrine-immune interactions and, 285-288, 292-298
  nutrition and, 272
  thymosin-tuftsin conjugate and, 163, 164
Leukokinin, thymosin-tuftsin conjugate and, 163
Levamisole, immunomodulators and, 24, 25, 28, 29, 34, 35
Levamisole, immunomodulators and
  chemical induction, 105-108
  mechanism of action, 72-76
Ligands
  cytokines and, 205
  neuroendocrine-immune interactions and, 286, 287
Lipids
  adjuvants and, 129, 131, 138, 141
  nutrition and, 264, 272
Lipocortin, immunomodulators and, 69, 71
Lipophilic amines, adjuvants and, 128-130, 146
Lipopolysaccharides
  adjuvants and, 144
  immunomodulators and, 57, 59, 65, 77, 85
  neuroendocrine-immune interactions and, 288
  nutrition and, 266
  thymosin-tuftsin conjugate and, 171
Liposomes
  adjuvants and
    ISCOMS, 138, 139
    muramyldipeptides, 142
    oil emulsions, 126
    surface active agents, 128-131, 137
  immunomodulators and, 85, 86, 108
Livestock
  modulation of behavior and, 314
  neuroendocrine-immune interactions and, 284, 289, 291
  nutrition and, 255, 256, 266, 268
Lung, immunomodulators and, 9, 12, 14
  mechanism of action, 68, 82, 83, 86

Lymph nodes
  adjuvants and, 136, 137, 144
  neuroendocrine-immune interactions and, 285, 299
  nutrition and, 263
Lymphocytes
  adjuvants and, 123, 127, 130, 144
  cytokines and, 182
  immunomodulators and, 6-9, 12
    chemical induction, 106-108, 110, 111, 113, 114
    mechanism of action, 49, 50, 55, 57, 88
    model systems, 24, 26, 28-30, 34-36
    physiology, 58-61, 64-66, 69-72
    synthetic compounds, 73, 75-78, 80
  interferon immunomodulators and, 218, 219
  interleukins and, 231, 235, 237, 239, 240, 244
  modulation of behavior and, 310-313
  neuroendocrine-immune interactions and, 285-293, 295
  nutrition and, 257-260, 262
    minerals, 269, 271, 273
    vitamins, 263, 264, 266-268
  thymosin-tuftsin conjugate and, 165-168, 170, 172, 173
Lymphoid cells
  immunomodulators and, 14
    mechanism of action, 43, 44, 46, 47, 49, 84
  interleukins and, 244
  neuroendocrine-immune interactions and, 283, 286, 287, 290, 293, 294
Lymphokines
  cytokines and, 182
  immunomodulators and
    chemical induction, 111, 115
    liposomes, 85
    mechanism of action, 48, 50
    microbial products, 84
    model systems, 29
    physiology, 59, 63-65, 68, 71
    synthetic compounds, 75, 76, 78, 80
  interferon immunomodulators and, 216, 219
  interleukins and, 231, 232, 235, 237, 241, 242

neuroendocrine-immune interactions and, 285, 293, 296, 298
nutrition and, 274
thymosin-tuftsin conjugate and, 166, 169, 172, 173

M

Macrophages
  adjuvants and, 123, 127, 141, 144–146
  cytokines and, 184, 186, 187, 190, 204
  immunomodulators and, 7, 9, 12–14
    chemical induction, 105, 106, 110, 111, 114, 115
    liposomes, 85, 86
    mechanism of action, 44, 47–50, 55, 57, 88
    microbial products, 81–84
    physiology, 59, 63, 64, 67, 68, 71
    synthetic compounds, 73–79
  interferon immunomodulators and, 217–219
  interleukins and, 232, 234, 244
  neuroendocrine-immune interactions and, 285–289, 291, 295, 296
  nutrition and, 256, 263
  thymosin-tuftsin conjugate and, 162–165
Major histocompatibility complex, immunomodulators and, 47, 48, 67
Mannitol, adjuvants and, 124, 125
Mastitis
  immunomodulators and, 4, 5, 12
    chemical induction, 105, 107
    mechanism of action, 53, 73, 74
    model systems, 35, 36
  interleukins and, 244
  nutrition and, 262, 265
Methylfurylbutyrolactones, immunomodulators and, 111
Mice
  adjuvants and, 129, 131, 133, 134, 136, 137
  cytokines and, 184, 191
  immunomodulators and
    chemical induction, 105, 108, 112, 114, 115
    mechanism of action, 71, 76–78, 85, 87

interleukins and, 237, 241, 245
Microbial products, immunomodulators and, 80–85
Migration
  cytokines and, 186
  immunomodulators and, 46, 47, 49, 50, 70–72
  interferon immunomodulators and, 217–219
  interleukins and, 240
  nutrition and, 269
  thymosin-tuftsin conjugate and, 164, 165
Migration inhibition factor, thymosin-tuftsin conjugate and, 163, 167
Milk
  adjuvants and, 135
  immunomodulators and, 5
    chemical induction, 105, 107, 110
    model systems, 36
  modulation of behavior and, 313
  nutrition and, 257, 261, 270
Mitogens
  adjuvants and, 144
  immunomodulators and
    chemical induction, 106, 109, 110, 113, 114
    mechanism of action, 48
    model systems, 25, 26, 28, 35, 36
    physiology, 60, 62, 64–66, 70
    synthetic compounds, 74, 75, 77, 78
  interleukins and, 235, 237, 239, 240
  nutrition and, 258, 262, 263, 266, 269, 273
  thymosin-tuftsin conjugate and, 167, 169, 172
Mixed lymphocyte reaction, thymosin-tuftsin conjugate and, 169–172
Molecular biology of cytokines, 181–189, 205, 207
Monoclonal antibodies
  adjuvants and, 136, 138, 147
  cytokines and, 185
  immunomodulators and, 68
Monocytes
  cytokines and, 182, 188, 189

immunomodulators and
    chemical induction, 109, 110
    liposomes, 85
    mechanism of action, 44, 49, 55, 57
    physiology, 60, 64, 67, 70–72
    synthetic compounds, 76
  interleukins and, 232, 234
  neuroendocrine-immune interactions
    and, 293, 295
  nutrition and, 263
  thymosin-tuftsin conjugate and, 163, 170–173
Monokines
  interleukins and, 232
  nutrition and, 274
Mortality, nutrition and, 256, 270, 272, 273
mRNA
  cytokines and, 188, 190, 193, 198, 204
  immunomodulators and, chemical induction, 104
  interleukins and, 234
Muramyldipeptide
  adjuvants and, 131, 141, 142
  immunomodulators and, 85, 113
Myelin-associated glycoprotein, adjuvants and, 139
Myeloid cells
  cytokines and, 188
  interleukins and, 234
  neuroendocrine-immune interactions and, 283, 286, 287, 293

N

Natural killer cells
  cytokines and, 184
  immunomodulators and, 8, 9
    chemical induction, 108, 113–115
    liposomes, 86
    mechanism of action, 44, 49, 55
    microbial products, 81, 83, 84
    physiology, 60, 63–68, 71
    synthetic compounds, 76, 78–80
  interleukins and, 235, 239, 240
  modulation of behavior and, 312, 313
  neuroendocrine-immune interactions and, 288, 290, 292, 295
  thymosin-tuftsin conjugate and, 167

Neonatal period, immunomodulators and, 6–9, 14
Neoplasms, immunomodulators and, 55, 56, 59
Nerve growth factor, neuroendocrine-immune interactions and, 296
Neuroendocrine hormones, immunomodulators and, 58–61
Neuroendocrine-immune interactions, 283–285, 297–299
  brain lesions, 295
  cells, 287–293
  cytokines, 296, 297
  innervation, 285, 286
  leukocytes, 293–295
  lymphoid cells, 286, 287
  modulation of behavior and, 312
Neurohormones, immunomodulators and, 12
Neuropeptides, neuroendocrine-immune interactions and, 283–287, 293, 294, 298
Neurotransmitters, immunomodulators and, 58, 66
Neutrophils
  adjuvants and, 130
  cytokines and, 186, 187, 189
  immunomodulators and, 12
    chemical induction, 107, 108, 110–112
    mechanism of action, 58
    model systems, 24, 26–28
    physiology, 63, 64, 70, 72
    synthetic compounds, 76–78
  interferon immunomodulators and, 217, 218
  interleukins and, 239, 240
  neuroendocrine-immune interactions and, 288, 290, 291, 293
  nutrition and, 256, 259, 260
    minerals, 269, 272, 274
    vitamins, 263, 266
  thymosin-tuftsin conjugate and, 164, 165
Newcastle disease virus
  adjuvants and, 129
  immunomodulators and, 59, 60, 106

Nitroblue tetrazolium, thymosin-tuftsin
  conjugate and, 165, 171
Nonionic block polymers, adjuvants and,
  130, 131
Nucleotides
  cytokines and, 191, 193, 197–199,
    202–204
  immunomodulators and, 57, 66, 77
  neuroendocrine-immune interactions
    and, 294
Nutritional modulation of immunity,
  255–260, 274
  minerals
    cobalt, 273, 274
    copper, 272, 273
    iron, 270, 271
    selenium, 268–270
    zinc, 271, 272
  protein and energy, 257, 261, 262
  vitamins
    B-complex vitamins, 266, 267
    vitamin A, 262, 263
    vitamin C, 267, 268
    vitamin D, 263
    vitamin E, 264–266

O

Oil emulsions, adjuvants and, 124–128
Opioid peptides, immunomodulators and,
  58, 59, 61
Opioids, neuroendocrine-immune
  interactions and, 292, 293
Oxamisole, immunomodulators and, 114
Oxygen
  cytokines and, 188
  immunomodulators and, 111
  nutrition and, 273

P

Pantothenic acid, modulation of
  immunity and, 267
Parasites
  adjuvants and, 129, 135
  immunomodulators and, 12, 47, 57, 84
  interferon immunomodulators and,
    221, 222, 224

  interleukins and, 237
Pasteurella haemolytica,
  immunomodulators and mechanism
    of action, 68, 82
  model systems, 33, 34
Pathogens
  immunomodulators and, 4, 6–8, 12–14
    chemical induction, 104–107
    mechanism of action, 44, 50, 53, 87
    model systems, 21, 30, 33, 35, 36
  interleukins and, 237, 241
  modulation of behavior and, 307, 313
  neuroendocrine-immune interactions
    and, 297
  nutrition and, 270, 271
  thymosin-tuftsin conjugate and, 162,
    168, 173
Penmates, modulation of behavior and,
  311
Peptides
  adjuvants and, 122, 147
  cytokines and, 182, 184, 187, 190, 207
  immunomodulators and
    chemical induction, 113
    mechanism of action, 58–60, 62, 69
  modulation of behavior and, 313
  neuroendocrine-immune interactions
    and, 286, 287, 292–295
  thymosin-tuftsin conjugate and, 163,
    164, 166, 168, 169
Peripheral blood lymphocytes
  immunomodulators and
    chemical induction, 106, 109, 114
    mechanism of action, 73, 74
  thymosin-tuftsin conjugate and, 170,
    172, 173
Peripheral blood mononuclear cells
  immunomodulators and, 6
  interferon immunomodulators and,
    218, 219
  interleukins and, 239, 241, 242
Peripheral nervous system,
  neuroendocrine-immune
    interactions and, 285, 286, 293
Phagocytes
  adjuvants and, 123, 130, 144–146
  immunomodulators and, 7, 12
    chemical induction, 111, 112
    liposomes, 85, 86

mechanism of action, 44, 46, 47, 49, 50, 88
microbial products, 81, 83
physiology, 60, 71
synthetic compounds, 73, 76–78
interferon immunomodulators and, 217
neuroendocrine-immune interactions and, 289, 290
nutrition and, 260, 268, 269
thymosin-tuftsin conjugate and, 163–165, 169–171, 173
Pharmacology
  adjuvants and, 132, 142, 146
  immunomodulators and
    chemical induction, 104
    mechanism of action, 55, 58, 61, 70, 72, 87
Phenotype, interferon immunomodulators and, 219, 220
Phospholipids
  adjuvants and, 125, 126
  immunomodulators and, 69, 85
Phosphorylation, cytokines and, 183, 185–188, 207
Physiology
  immunomodulators and, 11
  cytokines, 63–68
  glucocorticoids, 68–72
  mechanism of action, 54, 55, 57
  neuroendocrine hormones, 58–61
  thymic hormones, 61–63
  interferon immunomodulators and, 219, 220
Phytohemagglutinin
  cytokines and, 193
  immunomodulators and
    chemical induction, 106, 109, 110, 114
    mechanism of action, 60, 74, 76, 79
    model systems, 24, 29
  nutrition and, 266, 269, 271
  thymosin-tuftsin conjugate and, 170–172
Pigs
  adjuvants and, 125–127, 129, 134
  immunomodulators and, 6–8, 12
    chemical induction, 108–112
    mechanism of action, 74, 77, 80, 82, 86
    model systems, 23, 24, 26, 33

interferon immunomodulators and, 220
interleukins and, 237–239, 245, 246
modulation of behavior and, 307, 309–313
neuroendocrine-immune interactions and, 288
nutrition and, 257–261
  minerals, 270–272
  vitamins, 263–265, 267, 268
Pituitary, modulation of behavior and, 312, 313
Pituitary hormones, neuroendocrine-immune interactions and, 293–295, 298
Plasma cells, immunomodulators and, 7, 9
  chemical induction, 109
  mechanism of action, 44, 46, 84
Plasmids, cytokines and, 190, 191, 193, 196–200, 202, 204
Platelet-derived growth factor, cytokines and, 182, 183, 207
Pneumonia
  immunomodulators and, 12
  mechanism of action, 45, 74
  model systems, 30–33
  interferon immunomodulators and, 216, 217, 220
  thymosin-tuftsin conjugate and, 162
Polymeric adjuvants, 130, 131, 142–145
Polymorphonuclear leukocytes
  adjuvants and, 141
  immunomodulators and, mechanism of action, 44, 63, 70
Polynucleotides, immunomodulators and, 78–80
Polypeptides
  cytokines and, 186
  immunomodulators and, 48, 58, 62–64
  thymosin-tuftsin conjugate and, 166
Polysaccharides
  adjuvants and, 122, 136, 143–145
  immunomodulators and, 83, 84
Polyunsaturated fatty acids, nutrition and, 264
Porcine interferon-α, immunomodulators and, 216
Poultry
  adjuvants and, 121, 127

immunomodulators and, 53, 86, 105, 106
Prolactin, neuroendocrine-immune interactions and, 286, 289, 291, 294
Proliferation
  adjuvants and, 132, 137, 139
  cytokines and, 207
    biology, 183, 185–187
    recombinant bovine, 193, 198, 201, 202
  immunomodulators and, 10, 12, 13
    chemical induction, 108–111, 113, 114
    mechanism of action, 48
    physiology, 60, 65, 66, 69–71
    synthetic compounds, 74, 75, 77
  interferon immunomodulators and, 218, 219, 221
  interleukins and, 231, 236, 238–240
  neuroendocrine-immune interactions and, 287, 288, 290, 293
  nutrition and, 258–260, 262
    minerals, 269, 271, 273
    vitamins, 263, 268
Proopiomelanocortin, neuroendocrine-immune interactions and, 286, 294
Propionibacterium acnes, immunomodulators and, 81–83
Prostaglandins, interferon immunomodulators and, 217, 223
Protein
  adjuvants and, 123, 129–131, 140, 142
  cytokines and, 204, 207
    biology, 182, 183, 185–188
    recombinant bovine, 191, 193, 197–202
  immunomodulators and, 104, 107, 111, 113
  interferon immunomodulators and, 215, 223
  interleukins and, 231, 232, 234, 235, 238, 245
  neuroendocrine-immune interactions and, 296
  nutrition and, 256–258, 261, 262, 271
  thymosin-tuftsin conjugate and, 168
Protein-energy malnutrition, 257
Protein kinase, cytokines and, 182, 185, 187, 188, 207

Pseudorabies
  adjuvants and, 143
  immunomodulators and, 7, 9, 12, 13, 109, 110
  interleukins and, 238–240

Q

Quil A, adjuvants and, 133–138, 141

R

Rabbits, adjuvants and, 125, 134
Radiotherapy, thymosin-tuftsin conjugate and, 167, 168
Rat
  adjuvants and, 137
  immunomodulators and, 111
Reactive oxygen species, interferon immunomodulators and, 217, 218
Recombinant bovine GM-CSF, biology of, 190, 191, 198–202, 205
Recombinant bovine interferon-τ
  biology of, 190, 191, 202, 203, 205
  immunomodulators and, 29–32
Recombinant bovine interferon-α, immunomodulators and, 216–219, 221–224
Recombinant bovine interleukin-1
  biology of, 189–196, 205, 206
  in vivo use of, 244–246
Recombinant bovine interleukin-2
  biology of, 190, 191, 193, 196–198, 205
  in vivo use of, 241–244, 246
Recombinant human interferon-α, immunomodulators and, 34, 216
Recombinant human interleukin-1, biology of, 189
Recombinant human interleukin-2, *in vivo* use of, 237–240, 242, 246
Recombinant interleukin, *in vivo* use of, 234, 235, 237
Recombinant porcine interferon-τ, immunomodulators and, 220, 222
Recombinant porcine interleukin-1, biology of, 190, 191, 204–206
Replication, immunomodulators and
  chemical induction, 107
  mechanism of action, 76, 78

Resistance
  adjuvant and, 130
  immunomodulators and, 11
    chemical induction, 106, 113
    mechanism of action, 50
    model systems, 21, 33
  nutrition and, 256, 265, 270, 272, 274
Respiratory disease, *see also* Bovine respiratory disease
  immunomodulators and, 106
  interferon immunomodulators and, 217, 220
  nutrition and, 268
Respiratory infection, immunomodulators and, 7, 9, 12
Respiratory syncytial virus, adjuvants and, 139
Respiratory tract, immunomodulators and, 47, 77, 87
Riboflavin, modulation of immunity and, 267
RNA
  adjuvants and, 130
  cytokines and, 188
  immunomodulators and, 76, 78, 79, 113

S

Salmonella pullorum, nutrition and, 261, 263, 267, 272
Saponins, adjuvants and, 132–138
SDS-PAGE, cytokines and, 193, 197, 199, 200
Second messengers, cytokines and, 183, 185, 187, 205
Selenium, modulation of immunity and, 259, 265, 268–270
Serine kinase, cytokines and, 183, 185
Serum glutamic oxalacetic transaminase, nutrition and, 264
Sheep
  adjuvants and, 125, 127, 135, 136, 143
  immunomodulators and
    chemical induction, 105, 110
    mechanism of action, 74, 76, 78, 84
  nutrition and, 258–260, 264, 269, 272, 274
Shipping fever
  interferon immunomodulators and, 216
  thymosin-tuftsin conjugate and, 162, 174
Social behavior, modulation of immune function and, 309–311
Social order, modulation of immune function and, 308
Soy protein, nutrition and, 257, 261, 262
Spleen
  adjuvants and, 136, 137, 141
  immunomodulators and
    chemical induction, 114
    mechanism of action, 46
    microbial products, 82, 83, 86
    physiology, 58–61, 65
    synthetic compounds, 74
  modulation of behavior and, 312
  neuroendocrine-immune interactions and, 285, 286, 292, 295
  nutrition and, 264
  thymosin-tuftsin conjugate and, 165, 167
Staphylococcus aureus
  immunomodulators and, 35, 36
  interleukins and, 244
  thymosin-tuftsin conjugate and, 171
Staphylococcus haemolyticus, immunomodulators and, 110
Stem cells, immunomodulators and, 44–46, 48, 49
Steroids
  adjuvants and, 132, 137
  immunomodulators and, 68–71
Stress
  immunomodulators and, 4, 6, 9–12, 14
    chemical induction, 105, 108
    mechanism of action, 53, 54, 56, 86
    model systems, 21, 23–25, 31, 33, 36
    physiology, 60, 61
    synthetic compounds, 73
  interleukins and, 236, 237
  modulation of behavior and, 307–309, 311, 313
  neuroendocrine-immune interactions and, 292, 297
  nutrition and, 256, 261, 270
  thymosin-tuftsin conjugate and, 162, 173, 174
Subordinates, modulation of behavior and, 309–311
Sugar, adjuvants and, 133, 142

Sulpholipopolysaccharides, adjuvants and, 131, 132
Surface active agents, adjuvants and, 128–138
Susceptibility
  immunomodulators and, 6, 8–12
    mechanism of action, 46, 53–55
    model systems, 26, 35
  interferon immunomodulators and, 219
  interleukins and, 235, 237, 240
  nutrition and, 271
  thymosin-tuftsin conjugate and, 162, 173
Swainsonine, immunomodulators and, 113, 114
Swine
  adjuvants and, 127
  cytokines and, 184, 190, 207
  immunomodulators and, 105, 106
  interferon immunomodulators and, 216, 220, 225
  nutrition and, 264
Synthetic polynucleotides, immunomodulators and, 78–80

T

T cells
  adjuvants and, 137, 139, 141, 144, 147
  cytokines and, 184, 185
  immunomodulators and
    chemical induction, 105, 106, 109, 113–115
    mechanism of action, 44, 46–49, 52, 55
    microbial products, 81–85
    physiology, 59, 61, 62, 64, 65, 67, 69–72
    synthetic compounds, 75, 78–80
  interferon immunomodulators and, 218–220
  interleukins and, 232–235, 245
  neuroendocrine-immune interactions and, 284, 287, 288, 290, 292, 294, 296
  nutrition and, 256, 266
  thymosin-tuftsin conjugate and, 163, 165–169, 172, 173
T lymphocytes, immunomodulators and
  chemical induction, 108, 109, 111, 113

mechanism of action, 44, 46–49
microbial products, 84
physiology, 63, 68
synthetic compounds, 77
Thiabendazole, immunomodulators and
  chemical induction, 106, 108
  model systems, 25, 28
Thymosin-α, 163, 165–168
Thymosin-tuftsin conjugate, 161–163, 168–174
Thymulin
  immunomodulators and, 62, 63
  neuroendocrine-immune interactions and, 289, 290, 292
Thymus
  cytokines and, 189, 193, 196, 204
  immunomodulators and
    chemical induction, 114
    mechanism of action, 44, 47, 58, 60–63, 82
  modulation of behavior and, 312
  neuroendocrine-immune interactions and, 284–286, 289, 290, 292
  nutrition and, 263, 271, 272
  thymosin-tuftsin conjugate and, 165, 166, 168, 169
Thyroid stimulating hormone
  immunomodulators and, 59, 60
  neuroendocrine-immune interactions and, 291, 292
Toxicity, immunomodulators and, 55, 85, 115
Toxins
  adjuvants and, 132
  immunomodulators and, 47, 64, 68
Transcription
  cytokines and, 185, 191
  immunomodulators and, 67, 72
Transforming growth factor-β_2, neuroendocrine-immune interactions and, 288, 289
Tuftsin, 161–165, 168–174
Tumor necrosis factor, neuroendocrine-immune interactions and, 284, 287, 288, 291, 293, 296, 297
Tumors
  cytokines and, 187, 188
  immunomodulators and, 8
    chemical induction, 113, 115

liposomes, 85
mechanism of action, 54
microbial products, 81–83
physiology, 59, 62, 64, 65
synthetic compounds, 79
interleukins and, 235
neuroendocrine-immune interactions and, 287, 289, 291
thymosin-tuftsin conjugate and, 167, 172
Turkey, immunomodulators and, 105, 106
Tyrosine kinase, cytokines and, 182, 183

V

Vaccination
  adjuvants and, 122, 147
    aluminum salts, 122, 123
    ISCOMS, 140, 141
    oil emulsions, 124–128
    polymeric adjuvants, 143
    surface active agents, 128, 132–136
  cytokines and, 185
  immunomodulators and, 4–6
    chemical induction, 105–108
    liposomes, 85
    mechanism of action, 50, 53–56, 70, 86, 88
    microbial products, 82
    synthetic compounds, 72, 74
  interferon immunomodulators and, 221
  interleukins and, 237–239, 241, 244–246
  nutrition and, 264, 265
  thymosin-tuftsin conjugate and, 162
Vasopressin, neuroendocrine-immune interactions and, 294, 295
Virulence, immunomodulators and, 50, 82
Virus
  adjuvants and, 122, 147
    ISCOMS, 138–140

oil emulsions, 127
    polymeric adjuvants, 143
    surface active agents, 129, 132, 135
  cytokines and, 189, 202
  immunomodulators and, 4, 6, 8, 9, 12, 13
    chemical induction, 106, 107, 109
    mechanism of action, 44, 46, 47, 53, 55, 57, 85, 86
    microbial products, 81, 84
    model systems, 21, 32–34
    physiology, 66, 70
    synthetic compounds, 74, 76–80
  interferon immunomodulators and, 216, 218, 219, 221, 224, 225
  interleukins and, 237, 239, 241, 244, 245
  nutrition and, 263, 271
Vitamin A, modulation of immunity and, 258, 262, 263
Vitamin B_{12}, nutrition and, 273, 274
Vitamin C
  immunomodulators and, 111
  modulation of immunity and, 259, 267, 268
Vitamin D, modulation of immunity and, 258, 263
Vitamin E, modulation of immunity and, 258, 264–266, 271

W

Weaning
  immunomodulators and, 23–25, 105
  nutrition and, 261, 270
  thymosin-tuftsin conjugate and, 162

Z

Zinc, modulation of immunity and, 260, 271–273

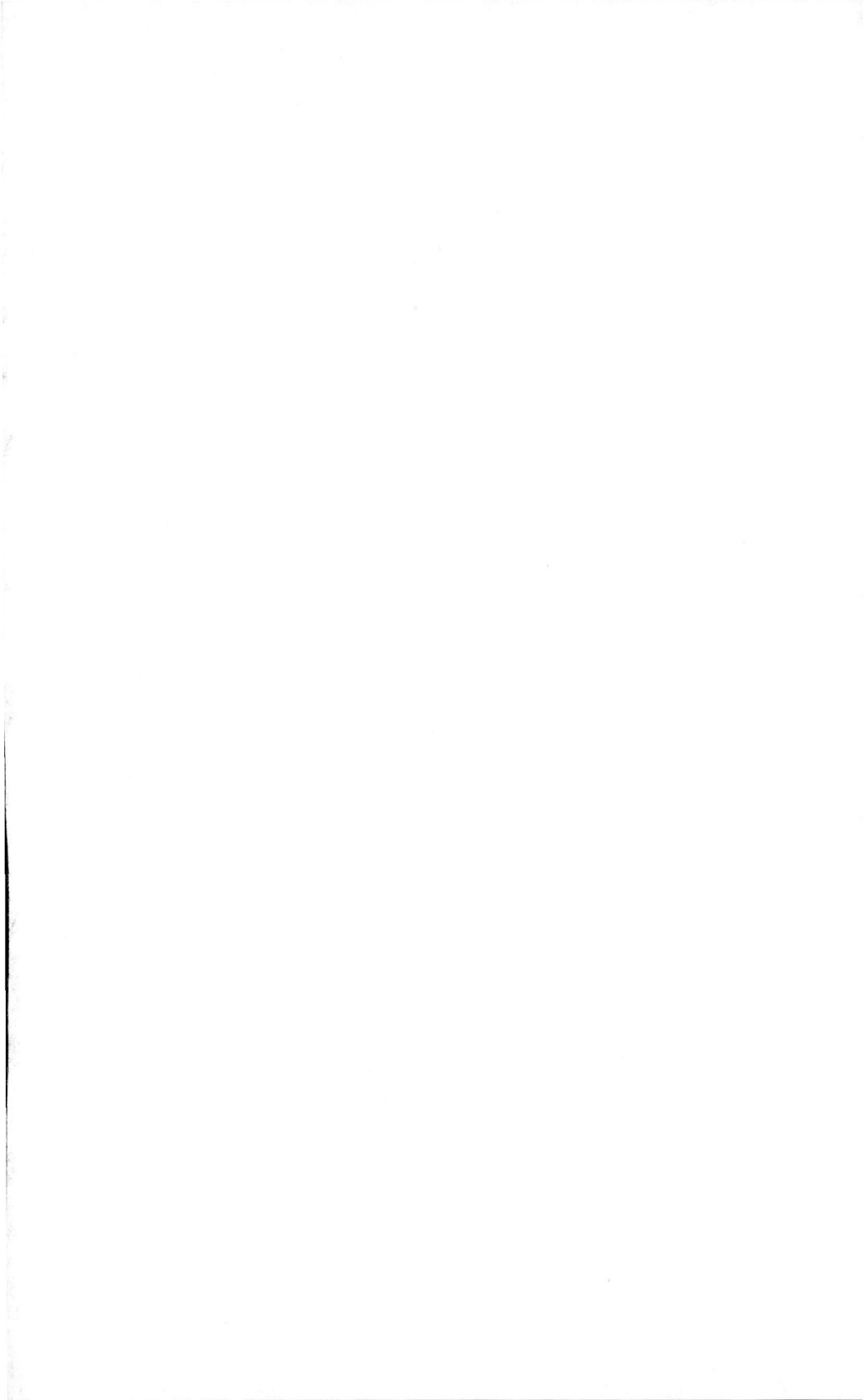